2009
YEAR BOOK OF
PATHOLOGY
AND LABORATORY
MEDICINE®

The 2009 Year Book Series

Year Book of Anesthesiology and Pain Management™: Drs Chestnut, Abram, Black, Gravlee, Lee, Mathru, and Roizen

Year Book of Cardiology®: Drs Gersh, Cheitlin, Elliott, Graham, Sundt, and Waldo

Year Book of Critical Care Medicine®: Drs Dellinger, Parrillo, Balk, Bekes, Dorman, and Dries

Year Book of Dentistry®: Drs Olin, Belvedere, Davis, Henderson, Johnson, Ohrbach, Scott, Spencer, and Zakariasen

Year Book of Dermatology and Dermatologic Surgery™: Drs Thiers and Lang

Year Book of Diagnostic Radiology®: Drs Osborn, Abbara, Birdwell, Elster, Gardiner, Levy, Manaster, Oestrich, and Rosado de Christenson

Year Book of Emergency Medicine®: Drs Hamilton, Handly, Quintana, Werner, and Bruno

Year Book of Endocrinology®: Drs Mazzaferri, Bessesen, Clarke, Howard, Kennedy, Leahy, Meikle, Molitch, Rogol, and Schteingart

Year Book of Gastroenterology™: Drs Lichtenstein, Dempsey, Drebin, Jaffe, Katzka, Kochman, Makar, Morris, Osterman, Rombeau, and Shah

Year Book of Hand and Upper Limb Surgery®: Drs Chang and Steinmann

Year Book of Medicine®: Drs Barkin, Berney, Frishman, Garrick, Loehrer, Phillips, and Khardori

Year Book of Neonatal and Perinatal Medicine®: Drs Fanaroff, Ehrenkranz, and Stevenson

Year Book of Neurology and Neurosurgery®: Drs Kim and Verma

Year Book of Obstetrics, Gynecology, and Women's Health®: Drs Dungan and Shulman

Year Book of Oncology®: Drs Loehrer, Arceci, Glatstein, Gordon, Hanna, Morrow, and Thigpen

Year Book of Ophthalmology®: Drs Rapuano, Cohen, Eagle, Flanders, Hammersmith, Myers, Nelson, Penne, Sergott, Shields, Tipperman, and Vander

Year Book of Orthopedics®: Drs Morrey, Beauchamp, Huddleston, Peterson, Swiontkowski, and Trigg

Year Book of Otolaryngology-Head and Neck Surgery®: Drs Balough, Gapany, Keefe, and Sindwani

Year Book of Pathology and Laboratory Medicine®: Drs Raab, Parwani Bejarano, and Bissell

Year Book of Pediatrics®: Dr Stockman

Year Book of Plastic and Aesthetic Surgery™: Drs Miller, Bartlett, Garner, McKinney, Ruberg, Salisbury, and Smith

Year Book of Psychiatry and Applied Mental Health®: Drs Talbott, Ballenger, Buckley, Frances, Markowitz, and Sarles

Year Book of Pulmonary Disease®: Drs Phillips, Barker, Lewis, Maurer, Tanoue, and Willsie

Year Book of Sports Medicine®: Drs Shephard, Cantu, Feldman, Jankowski, McCrory, Nieman, Pierrynowski, Rowland, and Shrier

Year Book of Surgery®: Drs Copeland, Bland, Daly, Eberlein, Fahey, Jones, Mozingo, Pruett, and Seeger

Year Book of Urology®: Drs Andriole and Coplen

Year Book of Vascular Surgery®: Dr Moneta

2009

The Year Book of PATHOLOGY AND LABORATORY MEDICINE®

Editors-in-Chief

Stephen S. Raab, MD
Professor of Pathology and Vice Chair of Quality, Department of Pathology, University of Colorado, Denver

Anil V. Parwani, MD, PhD
Assistant Professor of Pathology, Director, Division of Pathology Informatics, University of Pittsburgh School of Medicine; Staff Pathologist, University of Pittsburgh Medical Center Shadyside, Pittsburgh, Pennsylvania

Editor

Pablo A. Bejarano, MD
Assistant Professor and Director of Surgical Pathology, University of Miami School of Medicine; Pathologist, Jackson Memorial Hospital, Miami, Florida

Editor-in-Chief, Laboratory Medicine

Michael G. Bissell, MD, PhD, MPH
Professor of Pathology, Ohio State University; Director of Clinical Chemistry and Toxicology, Ohio State University Medical Center, Columbus, Ohio

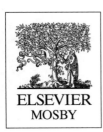

ELSEVIER
MOSBY

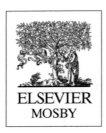

ELSEVIER
MOSBY

Vice President, Continuity: John A. Schrefer
Editor: Joanne Husovski
Production Supervisor: Donna M. Skelton
Electronic Article Manager: Travis L. Ross
Illustrations and Permissions Coordinator: Dawn Vohsen

2009 EDITION

Printed in the United States of America
Composition by TNQ Books and Journals Pvt Ltd, India
Printing/binding by Sheridan Books, Inc.

Editorial Office:
Elsevier
Suite 1800
1600 John F. Kennedy Blvd.
Philadelphia, PA 19103-2899

International Standard Serial Number: 1077-9108
International Standard Book Number: 978-1-4160-5725-3

Contributing Editors

Gissou Azabdaftari, MD
Department of Pathology, University of Colorado; Denver Health Science Center-Anschutz Medical Campus, Aurora, Colorado

Philip Boyer, MD, PhD
Assistant Professor, Department of Pathology, University of Colorado Health Sciences, Aurora, Colorado

Miroslav Djokic, MD
Associate Professor of Pathology, University of Pittsburgh School of Medicine; University of Pittsburgh Medical Center, Pittsburgh, Pennsylvania

Rajiv Dhir, MD
Associate Professor of Pathology; University of Pittsburgh School of Medicine; Chief of Pathology, Shadyside Hospital, University of Pittsburgh Health Systems; Director, Division of Genitourinary Pathology, University of Pittsburgh Medical Center Shadyside, Pittsburgh, Pennsylvania

Csaba Galambos, MD
Division of Pediatric Pathology, Children's Hospital of Pittsburgh, University of Pittsburgh Medical Center, Pittsburgh, Pennslyvania

Drazen M. Jukic, MD
Assistant Professor, Department of Dermatopathology and Pathology, University of Pittsburgh School of Medicine; Director, Dermatopathology, Medical Director, Histology and Immunohistochemistry, University of Pittsburgh Medical Center Shadyside, Pittsburgh, Pennsylvania

Federico A. Monzon, MD
Medical Director of Molecular Diagnostics, The Methodist Hospital; Houston, Texas

Raja Seethala, MD
Assistant Professor of Pathology, University of Pittsburgh School of Medicine; University of Pittsburgh Medical Center-PUH, Pittsburgh, Pennsylvania

Joshua Wisell, MD
Assistant Professor, Surgical Pathology, University of Colorado Health Sciences, Aurora, Colorado

Table of Contents

Journals Represented

Journals represented in this YEAR BOOK are listed below.

Acta Obstetricia et Gynecologica Scandinavica
American Heart Journal
American Journal of Cardiology
American Journal of Clinical Pathology
American Journal of Epidemiology
American Journal of Gastroenterology
American Journal of Pathology
American Journal of Respiratory and Critical Care Medicine
American Journal of Surgery
American Journal of Surgical Pathology
Annals of Surgery
Annals of Thoracic Surgery
Archives of Pathology and Laboratory Medicine
Blood
British Journal of Haematology
Cancer
Cancer Research
Chest
Clinical Chemistry
Clinical Infectious Diseases
Critical Care Medicine
Diagnostic Cytopathology
Digestive Diseases and Sciences
European Journal of Cancer
European Journal of Obstetrics, Gynecology and Reproductive Biology
Fertility and Sterility
Gastroenterology
Gastrointestinal Endoscopy
Genes Chromosomes and Cancer
Gut
Human Molecular Genetics
Human Pathology
Intensive Care Medicine
International Journal of Cardiology
Journal of Clinical Endocrinology and Metabolism
Journal of Clinical Microbiology
Journal of Clinical Oncology
Journal of Cutaneous Pathology
Journal of Hepatology
Journal of Pathology
Journal of Urology
Kidney International
Modern Pathology
Nature
Nature Medicine
Neuron
New England Journal of Medicine

Advances in Anatomic Pathology
American Journal of Clinical Pathology
American Journal of Kidney Diseases
Annals of Diagnostic Pathology
Annals of Surgical Oncology
BJU International
BMC Family Practice
Canadian Journal of Anesthesia
Cancer Epidemiology Biomarkers & Prevention
Clinical Cancer Research
Cytopathology
Heart
Journal of Clinical Anesthesia
Journal of Clinical Pathology
Journal of Cutaneous Pathology
Journal of Lower Genital Tract Disease
Journal of Molecular Diagnostics
Journal of the American Medical Association
Journal of Urology
Leukemia
Medicina Oral, Patología Oral y Cirugía Bucal
Modern Pathology
Nature Methods
New England Journal of Medicine
Pediatric Infectious Disease Journal
Plos One
Southern Medical Journal Thyroid
Transfusion
Transplantation
Transplantation Proceedings
Thorax
Thrombosis Research
Thyroid
Virchows Archiv
World Journal of Surgery

STANDARD ABBREVIATIONS

The following terms are abbreviated in this edition: acquired immunodeficiency syndrome (AIDS), cardiopulmonary resuscitation (CPR), central nervous system (CNS), cerebrospinal fluid (CSF), computed tomography (CT), deoxyribonucleic acid (DNA), electrocardiography (ECG), health maintenance organization (HMO), human immunodeficiency virus (HIV), intensive care unit (ICU), intramuscular (IM), intravenous (IV), magnetic resonance (MR) imaging (MRI), ribonucleic acid (RNA), ultrasound (US), and ultraviolet (UV).

NOTE

editors' comments are their own opinions. Mention of specific products within this publication does not constitute endorsement.

To facilitate the use of the YEAR BOOK OF PATHOLOGY AND LABORATORY MEDICINE as a reference tool, all illustrations and tables included in this publication are now identified as they appear in the original article. This change is meant to help the reader recognize that any illustration or table appearing in the YEAR BOOK OF PATHOLOGY AND LABORATORY MEDICINE may be only one of many in the original article. For this reason, figure and table numbers will often appear to be out of sequence within the YEAR BOOK OF PATHOLOGY AND LABORATORY MEDICINE.

Introduction

Welcome to the 2009 YEAR BOOK OF PATHOLOGY AND LABORATORY MEDICINE! The long-awaited online format of the YEAR BOOK became a reality last year as part of the new Elsevier product eClips Consult, which provides readers with more up-to-date and timely articles. The 2009 YEAR BOOK OF PATHOLOGY AND LABORATORY MEDICINE has a range of insightful and outstanding abstracted articles. Many selections have focused on advances in molecular pathology and diagnostic pathology with an emphasis on more practical articles dealing with the contemporary practice data highlighting the significant advances occurring in pathology and laboratory medicine this past year. This year we have continued with our trend of highlighting the best articles in the field of outcome analysis, cytology, and anatomical pathology.

Our team of contributing editors excels in these areas and has once again provided comprehensive and educational overviews of these articles.

These articles were chosen by the editors to focus on the major advances and highlights in these subspecialties. The editors include Drs Michael Bessel (Ohio State University) and Pablo Bejarno (University of Miami). Other contributing editors include Drs Miroslav Djokic, Rajiv Dhir, Drazen Jukic, Federico Bordonaba, Raja Seethala, Joshua Wisell, Gissou Azabdaftari, Philip Boyer and Csaba Galambos. We hope you find these articles and the accompanying summaries useful in your everyday practice and this gives you an expedited view of the most current literature, highlighted and comprehensively reviewed. Please feel free to provide either of us with feedback: (raabss@upmc.edu or parwaniav@upmc.edu). Thank you and enjoy the reading!

Stephen S. Raab, MD

Anil V. Parwani, MD, PhD

Editors-in-Chief

PART I

ANATOMIC PATHOLOGY

1 Outcomes Analysis

Effect of lean method implementation in the histopathology section of an anatomic pathology laboratory
Raab SS, Grzybicki DM, Condel JL, et al (Univ of Pittsburgh School of Medicine, PA; et al)
J Clin Pathol 2007 Aug 3, Epub ahead of print

Background.—In the United States, the lack of processes standardization in histopathology laboratories leads to less than optimal quality, errors, inefficiency, and increased costs. The effectiveness of large scale quality improvement initiatives rarely has been evaluated.

Aim.—To measure the effect of implementation of a Lean quality improvement process on the efficiency and quality of a histopathology laboratory section.

Methods.—We performed a non-concurrent interventional cohort study from January 1, 2003 to December 31, 2006 and implemented the Lean process on January 1, 2004. We also compared the productivity of the Lean histopathology section to a sister histopathology section that did not implement Lean processes. We measured pre- and post-Lean specimen turn-around time and productivity ratios (work units/full time equivalents). For 200 Lean interventions, we used a 5-part Likert scale to assess the impact on error, success, and complexity.

Results.—In the Lean laboratory, the mean monthly productivity ratio increased from 3,439 and 4,074 work units/full time equivalents ($P < 0.001$) as the mean daily histopathology section specimen turn-around time decreased from 9.7 to 9.0 hours ($P = 0.01$). The Lean histopathology section had a higher productivity ratio compared to a sister histopathology section (1,598 work units/full time equivalents, $P < 0.001$) that did not implement Lean processes. The mean impact, success, and complexity of interventions were 2.4, 2.7, and 2.5, respectively. The mean number of specific error causes affected by individual interventions was 2.6.

Conclusion.—We conclude that Lean process implementation improved histopathology section efficiency and quality.

► The application of industrial methods of quality control to laboratory medicine, or medicine in general, is not new. The application of Lean methods, with the Toyota Production System (TPS) being the prime example, is one of the currently applied industrial techniques of quality improvement. Some experts have argued that TPS originally focused on efficiency and that quality was observed as a secondary byproduct. Nonetheless, Lean consultants advertise their services to laboratories. Many in the field believe that the current application of Lean methods for improvement is extremely diverse. TPS methodology is relatively unique and rarely duplicated in medicine. In the Toyota system, learning lines involving trained individuals (ie, team leaders) completely devoted to problem solving are part of the work process; the front line worker to team leader ratio may be 4:1. Most medical systems currently are not willing to commit to this level of up-front investment. In Lean processes, there is a simultaneous focus on improving quality, efficiency, and cost, although much of the medical literature generally has reported on efficiency improvements and cost savings. These metrics are easier to evaluate than cost metrics, although the real goal, from the patient perspective, should be improving patient outcomes. The difficulty in evaluating patient outcomes, from the laboratory standpoint, is well known, as patient outcome data are a challenge to track. This article shows how efficiencies, cost, and quality were targeted by introducing Lean changes and a learning line.

For further reading on this subject I suggest articles by Condel et al[1] and Zarbo et al.[2]

S. S. Raab, MD

References

1. Condel JL, Sharbaugh DT, Raab SS. Error-free pathology: applying lean production methods to anatomic pathology. *Clin Lab Med.* 2004;24:865-899.
2. Zarbo RJ, D'Angelo R. Transforming to a quality culture: the Henry Ford Production System. *Am J Clin Pathol.* 2006;126:S21-S29.

Histological Grading of Colorectal Cancer: A Simple and Objective Method
Ueno H, Mochizuki H, Hashiguchi Y, et al (Natl Defense Med College, Tokorozawa, Saitama, Japan)
Ann Surg 247:811-818, 2008

Objective.—Tumor grade employed for colorectal cancer has long been based on the degree of differentiation, which is difficult to judge objectively. The aim of this study was to determine whether the extent of the *poorly* differentiated component (POR) could be a valuable criterion for a grading system.

Patients and Methods.—A total of 1075 patients with advanced colorectal cancer were pathologically reviewed. POR was newly defined as a region in which a cancer has no glandular formation, irrespective of a mucin-producing or invasive pattern, and we quantitatively classified the POR into 6 degrees using the microscopic field of an objective lens as a standard.

Results.—Survival analyses of the extent of POR demonstrated that a 3-category grading system provides the most efficient survival stratification. Grade III was applied to tumors (n = 339) for which the POR fully occupied the microscopic field of a 40× objective lens. For tumors having a smaller POR, cancer clusters without a gland structure composed of ≥ 5 cancer cells ("clusters") were counted in the microscopic field of a $4\times$ objective lens, where "clusters" were observed most intensively. Tumors with <10 "clusters" were classified as grade I (n = 161), and those with ≥ 10 "clusters" as grade II (n = 575). Patients classified as grade I demonstrated a very favorable prognosis, with a 99.3% cancer-related 5-year survival rate, whereas the survival was 86.0% for grade II and 68.9% for grade III ($P < 0.0001$ in each group). Multivariate analysis demonstrated that the grades of POR function as an independent prognosticator, as do T-stage and N-stage.

Conclusions.—The grading system utilizing POR is distinctive in terms of the simplicity of judgment based on its quantification and the ability to

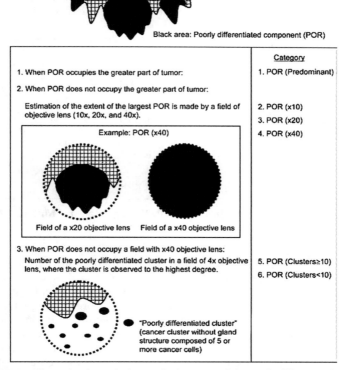

FIGURE 1.—Schema for the method to grade the extent of the poorly differentiated component. (Reprinted from Ueno H, Mochizuki H, Hashiguchi Y, et al. Histological grading of colorectal cancer: a simple and objective method. *Ann Surg.* 2008;247:811-818.)

determine which patients will likely be cured by surgery alone. It will aid in selecting postoperative treatment strategies (Fig 1).

▶ In the TNM classification system for colorectal adenocarcinomas, tumors are graded by their degree of differentiation and are classified as grade 1 (well differentiated) to grade 4 (undifferentiated). A problem with this system is that pathologists may disagree regarding individual tumor grades. Ueno et al write that there are 2 causes of this problem: 1) the distinctions between the tumor differentiation categories represent a continuum, and pathologists may disagree about individual tumor assessments, and 2) the least differentiated component has not been standardized. Ueno et al evaluated a proposed grading system that quantitatively measured the extent of the least differentiated tumor component. The value of this process is that a standardized method of tumor grading, using a microscopic field for measure, allows practicing pathologists to implement this grading system in daily practice. Fig 1 shows the application of using the poorly differentiated component to separate tumors into 3 grades. The article's photomicrographs are very useful for comparison. Although this grading system appears to correlate with patient outcomes, it will need to be confirmed in other pathology practices. In addition, even though this grading system has a quantitative component, its application still will have a qualitative component and the ability of pathologists to agree in individual assessments needs more formal application.

For further reading on this subject I suggest articles by Dukes et al[1] and Hamilton et al.[2]

S. S. Raab, MD

References

1. Dukes C. Histological grading of rectal cancer. *Proc R Soc Med.* 1937;30:371-376.
2. Hamilton SR, Vogelstein B, Kudo S. Carcinoma of the colon and rectum. In: Hamilton S, Aaltonen L, eds. *World Health Organization Classification of Tumors-Pathology and Genetics of Tumors of the Digestive System.* Lyon: IARC Press; 2000:105-119.

Mandatory Second Opinion in Surgical Pathology Referral Material: Clinical Consequences of Major Disagreements
Manion E, Cohen MB, Weydert J (Univ of Iowa Carver College of Medicine)
Am J Surg Pathol 32:732-737, 2008

Second opinion in pathology is intended to expose clinically significant errors that have a direct impact on patient care. Before definitive treatment of referred patients, our institution requires a second opinion of outside surgical pathology slides. We sought to determine if this local standard of practice has a measurable impact on patient care via clinical and pathologic follow-up. 5629 second opinion surgical pathology cases seen at the University of Iowa Hospitals and Clinics were studied. Each case was classified as: no diagnostic disagreement, minor diagnostic disagreement, or major diagnostic disagreement by the second opinion pathologist at the time of referral. A major diagnostic disagreement was defined as a change in pathologic diagnosis with potential for significant change in treatment or prognosis. Major diagnostic disagreements were categorized by organ system and according to the clinical significance of the changed diagnosis based on clinical and pathologic follow-up. Second opinion surgical pathology resulted in 132 (2.3% of total cases) major diagnostic disagreements and 507 (9.0%) cases with minor disagreements. The organ systems involved in the majority of the major disagreements were the female reproductive tract (32), gastrointestinal tract (27), and skin (24). Of the 132 major diagnostic disagreements, 68 (1.2% of total cases reviewed) prompted changes in the clinical management as a result of the second opinion interpretation. These findings support the idea that mandatory second opinion is an important part of patient care in the referral setting.

▶ Manion et al write that what exactly constitutes error in surgical pathology is debatable. The Institute of Medicine (IOM) defined a medical error to be the failure of a planned action to be completed as intended or the use of a wrong plan to achieve an aim. It would follow that a surgical pathology error occurs when the diagnostic test result does not correctly describe the disease process in the patient (ie, the planned action [the test] does not achieve the correct aim [making a correct diagnosis]). Thus, diagnostic disagreements are errors because they reflect differences in the diagnosis. Some authors have argued that diagnostic disagreements are a form of variation and not all variation affects patient care. In the IOM report, there was a careful distinction between error and patient outcome, which may be classified as no harm, harm, or near miss. The vast majority of medical errors are not associated with harm, but that does not mean that they are not errors. In surgical pathology, the vast majority of diagnostic variation also is not associated with harm, but similarly, the variation (or error) still exists. Manion et al classify errors as major and minor, which is a means of assessing potential harm. Minor errors supposedly do not affect patient treatment, but still presumably matter. Manion et al give an example that a minor error is a change in the Furman nuclear grade of a renal cell carcinoma from 2 to 1. It is true that this may not affect treatment, but presumably, Furman nuclear grading is nonetheless important (ie, for prognosis) or we would not be doing it in the first place. Thus, using better developed harm scales, we would still ascribe this error as causing harm, although not major or severe harm.

For further reading on this subject I suggest articles by Kohn et al.[1]

S. S. Raab, MD

Reference

1. Kohn LT, Corrigan JM, Donaldson MS, eds. To Err is Human: Building a Safer Health System. Washington, DC: National Academy Press; 1999.

Diagnostic Terminology and Morphologic Criteria for Cytologic Diagnosis of Thyroid Lesions: A Synopsis of the National Cancer Institute Thyroid Fine-Needle Aspiration State of the Science Conference

Baloch ZW, LiVolsi VA, Asa SL, et al (Univ of Pennsylvania Med Ctr, Philadelphia; Univ of Toronto, Canada; et al)
Diagn Cytopathol 36:425-437, 2008

The National Cancer Institute (NCI) sponsored the **NCI Thyroid Fine-needle Aspiration (FNA) State of the Science Conference** on October 22–23, 2007 in Bethesda, MD. The two-day meeting was accompanied by a permanent informational website and several on-line discussion periods between May 1 and December 15, 2007 (http://thyroidfna.cancer.gov). This document summarizes matters regarding diagnostic terminology/classification scheme for thyroid FNA interpretation and cytomorphologic criteria for the diagnosis of various benign and malignant thyroid lesions. (http://thyroidfna.cancer.gov/pages/info/agenda/).

▶ In October 2007, the National Cancer Institute (NCI) convened a state of the science conference to discuss issues in thyroid gland fine needle aspiration. The article by Baloch et al reports the proposed thyroid gland fine needle aspiration (FNA) classification scheme (Table 2 in the original article). This proposal represents a major step in standardizing how pathologists classify thyroid gland FNAs based on specific cytologic criteria. This standardization process will theoretically result in clinicians being able to formulate specific clinical management plans based on an accepted set of diagnoses, which are based on risk of cancer or neoplasia. I believe that a major problem in thyroid gland FNA is that pathologists tend to interpret less than optimal specimens and that these interpretations lead to false positive and false negative diagnoses. I think these less than optimal FNAs do not fall within the category of unsatisfactory, as this category represents the bare minimum in terms of cells and colloid that are necessary to make an interpretation. Therefore, I believe that pathologists should classify more FNAs as unsatisfactory (which may be difficult to do as clinicians may take issue with this) or use an alternative category, such as nonspecific specimen, which is not listed in this terminology.

For further reading on this topic I suggest articles by Raab et al,[1] and Zhu et al.[2]

S. S. Raab, MD

References

1. Raab SS, Grzybicki DM, Sudilovsky D, Balassanian R, Janosky JE, Vrbin CM. Effectiveness of Toyota process redesign in reducing thyroid gland fine needle aspiration error. *Am J Clin Pathol*. 2006;126:585-592.
2. Zhu W, Michael CW. How important is on-site adequacy assessment for thyroid FNA? An evaluation of 883 cases. *Diagn Cytopathol*. 2007;35:183-186.

Impact of Expected Changes in National Papanicolaou Test Volume on the Cytotechnology Labor Market: An Impending Crisis

Eltoum IA, Roberson J (Univ of Alabama at Birmingham)
Am J Clin Pathol 128:665-670, 2007

With the new screening and treatment guidelines and the prospect of human papillomavirus vaccination for adolescents, the current total volume of Papanicolaou (Pap) tests will be significantly reduced. We used available data to assess the current supply and demand in the cytotechnology labor market and how an expected change in Pap test volume impacts this market. Cytotechnologists' data were obtained from the American Society for Clinical Pathology (ASCP) Board of Registry and the Center for Medicare and Medicaid Services. Data for wages and vacancies were obtained from American Society for Cytotechnologists and ASCP Surveys. Cytotechnology training program data were obtained from annual reports of the Cytotechnology Programs Review Committee of American Society for Cytopathology. In the current market, the demand for cytotechnologists increases by 3.6% and the supply by 4.0% each year. At any given time, there is a vacancy rate of 3%. In the coming years, the demand will decrease remarkably with a projected total demand for cyto-technologists of 5,623 instead of 8,033 by the year 2010 and of 8,538 instead of 14,146 by the year 2026. The cytotechnology market faces an impending crisis. There is a high need for prospectively collected accurate data on demand for and supply of cytotechnologists.

▶ In the past, the backbone of cervical cancer prevention has always been the field of cytotechnology. A number of factors, including the relatively recent implementation of some new technologies, have resulted in major changes in which cervical cancer prevention is practiced. I believe that this trend is not only first appearing in cytotechnology, but will also ultimately alter how the rest of the field of pathology (cytopathology and surgical pathology) will be practiced. Eltoum and Roberson argue that the cytotechnology market faces an impending crisis as a result of the changes in the field of cervical cancer prevention. I believe that the long-term future of cytotechnology will need to transform if it is to thrive. Several potential options may be considered, and these generally include expanding the level of practice in other areas. Some have argued that cytotechnology should blend with the field of pathologists' assistants and become pathologist extenders in all areas of anatomic pathology. Others have argued that cytotechnologists should receive training in molecular biology, as cervical cancer screening (and nongynecologic testing) is becoming much more molecular in nature. As many cytotechnologists currently screen nongynecologic specimens, an alternative push would be to focus the field of cytotechnology on small tissue biopsies, nongynecologic cytology, and fine needle aspiration. Studies showing that cytotechnologist microscopic evaluation in these areas correlates with improved diagnosis would need to be conducted to document cytotechnologist value. This shift also would require a change in practice patterns and reimbursement structures. A third approach would be to transform cytotechnology into a field of quality improvement as cytotechnologists generally are well trained in quality assurance. Changes in cytotechnology will need to occur at the education (cytotechnology schools), practice, reimbursement, and social level for cytotechnology to remain as involved and critical as it has been in the past.

For further reading on this topic I suggest an article by Bedrosian et al.[1]

S. S. Raab, MD

Reference

1. Bedrosian UK, Zaleski S. Cytotechnologist productivity standards: monitoring performance in a TQM environment. *Diagn Cytopathol.* 1997;17:403-405.

Frequency and Outcome of Cervical Cancer Prevention Failures in the United States

Raab SS, Grzybicki DM, Zarbo RJ, et al (Univ of Pittsburgh School of Medicine, PA; Henry Ford Health System, Detroit, MI; et al)
Am J Clin Pathol 128:817-824, 2007

We measured the frequency and outcome of cervical cancer prevention failures that occurred in the Papanicolaou (Pap) and colposcopy testing phases involving 1,646,580 Pap tests in 4 American hospital systems between January 1, 1998, and December 31, 2004. We defined a screening failure as a 2-step or greater discordant Pap test result and follow-up biopsy diagnosis. A total of 5,278 failures were detected (0.321% of all Pap tests); 48% and 52% of failures occurred in the Pap test and colposcopy phases, respectively. Missed squamous cancers (1 in 187,786 Pap tests), glandular cancers (1 in 19,426 Pap tests), and high-grade lesions (1 in 6,870 Pap tests) constituted 4.1% of all failures. Unnecessary repeated tests or diagnostic delays occurred in 70.8% and 63.9% of failures involving high- and low-grade lesions, respectively. We conclude that cervical cancer prevention practices are remarkably successful in preventing squamous cancers, although a high frequency of failures results in low-impact negative outcomes.

▶ Cervical cancer screening services have long focused on improving preneoplastic lesion detection and eliminating specific types of false negative errors. This article indicates that cervical cancer screening has been highly successful in this endeavor, although a consequence has been that other types of errors are relatively prevalent. These errors result in overdiagnosis and overtreatment. The harm associated with these errors is not the catastrophic harm secondary to missed cancers, but a type of low-grade harm associated with overtesting, overtreatment, and patient anxiety. This article indicates that low-grade harm can occur in up to 1 in 10 women undergoing cervical cancer screening in their lifetime. These failures occur both in the Pap test screening phase and in the colposcopy phase of testing, and are secondary to a number of process breakdowns in interpretation and in specimen procurement. It is important to note that these failures are not solely occurring in Pap testing secondary to failures in interpretation or in clinical sampling. An important question is whether these errors are potentially reducible if we aim to maintain a high level of detection. I think the answer is uncertain. Standardizing processes would probably reduce these errors, although the fear of underdiagnosing disease probably plays a critical role in overdiagnosis. A national focus to reduce these errors probably would be necessary, although many believe that cervical cancer screening is exceptional as it helps in preventing cancer.

For further reading on this subject I suggest articles by Kitchener et al,[1] and Jones et al.[2]

S. S. Raab, MD

References

1. Kitchener HC, Castle PE, Cox JT. Chapter 7: achievements and limitations of cervical cytology screening. *Vaccine.* 2006;(24 Suppl 3):S63-S70.
2. Jones BA, Novis DA. Cervical biopsy-cytology correlation. A College of American Pathologists Q-Probes study of 22 439 correlations in 348 laboratories. *Arch Pathol Lab Med.* 1996;120:523-531.

A Contemporary Study Correlating Prostate Needle Biopsy and Radical Prostatectomy Gleason Score

Fine SW, Epstein JI (Memorial Sloan-Kettering Cancer Ctr, New York; Johns Hopkins Hosp, Baltimore, MD)
J Urol 179:1335-1339, 2008

Purpose.—We determined whether contemporary practice patterns of Gleason grading for prostate needle biopsy and radical prostatectomy have evolved.

Materials and Methods.—We correlated needle biopsy (assigned at Johns Hopkins Hospital and other institutions) and radical prostatectomy Gleason score for 1,455 men who underwent radical prostatectomy at Johns Hopkins Hospital from 2002 to 2003, and compared the results with those of a 1994 study of similar design.

Results.—Outside institutions diagnosed Gleason score 2–4 in 1.6% (23 of 1,455) of needle biopsies vs 22.3% (87 of 390) in 1994. Of needle biopsies labeled Gleason score 2–4, 30.4% revealed radical prostatectomy Gleason score 7–10. In 2002 to 2003 no Johns Hopkins Hospital needle biopsy was assigned Gleason score 2–4. Needle biopsies designated Gleason score 6 or less had 80.0% accuracy with regard to radical prostatectomy Gleason score vs 63% accuracy in older data. For needle biopsy Gleason score 7 or greater, 35.5% (outside institution) and 24.8% (Johns Hopkins Hospital) of radical prostatectomies displayed Gleason score less than 7. Overall, outside and Johns Hopkins Hospital needle biopsy diagnoses showed 69.7% and 75.9% agreement with radical prostatectomy Gleason score, respectively. Direct comparison of Johns

Hopkins Hospital and needle biopsy Gleason scores elsewhere revealed 81.8% agreement, with 87.1% for Gleason score 5–6, 68.1% for Gleason score 7 and 35.1% for Gleason score 8–10. For 59.4% of outside needle biopsies with Gleason score 8–10, Johns Hopkins Hospital Gleason score was 7 or less. Conversely, for 64.9% of Johns Hopkins Hospital needle biopsies with Gleason score 8–10, outside Gleason score was 7 or less. For needle biopsies with Gleason score 5–6, 7 and 8–10, the incidence of nonorgan confined disease at radical prostatectomy was 17.7%, 47.8% and 50.0%, respectively, for Johns Hopkins Hospital vs 18.2%, 44.6% and 37.5% for outside institutions.

Conclusions.—The last decade has seen the near elimination of once prevalent under grading of needle biopsy. All cases still assigned Gleason score 2–4 show Gleason score 5 or greater at radical prostatectomy and nearly a third reveal Gleason score 7–10, reaffirming that Gleason score 2–4 is a needle biopsy diagnosis that should not be made. As evidenced by variable over grading and under grading, as well as poor correlation with pathological stage, difficulties in the assignment of Gleason pattern 4 and overall Gleason score of 8–10 on needle biopsy remain an important issue.

▶ Fine and Epstein present convincing data that pathologists have shifted in the past decade to not using Gleason score 2-4 for prostate needle core biopsies. The authors argue that Gleason score 2-4 generally represents undergrading, as prostatectomy specimens show higher Gleason scores. A part of the problem relates to pathologist reproducibility and previously published studies reported that consensus diagnosis of Gleason Score 2-4 on prostate needle core biopsies is very rare. This study was performed at Johns Hopkins Hospital, and a secondary study finding was that there was improved correlation in Gleason grading between outside hospitals and Johns Hopkins Hospital in the study time frame. The authors argue that the community pathologists have undertaken a sustained effort in improving their Gleason grading. These findings are highly important, as they represent a standardization process that has been undertaken on a large scale. The lack of diagnostic reproducibility is not a good thing, as patients receive different diagnoses on the same specimen. This standardization effort, whether it came from community pathologists making a specific effort or for reasons unknown, reflects improvement on a large scale.

For further reading on this subject I suggest an important article by Bostwick.[1]

S. S. Raab, MD

Reference

1. Bostwick DG. Gleason grading of prostatic needle biopsies. Correlation with grade in 316 matched prostatectomies. *Am J Surg Pathol.* 1994;18:796-803.

Impact of Resection Status on Pattern of Failure and Survival After Pancreaticoduodenectomy for Pancreatic Adenocarcinoma

Raut CP, Tseng JF, Sun CC, et al (Univ of Texas M.D. Anderson Cancer Ctr, Houston, TX)
Ann Surg 246:52-60, 2007

Objective.—To better understand the impact of a microscopically positive margin (R1) on patterns of disease recurrence and survival after pancreaticoduodenectomy (PD) for pancreatic adenocarcinoma.

Summary Background Data.—A positive resection margin after PD is considered to be a poor prognostic factor, and some have proposed that an R1 margin may be a biologic predictor of more aggressive disease. The natural history of patients treated with contemporary multimodality therapy who underwent a positive margin PD has not been described.

Methods.—We analyzed our experience from 1990 to 2004, which included the prospective use of a standardized system for pathologic analysis of all PD specimens. All patients who underwent PD met objective computed tomographic criteria for resection. Standard pathologic evaluation of the PD specimen included permanent section analysis of the final bile duct, pancreatic, and superior mesenteric artery (SMA) margins. First recurrences (all sites) were defined as local, regional, or distant. Survival and follow-up were calculated from the date of initial histologic diagnosis to the dates of first recurrence or death and last contact, respectively.

Results.—PD was performed on 360 consecutive patients with pancreatic adenocarcinoma. Minimum follow-up was 12 months (median, 51.9 months). The resection margins were negative (R0) in 300 patients (83.3%) and positive (R1) in 60 (16.7%); no patients had macroscopically positive (R2) margins. By multivariate analysis (MVA), high mean operative blood loss and large tumor size were independent predictors of an R1 resection. Patients who underwent an R1 resection had a median overall survival of 21.5 months compared with 27.8 months in patients who underwent an R0 resection. After controlling for other variables on MVA, resection status did not independently affect survival. By MVA, only lymph node metastases, major perioperative complications, and blood loss adversely affected survival.

Conclusions.—There was no statistically significant difference in patient survival or recurrence based on R status. However, this series is unique in the incorporation of a standardized surgical technique for the SMA dissection, the prospective use of a reproducible system for pathologic evaluation of resection margins, the absence of R2 resections, and the frequent use of multimodality therapy (Fig 1).

▶ This article is important for several reasons. First, the ability to evaluate patient outcomes related to surgical procedures depends on developing standardized protocols of gross examination and histologic interpretation. Raut et al correctly point out that the lack of standardization of pathology margin

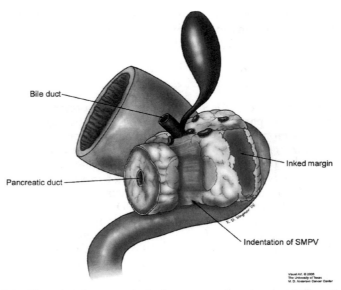

FIGURE 1.—Illustration of a pancreaticoduodenectomy specimen demonstrating how the superior mesenteric artery margin should be inked at the time of permanent section pathologic examination. This margin cannot be retrospectively evaluated if the margin was not inked for identification at the time of gross inspection. SMPV, superior mesentericportal vein. (Reprinted from Raut CP, Tseng JF, Sun CC, et al. Impact of resection status on pattern of failure and survival after pancreaticoduodenectomy for pancreatic adenocarcinoma. *Ann Surg.* 2007;246:52-60.)

reporting in pancreatic resections has limited the ability to truly evaluate the importance of microscopic tumor involvement of pancreatic margins. Raut et al clearly define the different margins (final bile duct, pancreatic, and superior mesenteric artery [SMA]) and then show that there was no statistically significant difference in patient survival or recurrence based on no microscopic involvement (R0) compared with microscopic involvement (R1) of margins. This evaluation depends on the ability to separate margin involvement into 3 categories: R0, R1, and R2 (macroscopic involvement). Thus, a second reason why this article is important is that pathologists need to formally assess margin status in this manner. The American Joint Committee on Cancer (AJCC) Cancer Staging Manual evaluates the soft tissue and perineural fibers adjacent to the right lateral border of the SMA and the margin should be obtained first by inking and then by sectioning in a perpendicular fashion (performed by the pathologist) (Fig 1).

For further reading on this subject I suggest articles by Sohn et al[1] and Willett et al.[2]

S. S. Raab, MD

References

1. Sohn TA, Yeo CJ, Cameron JL, et al. Resected adenocarcinoma of the pancreas-616 patients: results, outcomes, and prognostic indicators. *J Gastrointest Surg.* 2000;4:567-579.
2. Willett CG, Lewandrowski K, Warshaw AL, Efird J, Compton CC. Resection margins in carcinoma of the head of the pancreas: implications for radiation therapy. *Ann Surg.* 1993;217:144-148.

The frequency of missed test results and associated treatment delays in a highly computerized health system
Wahls TL, Cram PM (Iowa City Dept of Veterans Affairs (VA) Med Ctr; Univ of Iowa Carver College of Medicine; et al)
BMC Fam Pract 8:32, 2007

Background.—Diagnostic errors associated with the failure to follow up on abnormal diagnostic studies ("missed results") are a potential cause of treatment delay and a threat to patient safety. Few data exist concerning the frequency of missed results and associated treatment delays within the Veterans Health Administration (VA).

Objective.—The primary objective of the current study was to assess the frequency of missed results and resulting treatment delays encountered by primary care providers in VA clinics.

Methods.—An anonymous on-line survey of primary care providers was conducted as part of the health systems ongoing quality improvement programs. We collected information from providers concerning their clinical effort (e.g., number of clinic sessions, number of patient visits per session), number of patients with missed abnormal test results, and the number and types of treatment delays providers encountered during the two week period prior to administration of our survey.

Results.—The survey was completed by 106 out of 198 providers (54 percent response rate). Respondents saw an average of 86 patients per 2 week period. Providers encountered 64 patients with missed results during the two week period leading up to the study and 52 patients with treatment delays. The most common missed results included imaging studies (29 percent), clinical laboratory (22 percent), anatomic pathology (9 percent), and other (40 percent). The most common diagnostic delays were cancer (34 percent), endocrine problems (26 percent), cardiac problems (16 percent), and others (24 percent).

Conclusion.—Missed results leading to clinically important treatment delays are an important and likely underappreciated source of diagnostic error.

▶ The failure to communicate a diagnosis is a failure in the postanalytic phase of testing. Wahls and Cram use a survey method to assess the frequency of missed test results and resulting treatment delays. The authors found that over 30% of missed results were secondary to either clinical or anatomic pathology laboratory failures. These types of failures have a number of causes including delays in reporting, failures in transmission, failures in receipt, and failures in acting on results. Eliminating these failures requires system redesign that often involves a degree of standardization of process. These failures occur at the "hand-off" point between laboratory and clinical services, and often are difficult to address because neither service has complete control of the process. A limitation in this article is that there was no formal assessment of clinical consequences of delays. Other researchers have found that the major clinical consequence in a diagnostic delay is patient anxiety, although rarely more catastrophic events may occur.

For further reading on this subject I suggest articles by Raab et al.[1,2]

S. S. Raab, MD

References

1. Raab SS, Grzybicki DM, Janosky JE, et al. Clinical impact and frequency of anatomic pathology errors in cancer diagnosis. *Cancer.* 2005;104:2205-2213.
2. Raab SS, Grzybicki DM, Zarbo RJ, et al. Frequency and outcome of cervical cancer prevention failures in the United States. *Am J Clin Pathol.* 2007;128: 817-824.

2 Breast

Lobular Neoplasia on Core Needle Biopsy Does Not Require Excision

Nagi CS, O'Donnell JE, Tismenetsky M, et al (Mount Sinai School of Medicine, NY)

Cancer 112:2152-2158, 2008

Background.—Lobular neoplasia (LN), encompassing atypical lobular hyperplasia (ALH) and lobular carcinoma in situ (LCIS), is often an incidental finding on core needle biopsies (CNBs) performed in instances of radiologic densities and/or calcifications. Because LN is generally considered a risk factor for breast carcinoma, the utility of subsequent excision is controversial.

Methods.—The authors' database yielded 98 cases of LCIS and/or ALH. Cases containing LN accompanied by a second lesion mandating excision (eg, radial scar, atypical ductal hyperplasia [ADH]) and those failing to meet strict diagnostic criteria for LN (eg, atypical cells, mitoses, single-cell necrosis) were excluded. Radiographic calcifications were correlated with their histologic counterparts in terms of size, number, and pattern.

Results.—Ninety-one biopsies were performed for calcifications and 7 were performed for mass lesions. The ages of the patients ranged from 35 to 82 years. Fifty-three patients were followed radiologically without excision, 42 of whom had available clinicoradiologic information. The 45 patients who underwent excision were without disease at follow-up periods ranging from 1 to 8 years. Of these 45 patients, 42 (93%) had biopsy results demonstrating only LN. The remaining 3 patients had biopsies with the following findings: ADH in 1 biopsy, residual LCIS and a separate minute focus of infiltrating lobular carcinoma (clearly an incidental finding) in the second biopsy, and ductal carcinoma in situ admixed with LCIS in the third biopsy (a retrospective examination performed by 2 blinded breast pathologists revealed foci of atypical cells and mitoses).

Conclusions.—Excision of LN is unnecessary provided that: 1) careful radiographic-pathologic correlation is performed; and 2) strict histologic criteria are adhered to when making the diagnosis. Close radiologic and clinical follow-up is adequate.

▶ Atypical lobular hyperplasia and lobular carcinoma in situ are commonly considered risk factors for the development of breast carcinoma and not precursor lesions per se. As such, re-excision of these lesions, considered together as "lobular neoplasia," is not considered the optimal management strategy by many, as they consider the entire breast tissue to be at risk for development of invasive tumor. However, this viewpoint is not uniformly accepted, and others have suggested re-excision of such lesions,[1] including an article published the following month.[2] Of the 45 patients who underwent re-excision in this study, 2 had significant diagnostic changes in the re-excision specimen, both retrospectively were noted to have findings on the original core biopsy that were not initially appreciated, which may have mitigated the discrepancy.

Pathologists need to be aware that there is disagreement about how to treat these patients. Many may not undergo re-excision using strict criteria in the diagnosis of lobular neoplasia, including identifying cases with pleomorphic features, and maintaining close radiographic correlation are important recommendations.

G. Azabdaftari, MD

References

1. Elsheikh TM, Silverman JF. Follow-up surgical excision is indicated when breast core needle biopsies show atypical lobular hyperplasia or lobular carcinoma in situ a correlative study of 33 patients with review of the literature. *Am J Surg Pathol.* 2005;29:534-543.
2. Cangiarella J, Guth A, Axelrod D, et al. Is surgical excision necessary for the management of atypical lobular hyperplasia and lobular carcinoma in situ diagnosed on core needle biopsy?: a report of 38 cases and review of the literature. *Arch Pathol Lab Med.* 2008;132:979-983.

Heterogeneity of Breast Cancer Metastases: Comparison of Therapeutic Target Expression and Promoter Methylation Between Primary Tumors and Their Multifocal Metastases

Wu JM, Fackler MJ, Halushka MK, et al (Johns Hopkins Med Inst, Baltimore, MD; et al)
Clin Cancer Res 14:1938-1946, 2008

Purpose.—A comprehensive comparison of biomarker expression between patients' primary breast carcinoma (PBC) and their metastatic breast carcinomas (MBC) has not been done.

Experimental Design.—We did rapid autopsies (postmortem intervals, 1-4 hours) on 10 consenting patients who died of MBC. We constructed single-patient tissue microarrays from the patients' archived PBC and multiple different MBCs harvested at autopsy, which were immunohistochemically labeled for multiple biomarkers. Methylation of multiple gene promoters was assessed quantitatively on dissected PBC and MBC samples.

Results.—Extensive heterogeneity was observed between PBC and their paired MBC, as well as among multiple MBC from the same patient. Estrogen and progesterone receptors tended to be uniformly down-regulated in metastases. E-cadherin was down-regulated in a subset of the MBC of one case. Variable overexpression in MBC compared with the PBC was observed for cyclooxygenase-2 (five cases), epidermal growth factor receptor (EGFR; four cases), MET (four cases), and mesothelin (four cases). No case strongly overexpressed HER-2/neu by immunohistochemistry, but eight cases showed variable protein expression ranging from negative to equivocal (2+) in different MBC. In one case, variable low-level HER-2/neu gene amplification was found. EGFR and MET overexpression were restricted to the four basal-type cancers. EGFR protein overexpression did not correlate with EGFR gene amplification. Multigene promoter hypermethylation of *RASSF1a, HIN1, cyclin D2, Twist, estrogen receptor α, APC1, and RAR β* was overall very similar in the PBC and all MBCs in all cases.

Conclusions.—Therapeutic targets identified in the PBC or even some MBC may not reflect targets present in all metastatic sites.

▶ This study used a rapid autopsy protocol to study the biological changes between primary breast carcinomas and their associated metastatic deposits. With this methodology the investigators were able to construct tissue microarrays for each patient, which is composed of the primary tumor and metastases from different sites. This allowed direct evaluation and comparison of clinically important biomarker expression. Markers that are evaluated include estrogen receptor, progesterone receptor, E-cadherin, cyclooxygenase-2, epidermal growth factor receptor, mesothelin, and HER-2/neu. The important finding for the practicing pathologist is that metastatic lesions frequently demonstrate altered biological activity from the primary tumor. Some markers, notably ER and PR were often down-regulated in the metastatic disease, whereas others such as epidermal growth factor receptor (EGFR) and MET were often relatively overexpressed in the metastasis. Given the current use of therapeutic modalities targeted to specific proteins, these and similar findings will become important as pathologists evaluate samples from metastatic disease. The article also addresses fundamental issues in the biology of metastatic disease, notably that the promoter methylation profile for selected genes is not altered, thus the authors furthered the concept that "a cancer's genetic makeup and, therefore, its clinical behavior are likely determined at its primary site."

G. Azabdaftari, MD

Basal-Like Breast Cancer Defined by Five Biomarkers Has Superior Prognostic Value than Triple-Negative Phenotype
Cheang MCU, Voduc D, Bajdik C, et al (Univ of British Columbia; Cancer Control Res Program, British Columbia; et al)
Clin Cancer Res 14:1368-1376, 2008

Purpose.—Basal-like breast cancer is associated with high grade, poor prognosis, and younger patient age. Clinically, a triple-negative phenotype definition [estrogen receptor, progesterone receptor, and human epidermal growth factor receptor (HER)-2, all negative] is commonly used to identify such cases. EGFR and cytokeratin 5/6 are readily available positive markers of basal-like breast cancer applicable to standard pathology specimens. This study directly compares the prognostic significance between three- and five-biomarker surrogate panels to define intrinsic breast cancer subtypes, using a large clinically annotated series of breast tumors.

Experimental Design.—Four thousand forty-six invasive breast cancers were assembled into tissue microarrays. All had staging, pathology, treatment, and outcome information; median follow-up was 12.5 years. Cox regression analyses and likelihood ratio tests compared the prognostic significance for breast cancer death-specific survival (BCSS) of the two immunohistochemical panels.

Results.—Among 3,744 interpretable cases, 17% were basal using the triple-negative definition (10-year BCSS, 67%) and 9% were basal using the five-marker method (10-year BCSS, 62%). Likelihood ratio tests of multivariable Cox models including standard clinical variables show that the five-marker panel is significantly more prognostic than the three-marker panel. The poor prognosis of triple-negative phenotype is conferred almost entirely by those tumors positive for basal markers. Among triple-negative patients treated with adjuvant anthracycline-based chemotherapy, the additional positive basal markers identified a cohort of patients with significantly worse outcome.

Conclusions.—The expanded surrogate immunopanel of estrogen receptor, progesterone receptor, human HER-2, EGFR, and cytokeratin 5/6 provides a more specific definition of basal-like breast cancer that better predicts breast cancer survival.

▶ The concept of a distinct subtype of breast carcinoma with basal cell-like features first began 20 years ago.[1] From its inception, several features were noted to correlate including characteristic morphologic features, expression of basal-type cytokeratins, and poor prognosis. Additional features include the important observation that these tumors typically do not express estrogen and progesterone receptor or human epidermal growth factor receptor 2 (HER2/neu), resulting in a so-called triple negative phenotype. Despite 20 years of development of the basal-like carcinoma concept including the advent of gene expression pattern analysis,[2] a widely accepted consensus definition for basal cell carcinoma based on immunohistochemistry still does not exist. Some have proposed that the triple negative phenotype is sufficient to define basal-like carcinoma.[3] The authors of this study make an evidenced argument that using an expanded panel of immunohistochemical markers, a group of tumors can be identified that more closely approximates the basal-like carcinoma entity as defined by gene expression analysis. The practicing pathologist should remain aware of the basal-like carcinoma concept development, as it may ultimately become an important distinction with unique genetic, immunohistochemical, and prognostic implications.

G. Azabdaftari, MD

References

1. Dairkee SH, Puett L, Hackett AJ. Expression of basal and luminal epithelium-specific keratins in normal, benign, and malignant breast tissue. *J Natl Cancer Inst.* 1988;80:691-695.

2. Perou CM, Sorlie T, Eisen MB, et al. Molecular portraits of human breast tumours. *Nature.* 2000;406:747-752.
3. Kreike B, van Kouwenhove M, Horlings H, et al. Gene expression profiling and histopathological characterization of triple-negative/basal-like breast carcinomas. *Breast Cancer Res.* 2007;9:R65.

Lymphomas Involving the Breast: A Study of 106 Cases Comparing Localized and Disseminated Neoplasms

Talwalkar SS, Miranda RN, Valbuena JR, et al (Univ of Texas M.D. Anderson Cancer Ctr, Houston, TX; et al)
Am J Surg Pathol 32:1299-1309, 2008

Lymphomas involving the breast account for approximately 2% of extranodal and <1% of all non-Hodgkin lymphomas. Our aim in this study was to classify breast lymphomas using the World Health Organization classification and then compare this classification with clinical, histologic, and radiologic findings as well as survival. The study group included 106 patients with breast lymphoma (105 women and 1 man). The neoplasms were divided into 2 groups based on extent of disease at initial diagnosis: localized disease (n = 50) and disseminated disease (n = 56). The follow-up period ranged from 4 to 252 months (median, 49 mo). Almost all (97%) patients presented with a palpable breast mass or masses. In the localized group, diffuse large B-cell lymphoma (DLBCL) was most frequent (n = 32, 64%). In the disseminated group, follicular lymphoma was most frequent and exclusive to this group (*P* = 0.0004). Mucosa-associated lymphoid tissue lymphomas occurred in both groups without a significant difference in frequency. A variety of other types of B-cell and T-cell non-Hodgkin lymphomas and classical Hodgkin lymphoma involved the breast at much lower frequency; most of these neoplasms involved the breast as part of disseminated disease. The clinical presentation correlated with radiologic findings: localized lymphomas presented as solitary masses, whereas disseminated lymphomas commonly presented as multifocal masses. There was a significant difference in the disease-free survival between patients with localized and disseminated DLBCL (*P* = 0.003). In the disseminated group, patients with DLBCL had a worse disease-free survival compared with patients with mucosa-associated lymphoid tissue lymphoma or follicular lymphoma (*P* = 0.01).

▶ Lymphoma involving the breast is an uncommon and often surprising finding in general pathology practice, however, as it may be the primary or presenting site, practical knowledge in the accurate diagnosis of such lesions is important. This study collects the experience of The University of Texas MD Anderson Cancer Center over the last 20 years and classifies lesions according to the current World Health Organization system. Importantly, radiologic findings were also part of the study and were noted to correlate with the clinical findings; localized disease presented as solitary masses and secondary breast involvement presented as multiple masses. The authors note that the typical bimodal age distribution of breast lymphoma noted in previous studies was not present in their series. Also, the typical poor behavior of diffuse large B-cell lymphoma was not noted in their study. These differences may reflect the changes imposed by cancer screening programs. For the practicing pathologist this provides a useful and updated overview of breast-specific lymphoma with current WHO nomenclature.

G. Azabdaftari, MD

Prognostic differences of World Health Organization–assessed mitotic activity index and mitotic impression by quick scanning in invasive ductal breast cancer patients younger than 55 years

Skaland I, van Diest PJ, Janssen EAM, et al (Stavanger Unive Hospital, Norway; Univ Med Ctr, Utrecht, Netherlands)
Hum Pathol 39:584-590, 2008

The proliferation marker mitotic activity index is the strongest prognostic indicator in lymph node–negative breast cancer. The World Health Organization (WHO) 2003–defined procedure for determining WHO-mitotic activity index is often replaced by a quick scan mitotic impression. We evaluated the prognostic consequences of this practice in 433 $T_{1-3}N_0M_0$ lymph node–negative invasive ductal type breast cancers with long-term follow-up (median, 112 months; range, 12-187 months). Twenty-seven percent of the studied cases developed distant metastases, and 25% died of disease. Agreement between WHO-mitotic activity index (0-5 = 1, 6-10 = 2, >10 = 3) and mitotic impression (1, 2, 3) categories was 66% ($\kappa = 0.41$), including 85% for category 1, 26% for category 2, and 52% for category 3. The WHO-mitotic activity index was a much stronger prognosticator than the mitotic impression, and the 10-year survival rates of the same categories (eg, mitotic activity index and mitotic impression category both 2) differed greatly. When grade was assessed by combining WHO-mitotic activity index or mitotic impression with the same values for tubular formation and nuclear atypia, grades disagreed in 18% of the cases. Deviation from the formal WHO-mitotic activity index assessment guidelines in breast cancer often results in erroneous prognosis estimations with therapeutic consequences and may explain why the prognostic value of proliferative activity in breast cancer is not always confirmed.

▶ The proliferative activity of breast carcinoma is a well-known prognostic indicator; it is especially predictive in the absence of regional lymph node metastases. Although some now use the Ki-67 immunohistochemical marker, quantifying mitoses remains a proven mainstay for communicating the degree of proliferative activity and frequently functions as part of standardized pathology reporting. This study raises an important issue about the specific method by which this critical piece of data is collected by pathologists. The World Health Organization has recommended a specific method that involves counting mitoses in 10 high-powered fields in the most proliferative part of the tumor. As the authors of this study note, many pathologists have taken to a more efficient method where the rate of mitotic activity is quickly estimated often following a brief high-powered scan of a few areas of tumor. The authors performed both types of analyses and concluded that the formal WHO method was a stronger mitotic prognosticator than the quick impression method. The natural limitation to the study is the inherently subjective nature of the quick assessment. As pathologists approach this mitotic rate grading during daily surgical pathology differently, one might claim that the quick screen method used in the study is not generalizable to their practice. However, the predictive nature of the formal, WHO-defined method is supported by this study when compared with the alternative method. Pathologists should be aware of the methodology and established value of the WHO-defined method and realize the uncertainty of alternative methods.

G. Azabdaftari, MD

Refinement of breast cancer classification by molecular characterization of histological special types
Weigelt B, Horlings HM, Kreike B, et al (The Netherlands Cancer Inst, Amsterdam)
J Pathol 216:141-150, 2008

Most invasive breast cancers are classified as invasive ductal carcinoma not otherwise specified (IDC NOS), whereas about 25% are defined as histological 'special types'. These special-type breast cancers are categorized into at least 17 discrete pathological entities; however, whether these also constitute discrete molecular entities remains to be determined. Current therapy decision-making is increasingly governed by the molecular classification of breast cancer (luminal, basal-like, HER2+). The molecular classification is derived from mainly IDC NOS and it is unknown whether this classification applies to all histological subtypes. We aimed to refine the breast cancer classification systems by analysing a series of 11 histological special types [invasive lobular carcinoma (ILC), tubular, mucinous A, mucinous B, neuroendocrine, apocrine, IDC with osteoclastic giant cells, micropapillary, adenoid cystic, metaplastic, and medullary carcinoma] using immunohistochemistry and genome-wide gene expression profiling. Hierarchical clustering analysis confirmed that some histological special types constitute discrete entities, such as micropapillary carcinoma, but also revealed that others, including tubular and lobular carcinoma, are very similar at the transcriptome level. When classified by expression profiling, IDC NOS and ILC contain all molecular breast cancer types (ie luminal, basal-like, HER2+), whereas histological special-type cancers, apart from apocrine carcinoma, are homogeneous and only belong to one molecular subtype. Our analysis also revealed that some special types associated with a good prognosis, such as medullary and adenoid cystic carcinomas, display a poor prognosis basal-like transcriptome, providing strong circumstantial evidence that basal-like cancers constitute a heterogeneous group. Taken together, our results imply that the correct classification of breast cancers of special histological type will allow a more accurate prognostication of breast cancer patients and facilitate the identification of optimal therapeutic strategies.

▶ In 2000, Perou et al[1] published the results of a study subclassifying breast carcinomas based on the expression pattern of 8102 genes. Based on this molecular classification approach, 3 general categories of breast carcinoma have been proposed including luminal, basal-like, and HER2 +. This landmark study was, however, limited predominantly to invasive ductal carcinoma. This study applies the concept of gene expression profile-based taxonomy to include 11 subtypes of breast cancer, which are well known to pathologists, and of these only invasive lobular was included in the original Perou study. This wide reaching study suggests an overall classification scheme that could potentially encompass all epithelial breast neoplasms based on gene expression profiles. The practicing pathologist, who has relied on histopathologic and immunohistochemical features for classification, may find it interesting how the gene expression data validate the unique characterization of some subtypes (pleomorphic lobular) and demonstrate relationships between others (adenoid cystic, metaplastic, and basal-like). As acknowledged by the authors, this classification model is far from complete, but this study gives a workable indication of what a future arrangement may look like.

G. Azabdaftari, MD

Reference

1. Perou CM, Sorlie T, Eisen MB, et al. Molecular portraits of human breast tumours. *Nature*. 2000;406:747-752.

Atypical Vascular Lesions After Surgery and Radiation of the Breast: A Clinicopathologic Study of 32 Cases Analyzing Histologic Heterogeneity and Association With Angiosarcoma
Patton KT, Deyrup AT, Weiss SW (Emory Univ School of Medicine, Atlanta, GA)
Am J Surg Pathol 32:943-950, 2008

We report the clinicopathologic study of 32 cases of atypical vascular lesions (AVLs) after surgery and radiation of the breast, which were referred to us in consultation over a 17-year period. The patients, all women, ranged in age from 41 to 95 years (mean 61 y). The lesions developed within the radiation field from 1 to 12 years (median 6.0 y) after therapy. They occurred as one (n = 18) or more (n = 10) flesh-colored papules or erythematous patches/plaques ranging in size from 1 to 60 mm (mean 8.0 mm, median 4.0 mm). Tumors could be divided into 2 histologic types: a lymphatic type (LT) (n = 22) and a vascular type (VT) (n = 10). LT AVLs consisted predominantly of thin-walled, variably anastomosing lymphatic vessels that were usually confined to the superficial dermis but occasionally extended into the deep dermis and even subcutis. The VT (n = 10) typically consisted of small, irregularly dispersed, often blood-filled, pericyte-invested, capillary-sized vessels involving the superficial or deep dermis. VTs were often associated with extravasated erythrocytes, hemosiderin, and a surrounding minor LT component. In 4 cases, endothelial atypia, consisting of nuclear and nucleolar enlargement, was noted. Follow-up of 21 patients with LT AVLs (1 to 106 mo; mean 47 mo) disclosed recurrence/additional lesions in 6, all of whom had additional surgery. Of the 21 patients, 17 are alive without disease, 1 is alive with disease, 1 died of breast carcinoma, 1 died of unknown causes, and 1 showed progressive histologic changes in the AVLs over a period of 5 years resulting in a well-differentiated angiosarcoma. Follow-up in 8 patients with VT AVL (2 to 181 mo; mean 40 mo) disclosed that 6 were alive and well, but 2 of the 4 patients whose lesions displayed endothelial atypia had additional complications. One patient underwent a mastectomy that revealed extensive residual AVL and the second developed a high-grade angiosarcoma after 14 months. We conclude that AVLs encompass a wider spectrum of changes than previously appreciated, ranging from superficial lymphatic proliferations to more complex lymphatic and capillary vascular lesions. There seems to be an association of AVL with angiosarcoma that differs depending on the histologic features, with the VT AVLs having the higher risk. In the 2 patients who developed angiosarcoma, morphologic evidence suggested AVLs to be a precursor rather than simply a risk factor. Future outcome and management studies should take into account these differences.

▶ The vascular neoplasms most often associated with the treatment of breast carcinoma include those that arise as a complication of long-standing lymphedema (Stewart-Treves) and postirradiation angiosarcoma. Other vascular lesions have been noted to develop within previously irradiated fields that do not meet the criteria for angiosarcoma. Some have suggested that these were benign lesions.[1] However, only a small number of cases with follow-up data have been reported,[2] hence the significance of this study, which adds Dr Weiss's experience with these types of lesions. She expands the concept to include those composed of capillary vessels and those composed of lymphatic vessels. The significance of this distinction being that the lymphatic type may only rarely be associated with development of an angiosarcoma, whereas the vascular type may have a relatively increased risk of angiosarcoma development. The main caveat to the observations in this study and those of others are the still small collection of cases reported to date. Many uncertainties still exist, including the absolute risk of developing a truly aggressive vascular lesion following the diagnosis of an atypical vascular lesion, the relationship between the lymphatic and vascular types, and whether or not these atypical vascular lesions truly develop into more aggressive lesions or are markers of increased risk of developing such lesions.

J. Wisell, MD

References

1. Fineberg S, Rosen PP. Cutaneous angiosarcoma and atypical vascular lesions of the skin and breast after radiation therapy for breast carcinoma. *Am J Clin Pathol.* 1994;102:757-763.
2. Gengler C, Coindre JM, Leroux A, et al. Vascular proliferations of the skin after radiation therapy for breast cancer: clinicopathologic analysis of a series in favor of a benign process: a study from the French Sarcoma Group. *Cancer.* 2007;109: 1584-1598.

Aberrant Expression of E-cadherin in Lobular Carcinomas of the Breast
Da Silva L, Parry S, Reid L, et al (Univ of Queensland, Brisbane, Australia; et al)
Am J Surg Pathol 32:773-783, 2008

Invasive lobular carcinoma (ILC) and lobular carcinoma in situ characteristically show loss of E-cadherin expression and so immunohistochemistry for E-cadherin is being increasingly used as a tool to differentiate between lobular and ductal lesions in challenging situations. However, misinterpretation of "aberrant" positive staining may lead some to exclude a diagnosis of lobular carcinoma. E-cadherin and β-catenin immunohistochemistry was analyzed in 25 ILCs. E-cadherin "positive" ILCs were subjected to molecular analysis including comparative genomic hybridization. Different morphologic components of case 25, showing heterogenous E-cadherin expression, were analyzed by E-cadherin gene sequencing, methylation, and DASL gene expression profiling. Four ILCs were positive for E-cadherin, but each also had neoplastic cells with aberrant staining. Two of these ILCs were positive for β-catenin, again with some aberrantly stained neoplastic cells, and 2 were negative. The solid component of case 25 was positive for E-cadherin whereas the classic and alveolar areas were negative. All components harbored an inframe deletion in exon 7 (867del24) of the E-cadherin gene and loss of the wild type allele. Comparative genomic hybridization demonstrated evidence of clonal evolution from E-cadherin–positive to E-cadherin–negative components. E-cadherin downregulation seems to be through transcriptional repression via activation of transforming growth factor-β/SMAD2 rather than methylation. Positive staining for E-cadherin should not preclude a diagnosis of lobular in favor of ductal carcinoma. Molecular evidence suggests that even when E-cadherin is expressed, the cadherin-catenin complex maybe nonfunctional. Misclassification of tumors may lead to mismanagement of patients in clinical practice, particularly in the context of in situ disease at margins.

▶ E-cadherin is a molecule involved in cell-cell adhesion and has experienced widespread use as a marker to differentiate lobular from ductal carcinoma. More than a useful tool diagnostically, this pathway also likely has a major role in determining the histopathologic and clinical differences between lobular and closely related ductal carcinomas. This article confirms earlier reports of E-cadherin expression in cases diagnosed with routine histochemistry as lobular carcinoma. The genetic analysis performed in this article demonstrated nonfunctional, immunohistochemically viable E-cadherin protein. Recent studies[1] attempting to develop a breast carcinoma taxonomy are based on gene expression profiles. This study illustrates the point that the functional status of the protein ultimately determines the phenotype. Thus, any genetic-based classification may need further refinement by an understanding of the functional status of genes and post-translational modification events. For the diagnostic pathologist this is an important phenomenon to understand given the widespread diagnostic use of this particular molecular pathway.

G. Azabdaftari, MD

Reference

1. Weigelt B, Horlings HM, Kreike B, et al. Refinement of breast cancer classification by molecular characterization of histological special types. *J Pathol.* 2008;216: 141-150.

Distinction Between Isolated Tumor Cells and Micrometastases in Breast Cancer: is it Reliable and Useful?

de Mascarel I, MacGrogan G, Debled M, et al (Inst Bergonie, Bordeaux, France)
Cancer 112:1672-1678, 2008

Background.—In routine practice, the distinction between isolated tumor cells (ITC) and micrometastases (MIC) in patients with breast cancer is sometimes difficult to discern. The authors assessed differences in classifying patients according to the American Joint Commission on Cancer (AJCC) and the International Union Against Cancer (UICC) definitions and method of sizing.

Methods.—We assessed the characteristics of metastatic deposits in only 1 involved lymph node in 337 patients with operable breast cancer (median followup, 15.3 years). When sizing multiple clusters, either the diameter of the area with close clusters (Method 1) or the size of the largest cluster (Method 2) was taken into account. Patients were classified and their survival was assessed according to the 2 sizing methods and the criteria used for definitions (size in AJCC; size and topography in UICC).

Results.—With the AJCC definitions, 32 patients would be differently classified according to the method of sizing. With the UICC definitions, some patients with parenchymal ITC would be classified as pN1mi, 38 by Method 1 and 53 by Method 2. Some pathologists would classify the 66 patients who had isolated capsular vascular invasion as pN0. Classification was uncertain in 136 (40%) to 151 (45 %) patients. Survival was not significantly different between pN0(i+) and pN1(mi) patients.

Conclusions.—The distinction between ITC and MIC was often difficult and without any prognostic significance. Precise guidelines are more useful for staging than for therapy. Thus, complete axillary dissection is usually performed in pN0(i+) and pN1(mi) patients, whereas chemotherapy is not indicated or debatable when MIC is the only 1 pejorative criterion.

▶ Stratifying patients with metastatic carcinoma of the breast according to the degree of local regional lymph node involvement has proven useful in directing treatment and delineating prognosis.[1] However, defining the low end of this continuum, those patients with minimal metastatic tumor burden, poses challenges for pathologists. This study highlights 2 main areas where interpretations of these small deposits vary. First, how should one measure several small clusters of metastatic disease, together or separately? Second, should one take into account other features such as location of tumor within the lymph node and reaction when classifying, or should one rely solely on size? Despite the continued lack of consensus on these issues, pathologists may find the study authors' primary finding reassuring, as they found that "there was no significant difference in metastasis-free survival between pN0(i1) and pN1(mi) patients, whatever the method of sizing and the classification used." Practicing surgical pathologists should watch closely for further outcome data from similar studies and consensus recommendations that will hopefully follow.

G. Azabdaftari, MD

Reference

1. Nemoto T, Vana J, Bedwani RN, Baker HW, McGregor FH, Murphy GP. Management and survivial of female breast cancer: results of a national survey by the American Collage of Surgeons. *Cancer.* 1980;45:2917-2924.

Laminin 5 Expression in Metaplastic Breast Carcinomas
Carpenter PM, Wang-Rodriguez J, Chan OTM, et al (Univ of California, Irvine; Univ of California, San Diego; City of Hope Med Ctr, Duarte, CA)
Am J Surg Pathol 32:345-353, 2008

Metaplastic carcinoma of the breast shows squamous, sarcomatous, or chondromatous differentiation and has a poor prognosis. Laminin 5 is a heterotrimer of $\alpha3$, $\beta3$, and χ^2 chains and induces aggressive properties in cancer cells including motility, invasion, and epithelial to mesenchymal transition. Twenty-five cases included 7 squamous, 4 sarcomatous, 8 chondroid, 1 fibromatosislike metaplastic carcinomas, and 5 cases with 2 metaplastic components. Tumors were stained with laminin 5-specific β3 and χ^2 chain, p63, and cytokeratin 5/6 (CK 5/6) antibodies. All 4 antibodies stained normal myoepithelium. Both laminin 5 antibodies stained 24/25 (96%) of the tumors, with an identical distribution of the 2 chains in 87.5% of the positively staining cases. In contrast, p63 and CK 5/6 stained 68% and 64% of the tumors, respectively. By comparison, only 16% of high-grade carcinoma controls stained for laminin 5. Similar to the metaplastic carcinomas, all 12 triple negative tumors, those negative for estrogen receptor, progesterone receptor, and Her2/neu, expressed laminin 5. None of 4 breast sarcomas stained for either of the laminin 5 chains or CK 5/6, but 1 (25%) stained for p63. Laminin 5 expression in metaplastic and other basal-like carcinomas is of interest for several reasons. First, these data provide additional evidence of the myoepithelial and basal-like phenotype of these carcinomas. Second, these are the only breast carcinoma subtypes to demonstrate laminin 5 staining in a large proportion of cases. Third, expression of laminin 5 in metaplastic carcinomas may suggest a mechanism for their increased aggressiveness and epithelial to mesenchymal transition phenotype. Finally, compared with other myoepithelial markers, laminin 5 is more sensitive than those previously published. Thus laminin 5 may be helpful for making the diagnosis of metaplastic carcinomas in biopsies, allowing the potential for aggressive early treatment. Further study of other basal-like tumors for laminin 5 expression is warranted to determine the usefulness of laminin 5 in their diagnosis.

▶ The practicing surgical pathologist uncommonly encounters a metaplastic carcinoma of the breast, but the diagnosis should not be missed given their typically aggressive behavior relative to the more common types. Given the usual mesenchymal appearance and possible absence of an obvious epithelial component, such tumors may not be immediately recognized. The authors of this study have found that an immunohistochemical marker directed against Laminin 5 labels a large proportion of metaplastic breast carcinoma. This may have diagnostic use as commonly used current markers, such as p63 and high molecular weight cytokeratins, and are not entirely sensitive.[1] As Laminin 5 is expressed in normal basal layers of breast ducts and lobules, the findings of this study are also notable as they lend further support for classification of metaplastic carcinoma either as a basal-like carcinoma or as a closely related entity. The authors also raise the interesting issue of Laminin 5 stromal-related functions, roles in migration, invasion, and possible relevance in tumors with increased aggressiveness like metaplastic breast carcinoma.

For further reading on other uses for immunohistochemical studies in the diagnosis of breast cancer I suggest an important article by Yeh and Mies.[2]

G. Azabdaftari, MD

References

1. Leibl S, Gogg-Kammerer M, Sommersacher A, Denk H, Moinfar F. Metaplastic breast carcinomas: are they of myoepithelial differentiation?: immunohistochemical profile of the sarcomatoid subtype using novel myoepithelial markers. *Am J Surg Pathol.* 2005;29:347-353.
2. Yeh IT, Mies C. Application of Immunohistochemistry to Breast Lesions. *Arch Pathol Lab Med.* 2008;132:349-358.

3 Gastrointestinal System

Histologic Inflammation Is a Risk Factor for Progression to Colorectal Neoplasia in Ulcerative Colitis: A Cohort Study

Gupta RB, Harpaz N, Itzkowitz S, et al (Univ of Texas Southwestern, Dallas, TX; Mount Sinai School of Medicine, New York; et al)
Gastroenterology 133:1099-1105, 2007

Background & Aims.—Although inflammation is presumed to contribute to colonic neoplasia in ulcerative colitis (UC), few studies have directly examined this relationship. Our aim was to determine whether severity of microscopic inflammation over time is an independent risk factor for neoplastic progression in UC.

Methods.—A cohort of patients with UC undergoing regular endoscopic surveillance for dysplasia was studied. Degree of inflammation at each biopsy site had been graded as part of routine clinical care using a highly reproducible histologic activity index. Progression to neoplasia was analyzed in proportional hazards models with inflammation summarized in 3 different ways and each included as a time-changing covariate: (1) mean inflammatory score (IS-mean), (2) binary inflammatory score (IS-bin), and (3) maximum inflammatory score (IS-max). Potential confounders were analyzed in univariate testing and, when significant, in a multivariable model.

Results.—Of 418 patients who met inclusion criteria, 15 progressed to advanced neoplasia (high-grade dysplasia or colorectal cancer), and 65 progressed to any neoplasia (low-grade dysplasia, high-grade dysplasia, or colorectal cancer). Univariate analysis demonstrated significant relationships between histologic inflammation over time and progression to advanced neoplasia (hazard ration (HR), 3.0; 95% CI: 1.4–6.3 for IS-mean; HR, 3.4; 95% CI: 1.1–10.4 for IS-bin; and HR, 2.2; 95% CI: 1.2–4.2 for IS-max). This association was maintained in multivariable proportional hazards analysis.

Conclusions.—The severity of microscopic inflammation over time is an independent risk factor for developing advanced colorectal neoplasia among patients with long-standing UC.

▶ Although inflammatory activity may play a role in carcinogenesis, the progression to neoplasia in inflammatory bowel disease is likely multifactorial. There are molecular mechanisms that may explain the relationship between active chronic colitis and malignancy. However, the number of studies is small. In fact, 2 previous studies have not shown a relationship and, therefore, the conclusion in this article should be confirmed or refuted in the future with prospective studies, if possible. In addition, unified criteria among pathologists are needed because the inflammatory grading used by the pathologists at the authors' institution is not strictly applied by pathologists in other practices. The histologic activity index used in this study has 4 categories. Inactive, quiescent, or normal colon is when there is no infiltration by neutrophils. In mildly active disease, neutrophils are present in less than 50% of the crypts with no ulcers or erosions. Moderate activity shows neutrophils in greater than 50% of the crypts with no ulcers or erosions. Severe active disease is characterized by the presence of erosion or ulceration independent of other features that may be present or not. The degree of dysplasia was classified as negative, indefinite, low grade, high grade, and carcinoma. Unfortunately, not all patients' inflammatory activity was accurately identified before their inclusion in the surveillance period.

P. A. Bejarano, MD

Role of human papillomavirus in squamous cell metaplasia-dysplasia-carcinoma of the rectum

Kong CS, Welton ML, Longacre TA (Stanford Univ School of Medicine, CA)
Am J Surg Pathol 31:919-925, 2007

Primary colorectal squamous cell carcinoma (SCC) and squamous dysplasia are uncommon and little is known about their pathogenesis. Most have been reported in association with ulcerative colitis and other chronic disease states. Although cervical and anal SCC have been strongly linked to human papillomavirus (HPV) infection, the role of HPV in rectal squamous carcinoma has not been well-examined. We evaluated 3 cases of primary rectal SCC for the presence of high-risk HPV by immunohistochemistry for p16(INK4A), in situ hybridization, and polymerase chain reaction. HPV type 16 was detected by polymerase chain reaction in all cases. In addition, all cases exhibited diffuse strong reactivity for p16(INK4A) and punctate nuclear staining by Ventana HPVIII in situ hybridization. The presence of HPV 16 in all three cases suggests that high-risk HPV infection is a risk factor for rectal SCC, particularly in patients with underlying chronic inflammatory disease processes or altered immune status. Further studies are warranted to determine if SCC occurring more proximal in the colon are also HPV-dependent or occur via another, HPV-independent pathway.

▶ Most cases of squamous cell carcinomas (SCCs) of the colon and rectum are either metastasis or extension from an adjacent carcinoma. Primary SCCs of colon and rectum are extraordinarily rare, representing 0.1% of all colorectal carcinomas. The cases reported are associated to ulcerative colitis, schistosomiasis, amebiasis, and radiation therapy. This series of 3 cases adds to the 47 cases already reported in the literature. One of the patients had a long-standing history of ulcerative colitis. High-risk human papillomavirus (HPV) type 16 was identified in the 3 cases of this study by polymerase chain reaction, in-situ hybridization, and immunohistochemistry. It is important for clinicians treating patients with ulcerative colitis and history of cervical/anal HPV infection to be aware that SCCs of the rectum may develop. The overlying colonic mucosa may show squamous metaplasia. Because this squamous metaplasia is an immature mucosa it may become more susceptible to infection by HPV.

P. A. Bejarano, MD

High Intraepithelial Eosinophil Counts in Esophageal Squamous Epithelium Are Not Specific for Eosinophilic Esophagitis in Adults

Rodrigo S, Abboud G, Oh D, et al (Univ of Southern California, Los Angeles)
Am J Gastroenterol 103:435-442, 2008

Objectives.—The histologic criterion of >20 eosinophils per high power field (hpf) is presently believed to establish the diagnosis of idiopathic eosinophilic esophagitis (IEE). This is based on data that the number of intraepithelial eosinophils in gastroesophageal reflux disease (GERD) is less than 20/hpf. This study tests this belief.

Methods.—Pathology records were searched for patients who had an eosinophil count >20/hpf in an esophageal biopsy. This patient population was biased toward adults with GERD who had routine multilevel biopsies of the esophagus. The clinical, radiological, and manometric data and biopsies were studied.

Results.—Forty patients out of a total of 3,648 reports examined had an eosinophil count >20/hpf in squamous epithelium of an esophageal biopsy. Analysis of these 40 cases indicated that 6 (15%) patients had IEE, 2 (5%) had coincident IEE and GERD, 28 (70%) had GERD, and 2 (5%) each had achalasia and diverticulum. There was no significant difference among these groups in terms of maximum eosinophil number, biopsy levels with >20 esoinophils/hpf, presence of eosinophilic microabscesses, involvement of surface layers by eosinophils, and severity of basal cell hyperplasia and dilated intercellular spaces.

Conclusion.—All histologic features presently ascribed to IEE can occur in other esophageal diseases, notably GERD. As such, the finding of intraepithelial eosinophilia in any number is not specific for IEE. When a patient with GERD has an esophageal biopsy with an eosinophil count >20/hpf, it does not mean that the patient has IEE.

▶ Idiopathic eosinophilic esophagitis (IEE) is independent of eosinophilic gastroenteritis and tends to be observed more frequently in children than adults. However, this observation may be artifactual because it is much less likely for children to have gastroesophageal reflux. The symptoms of patients with IEE are dysphagia, food impaction, retrosternal pain heartburn, vomiting, and regurgitation. Endoscopically, the esophagus may be narrowed, show circumferential rings, exudates, fissures, and erythema. The treatment is topical corticosteroids. The histological definition of IEE has evolved since 1978 when the entity was first described. Without strong basis, eosinophilic esophagitis is currently defined by the presence of greater than 20 eosinophils per high power field in the epithelium. Men more frequently than women have tissue eosinophilia with counts greater than 20 eosinophils/hpf. The authors found that histological findings of IEE can occur in other esophageal diseases, in particular reflux. Those findings include not only the presence of > 20 eosinophils/hpf but also basal cell hyperplasia, intercellular edema, and eosinophilic microabscesses. Of the 40 patients whose biopsies had > 20 eosinophils/hpf, only 6(24%) had IEE clinically, whereas 28 (70%) had gastroesophageal reflux. The 2 additional patients have both entities. This is evidence of the lack of specificity of tissue eosinophilia for IEE.

P. Bejarano, MD

Calcifying fibrous tumor of small intestine
Emanuel P, Qin L, Harpaz N (Mount Sinai School of Medicine, New York)
Ann Diagn Pathol 12:138-141, 2008

Calcifying fibrous tumor (CFT) is a rare benign tumor with a predilection for children and young adults that usually arises in the subcutaneous and deep soft tissues, pleura, or peritoneum. It presents histologically as a well-circumscribed mass consisting of hyalinized, hypocellular lamellar collagen, bland spindle cells, chronic inflammatory cell infiltrates, and psammomatous or dystrophic calcifications. Calcifying fibrous tumor of the gastrointestinal tract is exceedingly rare and therefore prone to confusion with other spindle cell lesions more commonly encountered in this location. We describe 4 cases of calcifying fibrous tumor arising in the terminal ileum, one of which caused the heretofore unreported complication of intestinal intussusception, and discuss the differential diagnosis with other common and uncommon spindle cell lesions.

▶ These 4 new cases of CFT add to the previously 12 reported involving the gastrointestinal tract. The initial cases of calcifying fibrous tumor were found in the subcutaneous and deep soft tissues of the trunk and extremities, but it has been encountered in the thoracic and abdominal cavities and pelvis. This study does not describe the immunohistochemical profile of the 4 new cases. Nonetheless, this rare tumor needs to be distinguished from gastrointestinal stromal tumor (GIST), desmoid tumor, solitary fibrous tumor, inflammatory myofibroblastic tumor, and reactive nodular fibrous pseudotumor. In fact, being paucicellular, it has been postulated that calcifying fibrous tumor may be the sclerosing phase of inflammatory myofibroblastic tumor. However, the latter would not stain for anaplastic lymphoma kinase (ALK). The features of

GIST can be confirmed with immunostain for CD117 or platelet-derived growth factor receptor (PDGFR). A stain for CD34 would not distinguish both tumors. Desmoid tumor is usually infiltrative or cellular, but it can be circumscribed and paucicellular as well creating diagnostic difficulties. Nonetheless, desmoids tend to be positive for β catenin. Although solitary fibrous tumor is positive for CD34, it can express CD99 and bcl-2 as well.

P. A. Bejarano, MD

Aberrant Crypt Foci as Precursors of the Dysplasia-Carcinoma Sequence in Patients with Ulcerative Colitis

Kukitsu T, Takayama T, Miyanishi K, et al (Sapporo Med Univ School of Medicine, Japan; et al)
Clin Cancer Res 14:48-54, 2008

Purpose.—Long-standing ulcerative colitis (UC) predisposes patients to the development of colorectal cancer, but surveillance of colitis-associated cancer by detecting the precancerous lesion dysplasia is often difficult because of its rare occurrence and normal-looking appearance. In sporadic colorectal cancer, aberrant crypt foci (ACF) have been reported by many investigators to be precursor lesions of the adenoma-carcinoma sequence. In the present study, we analyzed the genetic background of ACF to determine whether they could be precursors for dysplasia, and we examined the usefulness of endoscopic examination of ACF as a surrogate marker for surveillance of colitis-associated cancer.

Experimental Design.—ACF were examined in 28 UC patients (19 patients with UC alone and 9 patients with UC and dysplasia; 2 of those patients with dysplasia also had cancer) using magnifying endoscopy. K-ras, APC, and p53 mutations were analyzed by two-step PCR RFLP, *in vitro* – synthesized protein assay, and single-strand conformation polymorphism, respectively. Methylation of p16 was analyzed by methylation-specific PCR.

Results.—ACF that appeared distinct endoscopically and histologically were identified in 27 out of 28 UC patients. They were negative for K-ras, APC, and p53 mutations but were frequently positive for p16 methylation (8 of 11; 73%). In dysplasia, K-ras and APC mutations were negative but p53 mutation (3 of 5; 60%) and p16 methylation (3 of 5; 60%) were positive. There was a significant stepwise increase in the number of ACF from patients with UC alone to patients with dysplasia and to patients with cancer. Univariate and multivariate analyses showed significant correlations between ACF and dysplasia.

Conclusions.—We have disclosed an ACF-dysplasia-cancer sequence in colitis-associated carcinogenesis similar to the ACF-adenoma-carcinoma sequence in sporadic colon carcinogenesis. This study suggests the use of ACF instead of dysplasia for the surveillance of colitis cancer and warrants

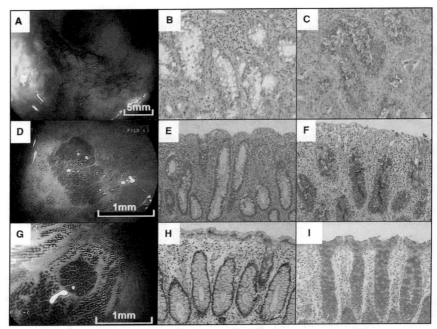

FIGURE 1.—Endoscopic and histologic features of dysplasia (*A-C*), ACF in a patient with UC (*D-F*), and ACF in a non-UC patient (*G-I*). *A*, dysplasia in a UC patient, which was not visible unless chromoendoscopy was done. *B*, the crypt was lined by columnar epithelia with some nuclear stratification, hyperchromatic nuclei, and loss of normal polarity (H&E; magnification, ×150). *C*, increased numbers of goblet cells were seen in the dysplasia of UC patients. Some dystrophic goblet cells were observed (Alcian blue; magnification, ×150). *D*, a representative ACF in a UC patient, which was characterized by darker staining with methylene blue and larger crypts with thicker epithelial lining than the background mucosa. The lining of each crypt was obscure and the boundaries of individual crypts were more unclear than in non-UC ACF (*G*). *E*, the colitis ACF showed marked infiltration of lymphocytes in the stroma, a more diverse range of crypt sizes, enlarged nuclei in epithelial cells, and increased chromatin staining compared with non-UC ACF (H&E; magnification, ×120). *F*, an increase in the number of goblet cells was seen in colitis ACF, similar to dysplasia in UC patients. Some dystrophic goblet cells were also identified (Alcian blue; magnification, ×120). *G*, a representative non-UC ACF consisting of crypts with round and oval lumens and with a wide pericryptal space. *H*, non-UC ACF showed slight enlargement, irregularity, and elongation of the ducts (H&E; magnification, ×150). *I*, the number of goblet cells in non-UC ACF was apparently fewer than that in colitis ACF (Alcian blue; magnification, ×150). For interpretation of the references to color in this figure legend, the reader is referred to the web version of this article. (Reprinted from Kukitsu T, Takayama T, Miyanishi K, et al. Aberrant crypt foci as precursors of the dysplasia-carcinoma sequence in patients with ulcerative colitis. *Clin Cancer Res.* 2008;14:48-54, with permission from the American Association for Cancer Research.)

further evaluation of ACF as a surveillance marker in large-scale studies (Fig 1).

▶ Dysplasia is a precancerous lesion that is easier to detect in nonulcerative colitis patients than in patients suffering from the disease. The difficulty is evident at endoscopy because dysplasia may appear as normal-looking mucosa. Several studies have documented the sequence of aberrant crypt foci-adenoma-carcinoma for sporadic colon carcinogenesis. This association has not been studied in detail on ulcerative colitis patients. Aberrant crypt foci is an endoscopic finding characterized by more darkly staining with methylene blue than the adjacent normal mucosa and have crypts with larger diameters, often showing oval or slit-like lumens and thicker epithelial linings. In this study, the aberrant crypt foci in patients with ulcerative colitis showed histologic features characterized by marked lymphocytic infiltrates of lamina propria accompanied by a wide range of crypt sizes, and enlarged and hyperchromatic nuclei (Fig 1). Gastroenterologist may target aberrant crypt foci in the surveillance for dysplasia in patients with ulcerative colitis requiring confirmation by pathologists on individual cases.

P. A. Bejarano, MD

Is Nonsmall Cell Type High-grade Neuroendocrine Carcinoma of the Tubular Gastrointestinal Tract a Distinct Disease Entity?

Shia J, Tang LH, Weiser MR, et al (Memorial Sloan-Kettering Cancer Ctr, NY; et al)
Am J Surg Pathol 32:719-731, 2008

Although small cell carcinoma of the gastrointestinal (GI) tract is well-recognized, nonsmall cell type high-grade neuroendocrine carcinoma (HGNEC) of this site remains undefined. At the current time, neither the World Health Organization nor American Joint Committee on Cancer includes this condition in the histologic classifications, and consequently it is being diagnosed and treated inconsistently. In this study, we aimed at delineating the histologic and immunophenotypical spectrum of HGNECs of the GI tract with emphasis on histologic subtypes. Guided primarily by the World Health Organization/ International Association for the Study of Lung Cancer criteria for pulmonary neuroendocrine tumors, we were able to classify 87 high-grade GI tract tumors that initially carried a diagnosis of either poorly differentiated carcinoma with or without any neuroendocrine characteristics, small cell carcinoma, or combined adenocarcinoma— neuroendocrine carcinoma into the following 4 categories. The first was small cell carcinoma (n = 23), which had features typical of pulmonary small cell carcinoma, although the cells tended to have a more round nuclear contour. The second was large cell neuroendocrine carcinoma (n = 31), which had a morphology similar to its pulmonary counterpart and showed positive immunoreactivity for either chromogranin (71%) or synaptophysin (94%) or both. The third was mixed neuroendocrine carcinoma (n = 11), which had intermediate histologic features (eg, cells with an increased nuclear/cytoplasmic ratio but with apparent nucleoli), and positive immunoreactivity for at least 1 neuroendocrine marker. The fourth was poorly differentiated adenocarcinoma (n = 17). In addition, 5 of the 87 tumors showed either nonsmall cell type neuroendocrine morphology (n = 3) or immunohistochemical reactivity for neuroendocrine markers (n = 2), but not both. Further analysis showed that most HGNECs arising in the squamous lined parts (esophagus and anal canal) were small cell type (78%), whereas most involving the glandular mucosa were large cell (53%) or mixed (82%)

type; associated adenocarcinomas were more frequent in large cell (61%) or mixed (36%) type than in small cell type (26%); and focal intracytoplasmic mucin was seen only in large cell or mixed type. As a group, the 2-year disease-specific survival for patients with HGNEC was 25.4% (median follow-up time, 11.3 mo). No significant survival difference was observed among the different histologic subtypes. In conclusion, our study demonstrates the existence of both small cell and nonsmall cell types of HGNEC in the GI tract, and provides a detailed illustration of their morphologic spectrum. There are differences in certain pathologic features between small cell and nonsmall cell types, whereas the differences between the subtypes of nonsmall cell category (large cell versus mixed) are less distinct. Given the current uncertainty as to whether large cell neuroendocrine carcinoma is as chemosensitive as small cell carcinoma even in the lung, our data provide further evidence in favor of a dichotomous classification scheme (small cell vs. nonsmall cell) for HGNEC of the GI tract. Separation of nonsmall cell type into large cell and mixed subtypes may not be necessary. These tumors are clinically aggressive. Prospective studies using defined diagnostic criteria are needed to determine their biologic characteristics and optimal management.

▶ There has been uncertainty on the histological features for the diagnosis of large cell neuroendocrine carcinoma of the intestine. Its definition is extrapolated from the better known cases observed in the lung. It is a tumor that has a diffuse growth pattern with neuroendocrine appearance that may include organoid, palisading, rosettes, or trabeculae. The cells are round to oval with visible cytoplasm, granular or vesicular nuclei with or without visible nucleoli, and mitosis. In addition, the cells are positive for cytokeratin and a neuroendocrine marker such as chromogranin or synaptophysin. The latter appears the most sensitive, and is preferred to CD56 because it is more specific. The use of cytokeratin may be useful as well to distinguish it from regular poorly differentiated adenocarcinomas with solid pattern of growth. Large cell carcinomas may show a perinuclear dot with cytokeratin. This article lends support to the view that despite similar behavior, small cell carcinoma should be separated from large cell neuroendocrine carcinomas. Additional studies are needed to assess differences in response to various therapeutic modalities.

P. Bejarano, MD

PDGFRA Immunostaining Can Help in the Diagnosis of Gastrointestinal Stromal Tumors

Miselli F, Millefanti C, Conca E, et al (Fondazione IRCCS Istituto Nazionale dei Tumori, Milano, Italy)
Am J Surg Pathol 32:738-743, 2008

Gastrointestinal stromal tumors (GISTs) are characterized by the presence of activating mutations affecting the *c-Kit* or the *PDGFRA* gene. Although these mutations are mutually exclusive, their proteins are coexpressed in many GISTs with various modulations of immunostaining depending on which gene is mutated. CD117 expression is currently considered a sensitive (although not entirely specific) marker of KIT activation, but there is no consensus concerning the reliability of PDGFRA antibody. Our database contains 236 molecularly analyzed GISTs, and we here describe the 180 cases that underwent KIT/PDGFRA immunophenotyping. By correlating the immunophenotype with the molecular status of the genes expected to be involved, we observed the coexpression of KIT and PDGFRA in the majority of the mutated *c-Kit* and wild-type *c-Kit/PDGFRA* GISTs, whereas the ± immunophenotype (0% vs. 48.6%) and PDGFRA dotlike immunostaining ($P < 0.005$) segregated with the PDGFRA-mutated GISTs. Taking either the dotlike decoration (26 cases) or ± immunophenotype (5 cases) as hallmarks of PDGFRA mutation, the presence of a *PDGFRA* mutation was predicted in 31 (83.8%) of the 37 *PDGFRA* mutated GISTs. Our findings suggest that, when critically applied, the routine use of CD117/PDGFRA immunophenotyping is a useful diagnostic tool (especially in CD117-negative cases) as it correctly predicts the presence of *PDGFRA* mutations in most cases.

▶ The diagnosis of gastrointestinal stromal tumor (GIST) is usually considered by pathologists when dealing with a spindle cell tumor of the gastrointestinal tract. After all, it is the most frequent mesenchymal tumor encountered in this organ system. The confidence in rendering a diagnosis of GIST is enhanced when the tumor shows immunoreactivity for CD117 (*c-Kit*). However, there are GISTs that do not express CD117. It has been postulated that an alternative stain is using an antibody against platelet-derived growth factor receptor alpha (PDGFRA). Unfortunately, it has not been entirely elucidated if immunostaining for PDGFRA could act as a diagnostic tool. Also, it is not clear if its expression indeed is associated with the mutation of the gene that leads to cell proliferation in the tumor. The authors found that PDGFRA immunoreactivity helps for diagnostic purposes and predicts mutation in 83.8% of cases. The pattern of immunoreactivity that the authors described is that of a dot-like pattern of stain.

P. Bejarano, MD

Multinucleate epithelial change in colorectal hyperplastic polyps: a review of 27 cases

Lambie DLJ, Brown IS (Dept of Histopathology, Sullivan Nicolaides Pathology, Queensland, Australia)
J Clin Pathol 61:611-614, 2008

Aim.—To document the histological features of multinucleated epithelial giant cells (MEGs) in colorectal hyperplastic polyps and determine a possible aetiological agent.

Methods.—Hyperplastic polyps were assessed for MEGs during the routine reporting at a private laboratory and public hospital laboratory. The histological features and clinical data were assessed, and immunohistochemical stains were performed to assess for viral infection (cytomegalovirus (CMV) and herpes simplex virus (HSV) 1 and 2) and to assist in the assessment of dysplasia (Ki-67, β-catenin and p53). Ultrastructural examination was performed in one case.

Results.—MEGs were identified in 27 polyps (24 patients). There was active inflammation in the polyps in nearly all cases (n = 24) and most showed changes in adjacent non-hyperplastic bowel mucosa such as focal basal cryptitis and apoptosis of crypt epithelium (16 patients). Immunohistochemistry for CMV, HSV and p53 was negative in all cases. The MEGs showed nuclear positivity for the proliferative marker Ki-67 and membranous positivity for β-catenin. Ultrastructural studies failed to reveal viral particles.

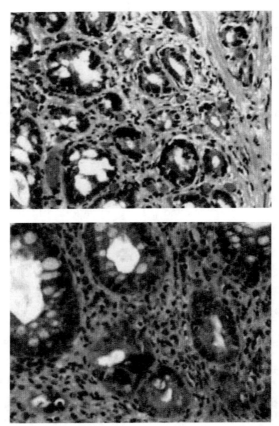

FIGURE 3.—Multinucleated epithelial giant cells with hyerchromatic nuclei. (A) Case 13. (B) Case 3. H&E, original magnification ×400. (Reprinted from Lambie DLJ, Brown IS. Multinucleate epithelial change in colorectal hyperplastic polyps: a review of 27 cases. *J Clin Pathol.* 2008;61:611-614.)

Conclusions.—All the polyps containing MEGs showed active inflammation and apoptosis, and in most there was also focal inflammation and apoptosis in the adjacent mucosa. Inflammation in conjunction with the increased epithelial proliferation characteristics of hyperplastic polyps could be the mechanism for the MEG formation. In this series, all the polyps were associated with sodium phosphate bowel preparation (NaP) and the pro-inflammatory properties of NaP may be a stimulus for the induction of giant cells (Fig 3).

► In the digestive tract, multinucleated epithelial cells may be observed in the squamous mucosal surface on the esophagus and hyperplastic polyps with serrated features of the large intestine. In the esophagus, it has been proven that it is a reactive change due to inflammation in most cases. As in the esophagus, the giant cells in hyperplastic polyps of the colon are not related to viruses and do not imply dysplastic changes (Fig 3A, B). Pre-endoscopic bowel preparation can be done using sodium phosphate or polyethylene glycol lavage. The former is a strong osmotic laxative. The authors made an unreported association between the use of sodium phosphate and the presence of multinucleated giant cells in colonic hyperplastic polyps. It is not clear what minimal time interval is required for giant cells to form after bowel preparation to support the authors' assertion, as their presence should occur within 24 hours. Other changes attributed to it include focal basal cryptitis and apoptosis at the base of the crypts. The few series of multinucleated epithelial change in colonic polyps have been described in hyperplastic polyps with serrated features. One wonders if the presence of multinucleated giant cells is a more prevalent feature in this type of polyps or can be seen equally in tubular adenomas. Also, it is not known if they can distinguish hyperplastic polyps from serrated adenomas.

P. Bejarano, MD

The natural history of aberrant crypt foci

Schoen RE, Mutch M, Rall C, et al (Univ of Pittsburgh, Pennsylvania, PA; Washington Univ, St Louis, MO; Marshfield Clinic, WI)
Gastrointest Endosc 67:1097-1102, 2008

Background.—Aberrant crypt foci (ACF) are the putative precursors to colorectal adenomas and may be useful as biomarkers. Knowledge of their natural history is essential to understanding their potential utility.

Objective.—Our purpose was to examine ACF detection 1 year after initial observation.

Design.—We conducted a multicenter study of ACF by using a standardized protocol. ACF in the rectum were assessed and subjects returned 1 year later to evaluate the natural history of the lesions.

Setting.—Ancillary study to the Prostate, Lung, Colorectal, and Ovarian Cancer Screening Trial.

Results.—Of 78 subjects enrolled, 64 (82%) returned for a repeat examination 1 year later. The mean age was 71 years, 70% were male, and 54% had a history of adenomatous polyps. At the initial examination, 66% of subjects had at least 1 ACF detected in the rectum, with a mean of 2.1 ± 2.3 per person. One year later, 60% of these subjects had at least 1 of the original ACF reidentified, but only 43% of all ACF were reidentified. A total of 56% of subjects had new ACF identified.

Limitations.—These results are generated from the pilot phase. Improvements or change in technique over time could have influenced the results.

Conclusions.—A total of 60% of subjects who had ACF continued to have at least one ACF 1 year later, but less than half the specific ACF could be reidentified, and more than 50% of subjects had new ACF. These results imply a considerable dynamic to ACF detection over a 1-year period of observation.

▶ Aberrant crypt foci are postulated to be the earliest morphological precursor of carcinoma of the large intestine. They may show dysplasia and genetic alterations that support the view that eventually they may progress to cancer. After preparing the colon for colonoscopy, several washings are performed and methylene blue is installed to coat the mucosal surface to identify aberrant crypt foci. In this study, aberrant crypt foci were defined endoscopically as colon crypts with a larger diameter than normal mucosa, having a thicker epithelium, and more darkly staining than normal crypts. In general, if the lesion is elevated more than 2 mm, it is considered a poly and not an aberrant crypt focus. Unfortunately, this article shows no microscopic photographs and it is not clear if pathologists were involved directly in the study. More informative articles on aberrant crypt foci addressed to pathologists are needed to better assess their significance for the daily practice of pathology.

P. Bejarano, MD

Nodular Gastritis: An Endoscopic Indicator of *Helicobacter Pylori* Infection

Chen M-J, Wang T-E, Chang W-H, et al (Nursing and Management College, Taipei, Taiwan)
Dig Dis Sci 52:2662-2666, 2007

We prospectively assessed the relationship between nodular gastritis and *Helicobacter pylori* infection. Of 1409 adults who underwent endoscopy for persistent dyspepsia between June 2004 and August 2005, 41 (2.9%) patients were diagnosed with nodular gastritis (11 [27%] men and 30 [73%] women). The mean age was 45.9 years. A control group of 65 patients without nodular gastritis was also evaluated. The prevalence of *H. pylori* infection was higher in patients with nodular gastritis than in controls (38/41 [93%] vs. 33/65 [51%]). Of 21 patients treated to eradicate *H. pylori*, the nodular gastritis pattern resolved or improved in 16 patients on subsequent endoscopy. This study suggests that a nodular pattern of the gastric mucosa on endocscopy is a good indicator for *H. pylori* infection in adults, with the high positive predictive value of 92.7%.

▶ This is a short but straightforward article with informative findings to clinicians and pathologists alike. Nodular gastritis appears to be more frequent in children. This study on adult patients found 2.9% incidence of nodular gastritis among 1409 patients. Nodular gastritis has an endoscopic miliary pattern with a cobblestone appearance involving predominately the antrum. Histologically, there are increased lymphoid follicles with germinal centers, thus the synonym of lymphonodular hyperplasia. This article found that nodular gastritis is a more specific finding for *Helicobacter pylori* infection than for chronic gastritis, ulcers, adenocarcinoma, and lymphoma of the stomach. Although *H. pylori* may be a risk factor for adenocarcinoma and lymphoma, it is not known if nodular gastritis by itself is a precursor of gastric malignancies. Endoscopists should inform pathologists if they observed features of nodular gastritis in their endoscopies to increase the awareness of the pathologist and likelihood of finding helicobacter organisms in individual cases.

P. Bejarano, MD

Is single-Cell Apoptosis Sufficient for the Diagnosis of Graft-Versus-Host Disease in the Colon?

Nguyen CV, Kastenberg DM, Choudhary C, et al (Thomas Jefferson Univ Hosp, Philadelphia, PA)
Dig Dis Sci 53:747-756, 2008

Low-grade lesions of graft-versus-host disease (GVHD) in the colon are not uncommon. To determine if minimal diagnostic criteria can be established in such biopsies, we correlated histologic findings with clinical history and investigated the role of endoscopy and electron microscopy in establishing GVHD. About 85 colonic biopsies that were histologically consistent with GVHD from 47 bone-marrow transplant recipients were reviewed retrospectively. Of nine cases showing only a single apoptotic cell in the intestinal epithelium, only four lacked any confounding factors of GVHD. These cases, while too few to assess the utility of finding one apoptotic cell with statistical significance, appear to support the idea that in the appropriate clinical setting, a single apoptotic cell could be reported as possibly representing early GVHD. Endoscopic findings did not reliably correlate with histology. Although electron microscopy can be a useful adjunct, it does not contribute to the diagnosis of GVHD (Fig 1).

▶ There is no question that examining an intestinal biopsy with the purpose of ruling out or documenting graft-versus-host disease (GVHD) is a cause of anxiety among pathologists. The therapeutic and prognostic implications are

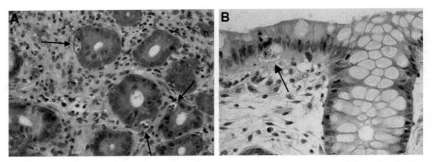

FIGURE 1.—(A) Single-cell apoptosis (arrows) within multiple crypts consistent with grade 1 GVHD. (B) Single apoptotic cell within the superficial mucosa (arrow). (Reprinted from the Nguyen CV, Kastenberg DM, Choudhary C, et al. Is single-cell apoptosis sufficient for the diagnosis of graft-versus-host disease in the colon? *Dig Dis Sci.* 2008;53:747-756, with permission from the Springer Science+Business Media.)

enormous and usually the clinicians are eager to know the findings as soon as possible. The diagnosis is straightforward when there are multiple apoptotic cells in several crypts in tissues obtained after 30 days of a bone marrow transplant. Unfortunately, this scenario is not very frequent. When the biopsy is obtained during the first 30 days after transplant the differential diagnosis must include a viral infection and, therefore, clinical correlation is needed. The most difficult scenario is when there is a single apoptotic cell in a crypt or on the superficial mucosa in biopsy tissues obtained after 30 days transplantation. An example of this can be seen in Fig 1. Although this study supports the view that minimal changes correspond to GVHD, it is also recommended that the findings be correlated with the clinical picture.

P. Bejarano, MD

4 Hepatobiliary System and Pancreas

WHO 2004 Criteria and CK19 are Reliable Prognostic Markers in Pancreatic Endocrine Tumors

Schmitt AM, Anlauf M, Rousson V, et al (Inst of Surgical Pathology, Zurich, Switzerland; Univ of Zurich, Switzerland; Univ of Kiel, Germany; et al)

Am J Surg Pathol 31:1677-1682, 2007

Background.—It is difficult to predict the biologic behavior of pancreatic endocrine tumors in absence of metastases or invasion into adjacent organs. The World Health Organization (WHO) has proposed in 2004 size, angioinvasion, mitotic activity, and MIB1 proliferation index as prognostic criteria. Our aim was to test retrospectively the predictive value of these 2004 WHO criteria and of CK19, CD99, COX2, and p27 immunohistochemistry in a large series of patients with long-term follow-up.

Design.—The histology of 216 pancreatic endocrine tumor specimens was reviewed and the tumors were reclassified according to the 2004 WHO classification. The prognostic value of the WHO classification and the histopathologic criteria necrosis and nodular fibrosis was tested in 113 patients. A tissue microarray was constructed for immunohistochemical staining. The staining results were scored quantitatively for MIB1 and semiquantitatively for CK19, COX2, p27, and CD99. The prognostic value of these markers was tested in 93 patients.

Results.—The stratification of the patients into 4 risk groups according to the 2004 WHO classification was reliable with regard to both time span to relapse and tumor-specific death. In a multivariate analysis, the CK19 status was shown to be independent of the WHO criteria. By contrast, the prognostic significance of COX2, p27, and CD99 could not be confirmed.

Conclusions.—The 2004 WHO classification with 4 risk groups is very reliable for predicting both disease-free survival and the time span until tumor-specific death. CK19 staining is a potential additional prognostic marker independent from the WHO criteria for pancreatic endocrine tumors.

▶ In general, pathologists are challenged on what terminology to use when they encounter a case of pancreatic endocrine tumor (PET). The uncertainty is based on part by the rarity of these tumors, which account for up to 2% of all pancreatic tumors. In addition, the behavior of them is difficult to predict.

In addition, the numbers of institutions where excision of these tumors are performed on a regular basis are not numerous. This limits the experience by pathologists and clinicians. The problem is compounded by the fact that there is no wide acceptance of the classification system proposed by the World Health Organization (WHO). This system divides PETs into 3 groups: benign, uncertain behavior, and carcinomas. The carcinomas are further subdivided into well and poorly differentiated. The lack of acceptance is that the system is based on the opinion of experts instead of data obtained from detailed studies. This article tries to document the validity of the WHO classification. The benign (WHO 1a) PET is confined to the pancreas, measures less than 2 cm, is nonangioinvasive, has less than 2 mitosis/10 HPF, and less than 2% of Ki-67-positive cells. PET of uncertain behavior (WHO 1b) is also confined to the pancreas and has at least one of the following: greater than 2 cm, 2 to 10 mitosis/10 HPF, greater than 2% Ki-67-positive cells, angioinvasion, or perineural invasion. Well-differentiated (WHO 2) pancreatic endocrine carcinoma is characterized by invasion of adjacent tissues or metastasis. Poorly differentiated (WHO 3) PETs have greater than 10 mitosis in 10 HPF. This article supports the WHO classification and sheds some light in particular for the WHO 1b tumors. Although disease-free survival is similar for WHO 1b and 2 tumors, their tumor-induced death are different with WHO 1b tumors progressing more slowly and deaths occurring less frequent than in WHO 2 tumors. This follow-up finding justifies their separation. The authors also found that CK19 positive tumors were associated with significantly shorter disease-free survival and tumor-induced death.

P. A. Bejarano, MD

Pathological classification of hepatic inflammatory pseudotumor with respect to IgG4-related disease

Zen Y, Fujii T, Sato Y, et al (Kanazawa Univ, Japan; et al)
Mod Pathol 20:884-894, 2007

Recently, much attention has focused on IgG4-related disease, which is characterized by abundant IgG4-positive plasma cell infiltration and high serum IgG4 levels. IgG4-related disease sometimes manifests as tumorous lesions, and its relationship to inflammatory pseudotumor has been suggested. In this study, we examined clinicopathological features of a total of 16 cases of hepatic inflammatory pseudotumor (11 men and 5 women with an average age of 67 years) with respect to IgG4-related disease. The tumors could be pathologically classified into two types: fibrohistiocytic (10 cases) and lymphoplasmacytic (6 cases). Fibrohistiocytic inflammatory pseudotumors were characterized by xanthogranulomatous inflammation, multinucleated giant cells, and neutrophilic infiltration, and mostly occurred in the peripheral hepatic parenchyma as mass-forming lesions. In contrast, lymphoplasmacytic inflammatory pseudotumors showed diffuse lymphoplasmacytic infiltration and prominent eosinophilic infiltration, and were all found around the hepatic hilum. In addition, venous occlusion with little inflammation and cholangitis without periductal fibrosis were frequently observed in the fibrohistiocytic type, whereas obliterative phlebitis and cholangitis with periductal fibrosis were common features of the lymphoplasmacytic type. Interestingly, IgG4-positive plasma cells were significantly more numerous in the lymphoplasmacytic than fibrohistiocytic type. However, two of the fibrohistiocytic inflammatory pseudotumors had relatively many IgG4-positive plasma cells. In conclusion, hepatic inflammatory pseudotumor could be classified into two types based on clinicopathological characteristics. The lymphoplasmacytic type is unique, and could belong to the so-called IgG4-related diseases. In contrast, the fibrohistiocytic type might still be a heterogeneous group of disorders. This latter type seems pathologically different from IgG4-related disease, although cases with relatively abundant IgG4-positive plasma cells should be differentiated from IgG4-related disease with secondary histopathologic modifications.

▶ There has been an increasing interest in studying the relationship between IgG4 and the development of autoimmune-driven mass-like inflammatory processes. Pancreatitis has been one of the more frequently analyzed and it has been shown that extensive IgG4 immunohistochemical expression in plasma cells is likely indicative of autoimmune pancreatitis. The expression is observed less in pancreatitis of other etiologies. Historically, the nomenclature of inflammatory pseudotumors has evolved to reflect the predominant cellular and architectural characteristics of individual cases. The 2 most frequent types include one that is fibrohistiocytic in which spindle myofibroblastic cells are present. The second type has a rich lymphoplasmacytic infiltrate creating a mass-like process. IgG4 expression in hepatic lesions of this nature is more striking in the lymphoplasmacytic type supporting the view that inflammatory pseudotumors may be having at least 2 different etiologic entities. The separation is also based on their different clinical manifestations. Whereas IgG4 lesions may be related to autoimmunity, the fibrohistiocytic variant may be a secondary change to a previous liver injury, such as cholangitis or infection. It would be interesting to study other liver diseases with IgG4 to see their evidence of autoimmunity.

P. A. Bejarano, MD

Ballooned hepatocytes in steatohepatitis: The value of keratin immunohistochemistry for diagnosis
Lackner C, Gogg-Kamerer M, Zatloukal K, et al (Med Univ of Graz, Austria; et al)
J Hepatol 48:821-828, 2008

Background/Aims.—Hepatocyte "ballooning" is an often used but ill defined term in liver pathology to designate a special form of liver cell degeneration associated with cell swelling and enlargement found particularly in steatohepatitis. Alterations of the intermediate filament cytoskeleton of the hepatocyte may contribute to the pathogenesis of this microscopic change. Ballooning degeneration is considered a hallmark of steatohepatitis, but enlarged hepatocytes may also be observed in a variety of other acute and chronic liver diseases.

Methods.—The intermediate filament cytoskeleton was investigated using keratin 8 and 18 immunohistochemistry in liver diseases associated with enlarged or ballooned hepatocytes.

Results.—Keratin 8/18 immunostaining was drastically reduced or lost in the cytoplasm of ballooned hepatocytes in alcoholic and non-alcoholic steatohepatitis, chronic cholestatic conditions, ischemia/reperfusion injury and in ballooned hepatocytes in chronic hepatitis C cases with concurrent steatohepatitis. In contrast, substantial decrease or loss of keratin 8/18 immunostaining was not noted in cases of acute hepatitis, giant cell hepatitis, chronic hepatitis B, or autoimmune hepatitis.

Conclusions.—Loss of keratin 8/18 immunostaining can serve as an objective marker of a specific type of ballooning degeneration of hepatocytes. Oxidative stress may be a common denominator in the pathogenesis of keratin filament alterations in these conditions.

▶ Ballooning of hepatocytes is a nonspecific finding, but is more associated with recent injury to the liver. However, it can be seen in chronic processes indicating ongoing insult. Thus, it can be seen in hepatitis, drug effect, preservation injury in transplantation, alcohol-induced liver disease and nonalcoholic steatohepatitis, among others. Ballooned hepatocytes represent hydropic degeneration with the accumulation of fluid in the cytoplasm. The cells are large, pale, and reticulated to clear cytoplasm. They are usually located in centrilobular areas. The cytoskeleton of hepatocytes and their organelles is composed of intermediate filaments made of keratins 8 and 18. These keratins are lost or diminished in ballooned hepatocytes and this negative finding can confirm the presence of ballooned hepatocytes. Alterations of cytoskeleton also account for the presence of Mallory bodies. However, the authors found that these are not always present in ballooned hepatocytes using CK8/18. Ubiquitin staining is used to highlight Mallory bodies when they are not readily observed in the hematoxylin and eosin sections.

P. A. Bejarano, MD

Histology Of Symptomatic Acute Hepatitis C Infection in Immunocompetent Adults
Johnson K, Kotiesh A, Boitnott JK, et al (Johns Hopkins Univ School of Medicine, Baltimore, MD)
Am J Surg Pathol 31:1754-1758, 2007

Acute hepatitis C in immunocompetent individuals is rarely symptomatic and rarely biopsied. Thus, the histologic descriptions of acute hepatitis

C remain limited. The histology of 5 cases of acute hepatitis C in adults were studied by selecting cases from the consult and surgical pathology files of a single institution. The 5 individuals, 3 males and 2 females, had an average age at biopsy of 50 ± 17 years. They presented with jaundice and other nonspecific abdominal symptoms. The time interval from clinical presentation to biopsy ranged from 2 to 18 weeks. The average alanine aminotransferase/aspartate aminotransferase/alkaline phosphatase at the time of biopsy was 308/73/85 U/L. The average total bilirubin was 5.2 mg/dL. Each individual had a single liver biopsy. The histologic findings of the 2 cases biopsied in close temporal proximity to the initial clinical presentation showed similar histologic findings of mixed portal infiltrates with lymphocytes and neutrophils along with bile ductular proliferation that raised the possibility of down stream biliary tract disease. The lobules showed canalicular cholestasis and mild to moderate inflammation. In the third and fourth case, obtained 8 weeks after presentation, the biopsies showed mild to moderate portal and lobular lymphocytic inflammation, findings that were also present in the last case, obtained 18 weeks after presentation. In conclusion, early after acute hepatitis C viral infection, biopsies can have a cholestatic pattern whereas later biopsies tend to show mild nonspecific portal and lobular lymphocytic inflammation. Proper histologic diagnosis can be aided by an awareness of the various histologic findings, which vary depending on the time interval from clinical symptoms to biopsy.

▶ This is a chronological evaluation of 5 immunocompetent patients who recently were infected with hepatitis C virus. The 5 liver biopsies were performed in 2 patients within 2 weeks of clinical presentation, in 2 other cases within 8 weeks. The last patient was biopsied at 18 weeks. Although rare, the patients acquired hepatitis C through contamination of radiopharmaceuticals, colonoscopy, and laboratory exposure. The only comparison on the histological findings with previous cases in the literature is with the liver post-transplant population. However, the latter group of individuals is immunosuppressed. There are differences between both groups. The number of immunocompetent patients with acute hepatitis C so far studied is very small. Hepatitis C is essentially recurrent in the large majority of transplanted patients and the biochemical manifestations arise around 3 to 4 months after the transplant. The histological features are spotty lobular necrosis and lymphocytic infiltrates. Thereafter, biopsies show portal and lobular infiltrates. Only in 4% to 7% of cases predominant cholestasis is present. On the other hand, the current study showed that cholestatic features are the main findings in the first 2 weeks after infection, and they even mimic bile duct obstruction. At 8 weeks it is somewhat subacute and resembles the initial post-transplant recurrent features. After that, both groups show typical features of chronic hepatitis.

P. A. Bejarano, MD

Pathology of Nonalcoholic Fatty Liver Disease

Yeh MM, Brunt EM (Univ of Washington School of Medicine, Seattle; Saint Louis Univ Health Sciences Ctr, MO)
Am J Clin Pathol 128:837-847, 2007

Nonalcoholic fatty liver disease (NAFLD) and nonalcoholic steatohepatitis (NASH) are gaining increasing recognition as components of the emerging epidemic of obesity in North America and in other parts of the world. These entities are considered the hepatic manifestations of the insulin resistance syndrome and represent the spectra of fatty liver disease associated with it. All features of metabolic syndrome are associated with NAFLD/NASH, including obesity, type 2 diabetes, arterial hypertension, and hyperlipidemia in the form of elevated triglyceride levels. NAFLD/NASH can progress to liver cirrhosis and has been reported as a cause of hepatocellular carcinoma. In this review, the histopathologic features of NAFLD/NASH and differential diagnostic considerations are discussed. In addition, grading and staging schema proposed and currently in use are reviewed. Finally, other aspects for consideration by practicing pathologists, such as sampling issues, histopathologic findings after therapeutic interventions, and recurrence after liver transplantation, are addressed.

▶ Nonalcoholic fatty liver disease (NAFLD) encompasses 2 processes. One is simple steatosis characterized by accumulation of fat in hepatocytes without additional tissue injury. The second is nonalcoholic steatohepatitis (NASH), which in addition to fat accumulation, the hepatocytes show injury that includes ballooning (hydropic degeneration), Mallory bodies, and pericellular fibrosis with or without inflammation. The prognostic significance of each is different. Distinguishing them is important because NASH is associated with chronic liver disease and cirrhosis more frequently than simple steatosis alone. At the present time, there is no clinical method to distinguish them. Only a pathologist has the ability to do it by assessing the morphologic features in a biopsy tissue. This article provides a nice review of the features of NASH in the adult and also compares them with those seen in children. In the pediatric population, steatosis has more affinity for periportal hepatocytes than centrilobular. In general, grading of NASH is still limited to clinicopathological studies and research clinical trials and it is not widely applied to daily practice. Because of the complex numerological approach of that grading system, it becomes cumbersome to apply. The current role of the diagnostic pathologist is to determine whether or not there are features of NASH. NASH may recur after transplantation. One of the aspects not reviewed is the combination of NASH and alcohol-induced liver disease in the same patient.

P. Bejarano, MD

Relevant Histopathologic Findings That Distinguish Acute Cellular Rejection From Cholangitis in Hepatic Allograft Biopsy Specimens

Bilezikçi B, Demirhan B, Kocbiyik A, et al (Başkent Univ School of Medicine, Ankara, Turkey)
Transplant Proc 40:248-250, 2008

Background and Aim.—Histopathologic differential diagnosis of acute cellular rejection (ACR) and cholangitis continue to pose important problems following liver transplantation. The purpose of the present study was to evaluate the histopathologic features of ACR versus cholangitis.

Methods.—The following variables were evaluated among 36 hepatic allograft biopsy specimens, consisting of 21 with ACR (group 1) and 15 with cholangitis (group 2) for ductal neutrophilic infiltration, presence/density of portal eosinophilia, centrilobular necrosis, central/portal vein endothelialitis, pericentral inflammation, hepatocyte ballooning, hepatocanalicular/ductular cholestasis, hepatocyte apoptosis, lobular inflammation, ductular proliferation, periductal fibrosis/edema, ductular epithelial damage, and portal inflammation. Only the first biopsy samples of the ACR group were included in this study.

Results.—The incidences of ductal neutrophilic infiltration (93.3% vs 19%), hepatocanalicular cholestasis (86.7% vs 47.6%), ductular cholestasis (60% vs 0%), ductular proliferation (93.3% vs 4.8%), and periductal fibrosis/edema (93.3% vs 19%) were significantly greater in group 2 than group 1 ($P < .05$). In contrasts the incidences of portal eosinophilia (mean ± SD, 3.37 ± 3.9 vs 0.73 ± 0.8), dense portal eosinophilia (mean ± SD, 0.33 ± 0.31 vs 0.11 ± 0.16), central vein endothelialitis (0% vs 57.1%), portal vein endothelialitis (20% vs 95.2%), apoptosis (40% vs 71.4%), and necroinflammation (0% vs 90.5%) were significantly higher in group 1 ($P < .05$). The other parenchymal histopathologic changes and features of portal inflammation were similar in the 2 groups.

Conclusion.—In the differential diagnosis, ductal changes (cholestasis, neutrophilic infiltration, proliferation, and periductal fibrosis/edema) favor cholangitis, whereas the presence and density of portal eosinophilia favor ACR. Portal inflammation is not a distinctive morphological finding.

▶ Distinguishing acute cellular rejection (ACR) from acute cholangitis in transplanted liver biopsy tissues may be difficult. However, this scenario is actually less complicated than when one is trying to deal with other diagnostic settings. For instance, separating ACR from mimickers of it such as recurrent hepatitis C, primary biliary cirrhosis, or autoimmune hepatitis can be more cumbersome. The presence of large number of neutrophils in or near portal tracts with or without edema favor cholangitis. If these features are accompanied by cholestasis, in particular canalicular cholestasis, the possibility of partial distal mechanical obstruction in the biliary tract is suggested and needs to be correlated with radiological studies. On the other hand, predominantly lymphocytic infiltrates favor rejection when bile duct epithelium is injured by lymphocytes. The confidence for a diagnosis of rejection over cholangitis is enhanced if eosinophils are present and also if endothelialitis of the branches of portal vein or centrilobular veins is observed.

P. Bejarano, MD

Absence of E-Cadherin Expression Distinguishes Noncohesive from Cohesive Pancreatic Cancer

Winter JM, Ting AH, Vilardell F, et al (The Johns Hopkins Univ School of Medicine, Baltimore, MD)
Clin Cancer Res 14:412-418, 2008

Purpose.—The role of E-cadherin in carcinogenesis is of great interest, but few studies have examined its relevance to pancreatic carcinoma.

Experimental Design.—We evaluated E-cadherin protein expression by immunohistochemistry in pancreatobiliary cancers having a noncohesive histologic phenotype (21 undifferentiated adenocarcinomas and 7 signet ring carcinomas), comparing the results with pancreatic cancers having a cohesive phenotype (25 moderately differentiated and 14 poorly differentiated adenocarcinomas).

Results.—Twenty of 21 undifferentiated cancers had complete absence of E-cadherin expression, as did two signet ring carcinomas. In contrast, cohesive cancers ($n = 39$) had E-cadherin labeling at the plasma membrane ($P < 0.001$). Subsets of cancers were also evaluated for β-catenin expression. All of the cohesive lesions ($n = 28$) showed a membranous β-catenin expression pattern, whereas noncohesive foci ($n = 7$) were characterized by either cytoplasmic labeling or complete absence of β-catenin protein expression, suggestive of a deficient zonula adherens in noncohesive cancers. E-cadherin promoter hypermethylation was observed in an undifferentiated pancreatic cancer cell line, MiaPaCa-2, whereas two pancreatic cancer cell lines derived from differentiated lesions lacked any evidence of E-cadherin promoter methylation. No pattern of E-cadherin promoter methylation could be determined in three primary cancers having mixed histologic patterns (contained both cohesive and noncohesive foci). No somatic mutations in E-cadherin were identified in noncohesive pancreatic cancers having inactivated E-cadherin.

Conclusions.—Noncohesive pancreatic cancers were characterized by the loss of E-cadherin protein expression. Promoter hypermethylation is a possible mechanism of E-cadherin gene silencing in a subset of these cancers.

▶ E-Cadherin is an adhesion molecule that serves to maintain the architectural integrity of certain types of epithelia. Immunohistochemical stain for E-Cadherin is mostly used to distinguish breast lobular carcinoma from invasive ductal adenocarcinoma. The latter keeps the expression of this molecule in contrast to lobular carcinomas, which lack it. Mutations and lack of expression of E-Cadherin have been identified in lobular carcinomas of the breast and signet ring cell carcinomas of the stomach. These tumors show discohesion of their cells with presence of single cell invasion. In this study, there was a correlation between discohesive tumors of the pancreas and poor survival. Carcinomas were classified as cohesive if the infiltrating glands were observed throughout the tumor. Noncohesive carcinomas meant that cancerous foci lacked infiltrating glands. This article did not analyze any correlation between the lack of expression of E-cadherin and histologic findings such as vascular invasion and infiltration of surrounding tissues. Therefore, a study correlating its presence or absence to multiple histologic features would be appropriate.

P. Bejarano, MD

Distinction of Hepatocellular Carcinoma From Benign Hepatic Mimickers Using Glypican-3 and CD34 Immunohistochemistry
Coston WMP, Loera S, Lau SK, et al (City of Hope Natl Medl Ctr, Duarte, CA; et al)
Am J Surg Pathol 32:433-444, 2008

Distinguishing a well-differentiated hepatocellular carcinoma (HCC) from normal and cirrhotic liver tissue or benign liver nodules, such as hepatic adenoma (HA) and focal nodular hyperplasia (FNH), may be very difficult in some cases, particularly in small needle core biopsies. We studied the expression of Glypican-3 (GPC3) and CD34 in 107 cases of HCC, 19 cases of HA, and 16 cases of focal nodular hyperplasia (FNH). In addition, we studied GPC3 expression in 225 cases of nonhepatic human tumors with epithelial differentiation. Ninety-four of 107 cases (88%) of HCC showed focal or diffuse cytoplasmic GPC3 staining, whereas all HA and FNH cases were GPC3-negative, and only 7 of 225 cases (3%) of nonhepatic tumors with epithelial differentiation expressed GPC3. The sensitivity and specificity of GPC3 for HCC was 88% and 97%, respectively. There were three CD34 staining patterns observed in hepatic tissue: negative, incomplete positive, and complete positive. In negative staining pattern, only blood vessels in portal triads or rare sinusoidal spaces immediately adjacent to portal tracts were positive. The negative staining pattern was seen in normal or cirrhotic liver tissue only. The complete CD34 staining pattern showed virtually all sinusoidal spaces with CD34-positive staining throughout the lesion. The complete CD34 staining pattern was seen in virtually all cases of HCC and in only some cases of HA and FNH. The incomplete CD34 staining pattern was characterized by either CD34 positivity in virtually all sinusoidal spaces in some but not all nodules or CD34 positivity in the peripheral sinusoidal spaces adjacent to portal triads. The incomplete CD34 staining pattern was seen in rare cases of HCC and in most cases of HA and FNH. We conclude that GPC3 is a very specific marker not only for differentiating HCC from nonhepatic tumors with epithelial differentiation, but also for differentiating HCC from HA and FNH. GPC3 immunoreactivity, in combination with a complete CD34 immunostaining pattern, greatly facilitates the accuracy of distinguishing between malignant hepatic lesions and benign mimickers.

▶ Distinguishing benign liver cell lesions such as adenoma and focal nodular hyperplasia from well-differentiated hepatocellular carcinoma may be very difficult on histologic grounds. This is a comprehensive study that not only analyzed benign liver lesions and hepatocellular carcinomas but also other types of tumors that have epithelioid appearances. Because of the poor sensitivity of alpha-feto protein staining for hepatocellular carcinoma, there has been a need for a marker that can distinguish carcinoma from other liver lesions, in particular adenoma. Although the combination of glypican-3 and CD34 is promoted in this article as specific markers in this setting, there are several aspects that make them not quite the silver bullet that pathologists were hoping they would be. For instance, only 11 of the 107 cases of hepatocellular carcinoma studied were biopsies. The large majority was resected specimens and, therefore, the interpretation of CD34 may be not entirely reliable on individual cases of needle biopsies where the limited sample is a problem. In addition, 37 of the 94 positive cases for glypican-3 showed < 50% immunoreactivity. In liver biopsies the percentage of positive cells could be less perhaps causing a high rate of false-negative results. Although other types of extrahepatic malignancies were studied, it would be appropriate to carry an analysis of metastatic carcinoma of the liver and stain them for glypican-3 to observe whether or not its specificity stands. Finally, it is becoming apparent that benign liver tumors with markedly inflammatory active hepatitis C tend to stain positive for glypican-3. Therefore, caution is necessary to not misinterpret those cells as carcinoma based just on a positive stain.

P. Bejarano, MD

Epstein-Barr Virus Hepatitis: Diagnostic Value of In Situ Hybridization, Polymerase Chain Reaction, and Immunohistochemistry on Liver Biopsy From Immunocompetent Patients
Suh N, Liapis H, Misdraji J, et al (Washington Univ School of Medicine; Massachusetts Gen Hosp/Harvard Med School, Boston, MA)
Am J Surg Pathol 31:1403-1409, 2007

Epstein-Barr virus (EBV) hepatitis is an uncommon, almost always self-limited disease in immunocompetent patients. Accurate diagnosis is imperative for appropriate clinical management. The aim of this study was to compare 3 available methods for EBV detection on routinely processed liver biopsies to determine their effectiveness in aiding the diagnosis. In 6 of the 8 cases of EBV hepatitis, EBV was detected by both polymerase chain reaction (PCR) for EBV DNA and in situ hybridization (ISH) for EBV early RNA (EBER). EBV was detected by PCR only in 1 case, and by ISH only in another. EBER-positive cells detected by ISH were typically few and individually distributed in the portal tracts and sinusoids. Immunohistochemical staining for EBV latent membrane proteins was negative in all 8 cases. Five cases of chronic hepatitis C used as negative controls were negative by all 3 detection methods for EBV. These data indicate that PCR and ISH are equally sensitive in detecting EBV in routinely processed liver biopsies. The ready implementation of ISH in pathology laboratories makes it a useful ancillary tool in confirming the diagnosis of EBV hepatitis in equivocal cases. However, EBER-positive cells can be sparse and easily overlooked. Immunohistochemistry for EBV latent membrane proteins apparently has no utility in the diagnosis of EBV hepatitis.

▶ This is the largest series of immunocompetent patients who had clinical manifestations of Epstein-Barr virus (EBV) hepatitis and who underwent liver biopsies. EBV infects greater than 90% of the world's population and persist for life in memory B lymphocytes. Most patients are asymptomatic, but the disease may become manifest in immunosuppressed individuals as a primary infection or as a reactivation. Immunocompetent patients include adolescent and young adults who develop infectious mononucleosis that may result in a self-limited hepatitis. Histopathological changes of EBV hepatitis are represented by mixed inflammatory cell infiltrates in the portal tracts with interface activity. Endophlebitis in portal veins is present and the sinusoids show lymphocytic infiltration with a beaded and single linear appearance. Some of the lymphocytes may be atypical. In addition, granulomas and bile duct injury can be observed. The latter feature could in part explain the elevation of alkaline phosphatase in some of the patients. The classical histological findings are not always present and, therefore, ancillary studies may be needed. In this study, the authors found that immunohistochemical staining is useless for diagnosis. However, the authors used only 1 type of antibody (DAKO), and it is not clear if using anti-EBV latent membrane proteins from other manufacturers will also yield similar negative results.

P. Bejarano, MD

Prognostic significance of immunohistochemical RhoA expression on survival in pancreatic ductal adenocarcinoma: a high-throughput analysis
Dittert D-D, Kielisch C, Alldinger I, et al (Univ Hosp Carl Gustav Carus, Dresden, Germany; Univ Hosp, Düsseldorf, Germany)
Hum Pathol 39:1002-1010, 2008

Among all human carcinomas, pancreatic cancer has one of the worst survival rates. Most patients will die of this cancer shortly after diagnosis, and currently, surgery is the only potential cure. Ductal adenocarcinoma is the most common histologic type. The search for prognostic parameters has progressed from mere physical or histomorphological tumor properties to molecular parameters. These, in turn, might point toward new therapeutic strategies. The *K-ras* oncogene is known to play a role in early stages of ductal adenocarcinoma carcinogenesis, and ras homologues are differentially expressed in cancerous versus normal ductal cells. RhoA belongs to a family of ras homologues comprising RhoA, RhoB, and RhoC. It is a guanosine triphosphatase associated with the cytoskeleton that seems to be involved in epithelial mesenchymal transition, a process of dedifferentiation. Immunohistologic RhoA expression was studied in a tissue microarray of 94 pancreatic ductal adenocarcinomas and correlated with clinicopathologic parameters and follow-up. RhoA protein expression, measured as labeling intensity or evaluated as percentage of reactive tumor cells, correlated with overall survival. A multivariate analysis demonstrated that RhoA protein expression is independent from other known prognostic parameters such as tumor size or grade. Moreover, a score combining RhoA expression with tumor size and grade resulted in a highly significant increase in the prognostic value for the overall survival of patients with pancreatic ductal adenocarcinoma.

▶ The survival of patients with pancreatic ductal adenocarcinoma (PDAC) is related to the size of the tumor and its respectability. Patients with nonresectable tumors usually die within a few months even if they are given chemotherapy or radiotherapy. It has been established that *K-ras* oncogene plays a role in carcinogenesis of PDAC. There are phosphatases that have homology to K-*ras*. These are guanosine triphosphatases (GTpases) called Rho. One of them is RhoA, which plays a role in the formation of stress fibers and intercellular adhesions. Its immunohistochemical expression is present in normal pancreas. In this study, RhoA strong positive staining in adenocarcinomas correlated with a better survival. A previous study on colorectal carcinomas showed that low expression of RhoA was related to a poor outcome. The mechanism by which patients with expression of RhoA in their tumors are at advantage is not known. Additional studies to elucidate this point and to confirm its value as a prognostic marker are needed.

P. A. Bejarano, MD

5   Dermatopathology

Collision tumor composed of Merkel cell carcinoma and lentigo maligna melanoma
Forman SB, Vidmar DA, Ferringer TC (Geisinger Med Ctr, Danville, PA; Lake Erie Dermatopathology, PA)
J Cutan Pathol 35:203-206, 2008

We report the case of an immunocompetent 79-year-old white man with a history of melanoma *in situ* on the back with a collision tumor composed of a Merkel cell carcinoma (MCC) and lentigo maligna melanoma on the left cheek. The cells of the MCC expressed cytokeratin 20 (CK 20) in a diffuse cytoplasmic pattern, AE1 and AE3 in a perinuclear dot-like pattern and diffusely with neuron-specific enolase. The tumor cells of the MCC failed to express thyroid transcription factor-1. The atypical melanocytes of lentigo maligna melanoma expressed Melan-A and S-100. At the same visit, a lentigo maligna was diagnosed by excisional biopsy on the right cheek. The variability in expression of CK 20, AE1 and AE3 in MCC are reviewed. Prior reports of MCC in collision with non-melanoma skin cancers are reviewed. Additionally, the role of immunosuppression in the development of MCC is considered.

▶ All in all, there are multiple "collision" tumors that have been reported in the literature, especially literature that deals with skin pathology. I chose to review this article because, as I learned from one of the greatest pathologists of our time, Dr. Juan Rosai, one often sees in the slides only what one expects. On the other hand, the devil is in the details, and in my practice I have seen several times cases of skin biopsy that included large specimens with 2 or more either separate or collided neoplastic processes, whereas only 1 was mentioned.

To applaud the authors, they have chosen to address this tumor (neoplasm) as a "collision" tumor, rather than employing such designation as "mixed" or "transitional" tumor/neoplasm. All in all, the article is somewhat well-written, but appears to be hampered by a relatively skimpy literature selection. For the most part, however, the images are excellent, although Fig 4 in the original article bears a somewhat cryptic title–"There is a junctional proliferation of atypical melanocytes"–rather than outlining the lesion as a melanoma in-situ.

This article was obviously written almost a year before the landmark article connecting a Merkel cell carcinoma with human polyoma virus, but the authors should have included the excellent article written by Miller[1] in 1999 that dealt with the similarities and differences of these 2 neoplasms. The authors did, however, include the excellent article by Howard et al.[2] Miller's article will help the practicing pathologist to understand what he or she can expect while examining the skin of an individual. To address the issue further one would be wise to review the articles outlined herein in addition to some case reports posted on the University of Pittsburgh Department of Pathology site,[3,4] which will considerably broaden the approach to the problem.

In summary, although the Merkel cell carcinoma is a rare disease, it is a one that you cannot allow yourself to miss, as it is perfectly treatable by surgery if caught early.

D. M. Jukic, MD, PhD

References

1. Miller RW, Rabkin C. Merkel cell carcinoma and melanoma: etiological similarities and differences. *Cancer Epidemiol Biomarkers Prev.* 1999;8:153-158. Erratum in: Cancer Epidemiol Biomarkers Prev 1999 May;8(5):485.
2. Howard RA, Dores GM, Curtis RE, Anderson WF, Travis LB. Merkel cell carcinoma and multiple primary cancers. *Cancer Epidemiol Biomarkers Prev.* 2006; 15:1545-1549.
3. University of Pittsburgh Department of Pathology. Multiple cutaneous malignancies and related fatal outcome, http://path.upmc.edu/cases/case398.html. Accessed October 6, 2008.
4. University of Pittsburgh Department of Pathology. An elderly man with a plaque-like crusted lesion of his right temple, http://path.upmc.edu/cases/case449.html. Accessed October 6, 2008.

Collagen-rich variant of benign epithelioid peripheral nerve sheath tumor of the skin
Jokinen CH, Wolgamot GM, Argenyi ZB (Univ of Washington, Seattle, WA)
J Cutan Pathol 35:215-219, 2008

Schwannoma and neurofibroma account for the majority of cutaneous benign peripheral nerve sheath tumors and usually pose little diagnostic difficulty in their classic forms. In rare instances, however, benign peripheral nerve sheath tumors may display epithelioid morphology and lack otherwise usual features of schwannoma or neurofibroma, making classification difficult. These unusual changes may prompt consideration of other benign neoplasms or a malignancy. Benign epithelioid peripheral nerve sheath tumor (BEPNST) is a somewhat non-specific term recently proposed to describe these neoplasms of imprecise histogenesis. Also diagnostically challenging, rare BEPNST with unusual arrangements of extracellular collagen have been described and reported as neuroblastoma-like schwannoma and collagenous spherulosis. We report a unique case of cutaneous BEPNST with a peculiar arrangement of abundant extracellular collagen, different than the previously observed patterns. Specifically, the neoplastic cells in this tumor were nearly obscured by the collagen, which formed large nodules and compressed the majority of the few remaining tumor cells to the periphery of the lesion. This excessive

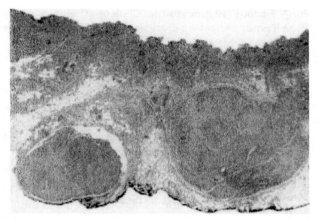

FIGURE 1.—Low magnification of the well-circumscribed mass in the deep dermis highlights the extensive eosinophilic collagenous material compared with the relatively few cells. A single hypercellular nodule is present (bottom left; higher magnification of this area depicted in Fig. 2C in the original article) (hematoxylin and eosin). (Reprinted from Jokinen CH, Wolgamot GM, Argenyi ZB. Collagen-rich variant of benign epithelioid peripheral nerve sheath tumor of the skin. *J Cutan Pathol.* 2008;35:215-219, with permission from Blackwell Munksgaard.)

collagen production emphasizes the importance of adequate sampling to ensure a correct diagnosis (Fig 1).

▶ When it comes to spindle cell neoplasms in skin, one always has to take a step back. What is it? Is it just a plain dermatofibroma, or perhaps blue nevus, or could it be a malignant peripheral sheath tumor, or even a much feared desmoplastic melanoma.

In this article, the authors outline an unusual entity of what they choose to consider a variant of benign epithelioid peripheral nerve sheath tumor. Indeed, the photographs in this article are commendable, especially Fig 1 which outlines the low-power architecture in a very nice way.

Although I would have probably broadened the immunoprofile and performed CD56, NK1-C3, PGP 9.5, CD 34, and some other stains, I do not think that these were a deal breaker. Of interest, I expected the p75 to be expressed in a much higher percentage of cells (80%-90%). The low expression indicated at only 50% is somewhat surprising. However, a practicing pathologist would do good to pay attention to this article, which can ultimately save a patient from unnecessary radical and heroic therapies if one starts considering every collagenous schwannoma a desmoplastic melanoma.

D. M. Jukic, MD, PhD

Deep "Benign" Fibrous Histiocytoma: Clinicopathologic Analysis of 69 Cases of a Rare Tumor Indicating Occasional Metastatic Potential

Gleason BC, Fletcher CDM (Harvard Med School, Boston, MA)
Am J Surg Pathol 32:354-362, 2008

Benign fibrous histiocytoma (FH) is one of the most common mesenchymal neoplasms of the skin. Several histologic variants of cutaneous FH have been described, some of which also have distinct clinical features including a propensity for local recurrence. Deep benign FH is an uncommon and poorly recognized clinical subtype that arises in subcutaneous or deep soft tissue. Only a single small series of these neoplasms has been published, and their clinical behavior is not well characterized. In this study, we report the clinicopathologic features of 69 deep FH retrieved from our consultation files. The patients included 41 males and 28 females, ranging in age from 6 to 84 years (median, 37 y). The most common anatomic location was the extremities (58%); the remainder arose on the head and neck (22%), trunk (11%), and in the deep soft tissue of the retroperitoneum, mediastinum, or pelvis (9%). All lesions arising in nonvisceral soft tissue were subcutaneous. The tumors ranged from 0.5 to 25 cm in size (median, 3.0 cm) and were well circumscribed grossly and microscopically. All tumors were composed of bland ovoid to spindle cells arranged in a storiform pattern with admixed lymphocytes. Multinucleate giant cells, osteoclastic giant cells, and/or foam cells were present in 59% of cases, whereas the other 41% were cytologically monomorphic, often resembling cellular FH. Other common findings included a hemangiopericytomalike vascular pattern (42%) and stromal hyalinization (39%). Four cases were classified as atypical deep FH due to the presence of scattered markedly pleomorphic spindle cells within an otherwise histologically typical lesion. The median mitotic rate was 3/10 HPF; 10 cases (14%) had >10 mitoses/10 HPF. Necrosis (2 cases) and lymphovascular invasion (1 case) were rare. Immunohistochemistry revealed expression of CD34 in 20/50 cases (40%), smooth muscle actin in 15/40 (38%), and focal desmin in 1/12 (8%). Of the 37 patients for whom clinical follow-up was available (median, 40 mo), 8 (22%) had a local recurrence; in all 8 cases, the tumor had been marginally or incompletely excised. Metastases occurred in 2 patients (5%), both of whom ultimately died of disease; however, this number is likely exaggerated due to consultation bias. The metastasizing tumors were large (6 and 9 cm) and 1 had tumor necrosis but they were otherwise histologically identical to the nonmetastasizing lesions. In summary, deep FH has many histologic features in common with cutaneous cellular FH; however, it usually has a more diffusely storiform pattern than the latter, is well circumscribed, and may have striking hemangiopericytomalike vessels. Similar to the cellular, aneurysmal, and atypical variants of FH, deep FH recurs in approximately 20% of cases and may rarely metastasize.

▶ If you observed Christopher Fletcher giving talks, you are likely to know about this entity. In summary, Dr Fletcher has long lectured about the significance of being able to identify the rare examples of fibrous histiocytomas (FHs) that do metastasize. I would argue that, at least for the practicing pathologist, it is even more important to be aware of this entity, but to be able to recognize the entities that will do just fine if left alone, or perhaps, as the case might be with more cellular entities, get re-excised.

The great strength of the article, and its biggest drawback, is the numbers. The authors have examined 69 cases; however, the long-term follow-up was available in only 37 cases, which, at least in my mind, somewhat limits the recommendations made in this article. Truthfully, 2 cases metastasized and ultimately killed the patients, but according to the authors there did not appear to be any distinguishing characteristics for these 2 cases. However, in everyday practice the presence of storiform growth pattern, cytological polymorphism, and increased mitotic rates, as well as foci of tumor necrosis in addition to the fact that these were the deep-seated FHs, should raise enough flags for the practicing pathologist to at least ask for a second opinion.

D. M. Jukic, MD, PhD

Confirmation of Sentinel Lymph Node Identity by Analysis of Fine-Needle Biopsy Samples Using Inductively Coupled Plasma–Mass Spectrometry
Beavis A, Dawson M, Doble P, et al (Univ of Technology, Sydney, New South Wales; et al)
Ann Surg Oncol 15:934-940, 2008

Background.—The sentinel lymph node (SLN) biopsy technique is a reliable means of determining the tumor-harboring status of regional lymph nodes in melanoma patients. When technetium 99 m-labeled antimony trisulfide colloid ($^{99\,m}Tc\text{-}Sb_2S_3$) particles are used to perform preoperative lymphoscintigraphy for SLN identification, they are retained in the SLN but are absent or present in only tiny amounts in non-SLNs. The present study investigated the potential for a novel means of assessing the accuracy of surgical identification of SLNs. This involved the use of inductively coupled plasma–mass spectrometry (ICP-MS) to analyze antimony concentrations in fine-needle biopsy (FNB) samples from surgically procured lymph nodes.

Methods.—A total of 47 FNB samples from surgically excised lymph nodes (32 SLNs and 15 non-SLNs) were collected. The SLNs were localized by preoperative lymphoscintigraphy that used $^{99\,m}Tc\text{-}Sb_2S_3$, blue dye, and gamma probe techniques. The concentrations of antimony were measured in the FNB samples by ICP-MS.

Results.—The mean and median antimony concentrations (in parts per billion) were .898 and .451 in the SLNs, and .015 and .068 in the non-SLNs, the differences being highly statistically significant ($P < .00005$).

Conclusions.—Our results show that ICP-MS analysis of antimony concentrations in FNB specimens from lymph nodes can accurately confirm the identity of SLNs. Used in conjunction with techniques such as proton magnetic resonance spectroscopy for the nonsurgical evaluation of SLNs, ICP-MS analysis of antimony concentrations in FNB samples could potentially serve as a minimally invasive alternative to surgery and histopathologic evaluation to objectively classify a given node as sentinel or nonsentinel and determine its tumor-harboring status.

▶ Superficially, it seems unusual that one would review an article about a technique of sentinel lymph node (SLN) procedure in a dermatopathology section of this publication. However, in most of the major centers and even tertiary hospitals we are frequently called to perform a sentinel node evaluation. Some of us more fortunate ones do it via evaluation of paraffin embedded sections, whereas the less fortunate ones do it via evaluation of frozen sections after being incessantly bullied by surgeons.

In effect, we spend countless hours evaluating lymph nodes that were not supposed to be removed in the first place, whereas (and especially after one reads this article) apparently the lymph nodes that were supposed to be removed are still in the patient. I, for one, would welcome a technique that would have enhanced the retrieval of "real" SLNs while avoiding the removal of "false positives." Although the authors claim that "inductively coupled plasma-mass spectrometry (ICP-MS) analysis of antimony concentrations in fine-needle biopsy (FNB) samples could potentially serve as a minimally invasive alternative to surgery and histopathologic evaluation to objectively classify a given node as sentinel or nonsentinel and determine its tumor-harboring status," only a part of this argument holds. Namely, once the lymph node is removed (or is under the suspicion to be removed) there is no alternative to a histopathologic examination. Even more interesting, although this would hardly encompass the realm of dermatopathology, it is quite possible that the pathologist skilled in performing fine-needle aspiration procedures could actually perform the FNBs in vivo. If I understood the authors correctly, the FNBs were performed postremoval for the sake of this protocol (article), but they should be quite feasible intraoperatively. Even though the authors do not delve into the exact time it takes to perform such a procedure, we are sincerely hoping that the procedure could be done expeditiously.

In the meantime, we all better invest into digital slide analyzers, which will allow us to examine the SLNs via the so-called "rare event protocols,' allowing us to miss virtually no positive cells.

For further reading on this subject I suggest an article by Mesker et al.[1]

D. M. Jukic, MD, PhD

Reference

1. Mesker WE, Doekhie FS, Vrolijk H, et al. Automated analysis of multiple sections for the detection of occult cells in lymph nodes. *Clin Cancer Res.* 2003;9: 4826-4834.

6 Lung and Mediastinum

Cysts of the posterior mediastinum showing müllerian differentiation (Hattori's cysts)
Thomas-de-Montpréville V, Dulmet E (Marie Lannelongue Surgical Ctr, France)
Ann Diagn Pathol 11:417-420, 2007

Cysts of probable müllerian origin have recently been recognized in the mediastinum by Hattori (*Virchows Arch.* 2005;446:82-84; *Chest.* 2005;128:3388-3390). In a retrospective study, we found 9 such cases, accounting for 5.5% of a series of 163 consecutive mediastinal nonneoplastic cysts operated in our institution. These cysts occurred in 9 women aged 40 to 58 years (mean, 50.6 years). These women often had overweight (n = 4) or various gynecologic history (n = 5). Cysts were paravertebral (n = 8) or prevertebral (n = 1). They were initially classified as bronchogenic or unspecified benign serous cysts. Their diameter measured 1.3 to 5 cm. Their thin wall contained smooth muscle. They were lined by a simple cylindrical or cuboidal, nonmucinous, and often ciliated epithelium resembling uterine tubal epithelium. This epithelium expressed cytokeratin 7, epithelial membrane antigen and estrogen and progesterone receptors. It was negative for cytokeratin 5/6. In the same series, there were 66 bronchogenic cysts, 6 being paravertebral. In conclusion, cysts with müllerian differentiation account for a small proportion of mediastinal cysts and have a usual but nonspecific paravertebral location.

▶ The authors describe the largest series of this unique type of cyst occurring in the mediastinum. It is interesting that, although the number of cases described in the literature is very small, the authors found 9 of these cysts among 163 consecutive mediastinal cysts. This number represents 5.5% of mediastinal cysts in their series, indicating that cysts with müllerian differentiation are not so rare. It is conceivable that cysts showing müllerian differentiation were in the past considered bronchogenic cysts without cartilage. Apart from their immunohistochemical expression for estrogen and progesterone receptors, their histological features would make them similar to other types of cysts. The photographs in this article show lesions that are architecturally reminiscent of fallopian tube as there is formation of papillary-like structures lined by cylindrical to cuboidal epithelium and containing bundles of smooth muscle fibers.

Because the histogenesis is not clear, the term cyst with müllerian differentiation is preferable to "müllerian cyst" or "cyst of müllerian origin."

P. Bejarano, MD

Effect of Formalin Fixation on Tumor Size Determination in Stage I Non-Small Cell Lung Cancer

Hsu P-K, Huang H-C, Hsieh C-C, et al (Taipei-Veterans General Hosp Natl Yang-Ming Univ, Taiwan)
Ann Thorac Surg 84:1825-1829, 2007

Background.—Tumor size is an important prognostic factor in non-small cell lung cancer (NSCLC), but the American Joint Committee on Cancer staging system does not mandate a specific measurement method. Moreover, measuring fresh specimens and formalin-fixed specimens may yield disparate results. Our goal was to evaluate this disparity for stage I NSCLC.

Methods.—We enrolled 401 patients with stage I NSCLC who underwent surgical interventions and follow-up in our hospital between 1993 and 2002. Tumors invading visceral pleura, involving the main bronchus, or associated with atelectasis or obstructive pneumonitis were excluded. Tumor size was measured immediately after resection by surgeons and after formalin fixation by pathologists. Patients were assigned to one of three groups. Group 1 included 201 patients with tumors of 3 cm or less as indicated by both operation notes and pathology reports. Group 2 included 160 patients with tumors larger than 3 cm by both records. Group 3 included 40 patients with tumors larger than 3 cm according to operation notes but 3 cm or less according to pathology reports. Survival rates were compared.

Results.—Mean follow-up was 58 months. Five-year survival was 70.1% in group 1, 49.1% in group 2, and 51.1% in group 3. As expected, there was a significant survival difference between groups 1 and 2 ($p < 0.001$); however, there was also a difference between groups 1 and 3 ($p = 0.006$).

Conclusions.—Formalin fixation may cause tumor shrinkage and migration from T2 to T1. For accurate tumor staging, size measurements should be performed immediately after resection instead of after formalin fixation. TNM staging should specify how to measure tumor size and the specimen status to be measured.

▶ The pathological staging of lung carcinoma is based on the size of the tumor. A pT1 tumor measures less than 3 cm, whereas a pT2 tumor is greater than 3 cm. Although the clinical implications of accurate measurement of a tumor are obvious, the American Joint Committee on Cancer (AJCC) staging system does not specify how this measurement should be obtained. The authors suggest that the surgeons should cut the specimen and expose the tumor and measure it immediately after surgery because there is considerable reduction in the size of the tumor after fixation in formalin. The mean size of the tumors changed from 4.01 cm to 2.85 cm in a sample of 40 tumors as reported by surgeons and pathologists, respectively. This shrinkage occurred in approximately 10% of all specimens among the 401 tumors when the measurements obtained in the operating room were compared with the sizes obtained by pathologists after formalin fixation. That the AJCC staining system is going to be changed based on these data remains to be seen.

P. Bejarano, MD

Immunohistochemical Detection of XIAP in Mesothelium and Mesothelial Lesions
Wu M, Sun Y, Li G, et al (Mount Sinai School of Medicine, New York; et al)
Am J Clin Pathol 128:783-787, 2007

We examined benign and malignant mesothelial tissue samples for the presence of X-linked inhibitor of apoptosis protein (XIAP), a potent constituent of the inhibitor of apoptosis family of caspase inhibitors.

We subjected 55 sections (31 malignant mesotheliomas, 2 well-differentiated peritoneal mesotheliomas, 13 pleural mesothelial hyperplasias, and 9 benign mesothelial tissues) from archival formalin-fixed, paraffin-embedded surgical tissue blocks to citrate-based antigen retrieval and then incubated them with monoclonal anti-XIAP (clone 48, dilution 1:250; BD Biosciences, San Jose, CA) at 4°C for 72 hours and developed them using EnVision-Plus reagents (DAKO, Carpinteria, CA) and diaminobenzidine as the chromogen. Particulate or nonhomogeneous cytoplasmic staining was considered positive.

All 9 normal mesothelial samples were negative for XIAP. Of 13 mesothelial hyperplasias, 1 (8%) was weakly positive in fewer than 10% of cells, as was 1 of 2 well-differentiated peritoneal mesotheliomas. Of 31 malignant mesotheliomas, 25 (81%) displayed XIAP positivity.

XIAP immunostaining, when strong, allows for distinction of malignant from benign and hyperplastic mesothelial cell populations and is a potentially useful immunodiagnostic marker in small samples and morphologically controversial cases. Elevated expression of XIAP could contribute to tumorigenesis in mesothelioma.

▶ Because reactive mesothelial proliferations may be difficult to distinguish from malignant mesotheliomas, the use of X-linked inhibitor of apoptosis protein (XIAP) is a welcome immunohistochemical marker to distinguish these 2 processes. A granular cytoplasmic pattern of stain is observed in malignant mesotheliomas, whereas it tends to be negative in reactive mesothelial hyperplasias. So far, the only markers that have been used to distinguish benign from malignant mesothelial proliferations, in particular in pleural effusions, have included p53 as well as epithelial membrane antigen showing strong, linear, and cellular membrane staining. However, the results are inconsistent. Other markers such as calretinin, CK5/6 and WT-1 do not separate malignant mesothelioma from reactive mesothelial hyperplasias. Although XIAP may be helpful in the epithelioid pattern of mesotheliomas (93% staining), its sensitivity decreases in sarcomatoid mesotheliomas as it stains only 40% of them. Therefore, spindle cell lesions of the pleura continue being difficult to diagnose with certainty. The diagnosis of pleural lesions should include morphology and a battery of immunostains. An interesting aspect of XIAP is that eventually it can be a target of therapeutic agents that may block its expression by restoring apoptotic activity, which is what occurs in several cancer therapy modalities.

P. Bejarano, MD

Malignant Pleural Mesothelioma: Surgical Management in 285 Patients
Schipper PH, Nichols FC, Thomse KM, et al (General Thoracic Surgery and Biostatistics, Rochester, MN)
Ann Thorac Surg 85:257-264, 2008

Background.—Malignant pleural mesothelioma is a rare, aggressive, and deadly malignancy. Despite increasing incidence, no treatment modality is accepted standard of care. This report analyzes our experience with surgical management of mesothelioma.

Methods.—All patients with surgery for mesothelioma from January 1985 through December 2003 were retrospectively reviewed.

Results.—There were 285 patients with a median age of 66 years (range, 26 to 91 years). One hundred forty-six patients (51%) had biopsy only, 73 (26%) had extrapleural pneumonectomy, 34 (12%) had subtotal parietal pleurectomy, 22 (8%) underwent exploration without resection, and 10 (3%) had total pleurectomy. Histopathology was epithelial, nonepithelial, and unclassified in 134, 108, and 43 patients, respectively. Twenty patients were stage IA, 82 patients were stage IB, 24 patients were stage II, 75 patients were stage III, 60 patients were stage IV, and 24 patients were of unknown stage. Fifty-three patients (19%) had chemotherapy alone, 16 (5.6%) had radiation alone, and 42 (14.7%) had both. Thirty-day operative mortality was 6.3% and was not significantly associated with the operative procedure ($p = 0.79$). Fifty-one percent of extrapleural pneumonectomy patients had major complications, significantly greater than patients having any other procedure ($p < 0.001$). Median follow-up was 11 months (range, 0 to 7 years). Overall median survival was 10.7 months; however, for patients having extrapleural pneumonectomy, median survival was 16 months. One-, 2-, and 3-year survival after extrapleural pneumonectomy was 61%, 25%, and 14%, respectively.

Conclusions.—Extrapleural pneumonectomy can be performed with similar 30-day mortality as other procedures for malignant pleural mesothelioma with a median survival better than subtotal pleurectomy, exploration without resection, and biopsy alone. However, extrapleural pneumonectomy has significant morbidity and a 3-year survival of only 14%.

▶ The incidence of malignant pleural mesotheliomas continues to rise worldwide. The peak of the number of cases predicted has not been reached yet as the latency period between occupational exposure and the development of malignant pleural mesothelioma range from 12 to 50 years. In the United States, about 3000 new cases occur each year, and most patients are men. Approximately 90% of patients with mesothelioma were exposed to asbestos. Patients undergoing extrapleural pneumonectomy have en bloc resection of the involved ipsilateral parietal pleura, lung, pericardium, and diaphragm. Usually, the diaphragm and pericardium are reconstructed with polytetrafluoroethylene soft-tissue patch. Total pleurectomy consists of a complete extrapleural stripping of the parietal and mediastinal pleura and involved visceral pleura. In this series, survival was lower for patients with nonepithelial type, such as sarcomatoid or desmoplastic mesotheliomas. This study confirms the dismal prognosis of malignant mesothelioma of the pleura, regardless of the surgical approach used.

P. Bejarano, MD

Epidermal Growth Factor Receptor Signaling in Adenocarcinomas With Bronchioloalveolar Components

Sarkaria IS, Zakowski MF, Pham D, et al (Memorial Sloan-Kettering Cancer Ctr, New York)
Ann Thorac Surg 85:216-223, 2008

Background.—Epidermal growth factor receptor (EGFR) has gained importance in non–small cell lung cancer given impressive responses to agents targeting this molecule, particularly in bronchioloalveolar carcinoma (BAC) and adenocarcinomas, mixed subtype, with BAC components (adeno/BAC). This study assesses EGFR signaling in these tumors.

Methods.—One hundred fifty tumors were classified as BAC or adeno/ BAC. Tumor marker expression was determined by immunohistochemistry. Correlations with expression were examined for all tumors (BAC and adeno/BAC), and by BAC and adeno/BAC subset analyses.

Results.—Positive immunophenotype was observed in 40.6% of tumors for EGFR, 51.3% for p-AKT, 58.7% for p-ERK, and 28.0% for PTEN, with increased overexpression of EGFR ($p = 0.025$) and p-AKT ($p < 0.0001$) in adeno/BAC. Epidermal growth factor receptor immunophenotype was greater in never-smokers ($p = 0.008$) and correlated with improved overall survival ($p = 0.018$). On subset analysis, EGFR correlated with improved overall survival ($p = 0.05$) and disease-free interval ($p = 0.044$) only in adeno/BAC. Epidermal growth factor receptor independently predicted improved disease-free interval in adeno/BAC ($p = 0.03$; hazard ratio, 0.47; 95% confidence interval, 0.23 to 0.94).

Conclusions.—Overexpression of EGFR in lung adenocarcinomas with components of BAC histology correlate with never-smoker status and improved overall survival and disease-free interval. Epidermal growth factor receptor immunophenotype may be a useful predictor of clinical outcomes in this tumor subset.

▶ This study does not analyze the response to tyrosine kinase inhibitor therapies. Instead, it only determines the prognosis of bronchioloalveolar adenocarcinomas and mixed adenocarcinomas containing both, bronchioloalveolar components and invasive areas. The assessment is based on the immunohistochemical expression of epidermal growth factor receptor (EGFR) and the intracellular signaling mechanism components that mediate the effects of EGFR in nonsmall cell carcinomas. Those mechanisms include RAS (rat sarcoma virus) dependent Raf (murine leukemia viral oncogene homolog)/MEK (mitogen activated protein kinase kinase)/ERK (extracellular signal related kinase) signaling, and activation of the AKT (murine thymoma viral oncogen homolog) serine/threonine kinase through PI3K (phosphatidylinositol 3 kinase) signaling. The overexpression of the markers in this study show increasing immunoreactivity from noninvasive bronchioloalveolar carcinoma (BACs) to invasive adenocarcinoma with areas of BAC suggesting that tumor progression starts from atypical adenomatous hyperplasia, to noninvasive BAC and mixed tumors, and eventually to frankly invasive adenocarcinomas. This article is addressed to surgeons and oncologists and thus, it is expected that pathologists be requested more frequently to perform stains for EGFR, not for therapeutic purposes, but to disclose a prognostic factor.

P. Bejarano, MD

Primary Mediastinal Seminoma: A Comprehensive Assessment Integrated With Histology, Immunohistochemistry, and Fluorescence In Situ Hybridization for Chromosome 12p Abnormalities in 23 Cases
Sung M-T, MacLennan GT, Lopez-Beltran A, et al (Chang Gung Univ College of Medicine, Kaohsiung, Taiwan; Case Western Reserve Univ, Cleveland, OH; Cordoba Univ, Spain; et al)
Am J Surg Pathol 32:146-155, 2008

Accurate diagnosis of mediastinal seminoma is critical because of its favorable response to radiation therapy and/or cisplatin-based chemotherapy. Immunohistochemical staining for OCT4 has recently been validated as a powerful tool for detecting gonadal seminoma. However, discrepancies between the genetic alterations and immunoprofiles of mediastinal and testicular seminomas have been reported, raising the question of whether techniques that are useful in the diagnosis of gonadal seminoma are applicable to its mediastinal counterpart. The present study was conducted to evaluate the morphologic and immunohistochemical characteristics and chromosomal abnormalities of 12p in 23 primary mediastinal seminomas and to compare their applicability as diagnostic tools. Dual-color fluorescence in situ hybridization (FISH) analyses for chromosome 12p and immunostains for OCT4, c-kit, placental-like alkaline phosphatase, CD30, and a panel of cytokeratins, including cytokeratin AE1/AE3 (AE1/3), high molecular weight cytokeratin (34βE12, HMWCK), CAM5.2, cytokeratin 7 (CK7), cytokeratin 20 (CK20), and epithelial membrane antigen were performed. Lymphocytic infiltration was found in all 23 cases (100%). The incidence of other histologic characteristics were as follows: fibrous septa/stroma (21 cases, 91%), prominent tumor cell nucleoli (21 cases, 91%), clear tumor cell cytoplasm (20 cases, 87%), distinct tumor cell borders (20 cases, 87%), granulomatous inflammation (17 cases, 74%), cellular pleomorphism (10 cases, 43%), necrosis (8 cases, 35%), prominent cystic change (2 cases, 8%), intercellular edema (1 case, 4%), and syncytiotrophoblasts (1 case, 4%). The mean mitotic count was 4.4 (range 0 to 16) per 10 high-power fields. Moderate to strong nuclear OCT4 staining was identified in all 23 cases (100%). Seventeen tumors (74%) showed membranous expression of c-kit, with variable staining intensity and percentages. Weakly to moderately intense immunostaining for placental-like alkaline phosphatase was identified in 10 cases (43%) with occasional background staining artifact. The incidences of positive staining were 43% for AE1/3, 39% for HMWCK, 48% for CAM5.2, 39% for CK7, and 9% for epithelial membrane antigen, respectively. In most cases, these epithelial markers highlighted only a small proportion of tumor cells with variable intensities. Immunostaining for CD30 and CK20 was completely negative in all seminomas. Twenty-two seminomas (96%) revealed chromosome 12p abnormalities, including 12p amplification in 20 cases (87%) or i(12p) in 15 cases (65%). Lymphocytic infiltration is the most common histologic feature observed in primary mediastinal seminoma and both OCT4 immunostain and FISH for 12p abnormalities can be very helpful in diagnosing mediastinal seminoma. The intense staining pattern of OCT4 and the high sensitivity of FISH make them superior to other auxiliary diagnostic utilities for detecting seminoma. In addition, the incidences of cytokeratin expression of primary mediastinal seminoma are similar to those of its gonadal counterpart and pathologists must exercise caution in the interpretation of epithelial markers in mediastinal neoplasms.

▶ Primary seminomas occur in the testicles, retroperitoneum, mediastinum, and pineal gland. The histogenesis of extragonadal seminomas is unknown. Mediastinal seminomas account for 3% to 4% of all mediastinal tumors in this site and their prognosis is good as they respond very well to radiation and/or chemotherapy using cisplatin. The diagnosis may be difficult in small biopsy tissues. They can be confused with other tumors that include embryonal carcinoma and yolk sac tumor. Because of the rich lymphocytic infiltrates in seminomas, benign inflammatory processes, lymphoma and thymic tumors enter in the differential diagnosis. This article offers information and strong evidence that OCT4 is a very helpful marker for mediastinal seminomas. It regulates cellular pluripotency of primordial germ cells and embryonic stem cells. As most transcription factors, its immunohistochemical expression is observed in the nuclei, and thus, it is easy to interpret rendering little to no background. In general, it appears to be a better marker than PLAP and c-kit. However, the number of studies is still small.

P. Bejarano, MD

Survival after Surgery in Stage IA and IB Non–Small Cell Lung Cancer

Ost D, Goldberg J, Rolnitzky L, et al (New York Univ School of Medicine, New York)

Am J Respir Crit Care Med 177:516-523, 2008

Rationale.—Whether histologic subtype of non–small cell lung cancer (NSCLC) has an important effect on prognosis after surgery is unknown.

Objectives.—We hypothesized that we could predict mortality more effectively by integrating precise tumor size and histology rather than relying on conventional staging.

Methods.—We used the SEER (Surveillance, Epidemiology, and End Results) registry. Inclusion criteria were as follows: (1) primary squamous cell or adenocarcinoma; (2) potentially curative surgery, defined as a lobectomy or bilobectomy; (3) lymph node dissection performed; and (4) pathologic stage IA or IB.

Measurements and Main Results.—From 1988 to 2000, 7,965 patients were included. For both all-cause and lung cancer–associated mortality, tumor size demonstrated the strongest association (log-rank $P < 0.0001$ for each). When tumors were small (≤ 2 cm), lung cancer-associated mortality was similar for adenocarcinoma when compared with squamous cell carcinoma. When tumors were 3 cm or larger in size, lung cancer–associated mortality was higher for adenocarcinoma. The increased risk of lung cancer–associated mortality with adenocarcinoma was more pronounced in those younger than 65 years. Survival prediction using precise size and histology had much better discriminatory power than conventional TNM (tumor-node-metastasis) staging ($P = 0.005$).

Conclusions.—Staging that takes into account size, histology, late recurrence risk, and patient age is more accurate than the current TNM system and is clinically relevant because improved prediction can facilitate better decisions on the use of adjuvant chemotherapy.

▶ The current pathological tumor-node-metastasis (TNM) staging system from The American Joint Committee on Cancer does not distinguish between histological subtypes of pulmonary nonsmall cell carcinomas. It considers only the tumor size and pleural invasion to separate T1 and T2 patients. The cutoff size is 3.0 cm, which may be arbitrary if the histological subtype is ignored. The authors belong to the group of splitters because they found that distinction between adenocarcinomas and squamous cell carcinomas (SCCs) have prognostic implications. Adenocarcinomas behave more aggressively and, therefore, these tumors need to be treated with different and/or stronger chemothera-peutic agents than those used to treat SCCs. The importance of the role pathol-ogists play to tell apart adenocarcinomas from SCCs is becoming more evident. When certain target therapies designed to treat adenocarcinomas are given to patients with SCCs, complications such as bleeding may occur. One issue not addressed in this article is the implications of large cell carcinoma of the lung. There are immunohistochemical markers such as TTF1, p63, and CK7 that have the ability to determine if a large cell carcinoma is, in reality, poorly differentiated carcinoma of squamous or glandular origin.

P. Bejarano, MD

Immunohistochemical detection of XIAP and p63 in adenomatous hyperplasia, atypical adenomatous hyperplasia, bronchioloalveolar carcinoma and well-differentiated adenocarcinoma

Wu M, Orta L, Gil J, et al (Mount Sinai School of Medicine, NY; et al)
Mod Pathol 21:553-558, 2008

The critical distinction of bronchioloalveolar carcinoma (BAC), well-differentiated adenocarcinoma (WDAC) of lung, adenomatous hyper-plasia (AH) and atypical adenomatous hyperplasia (AAH), is based on morphological criteria alone, and is therefore potentially subjective. We examined expression of two markers, X-linked inhibitor of apoptosis protein (XIAP), the most potent of the inhibitor of apoptosis protein (IAP) family, and p63, a marker of bronchial reserve cells (BRC) and squa-mous cells, in these entities. H&E slides of 37 tissue blocks from 27 patients were reviewed and classified as AH ($n = 7$), AAH ($n = 8$), BAC ($n = 9$) and WDAC ($n = 13$). Immunostaining was performed on 4 μm sections with monoclonal anti-XIAP and monoclonal anti-p63. Granular or heterogeneous cytoplasmic staining for XIAP and nuclear staining for p63 were considered positive. Neither XIAP nor p63 were detected in normal lung alveolar cells. All seven AHs were negative for XIAP and negative or focally positive for p63. All eight AAHs were positive for XIAP and displayed p63 positivity in scattered cells. All BACs displayed XIAP positivity, which ranged from focal/weak to diffuse/strong. p63 was negative in seven and focally positive in two of nine BACs. Twelve of 13 WDACs showed XIAP positivity in a similar pattern to BAC; all were negative for p63. One aberrant case diagnosed on H & E as WDAC was negative for XIAP but strongly positive for p63. Significant XIAP expression appears to be useful for distinguishing AAH from AH. Commonality of XIAP staining in AAH, BAC and WDAC supports the possibility that AAH may be a pre-malignant lesion. The rarity of p63 expression confirms previous reports and supports a nonbronchial histo-genesis of these entities. In contrast, diffuse p63 staining may facilitate the identification of rare cases that may have been misclassified as alveolar in origin based on morphology but may be of BRC origin.

▶ There is a group of alveolar lesions in the lung that are distinguished by the severity of the atypia they display. However, grading of atypia in those glandular lesions is subjective and its significance can be uncertain in individual cases. Clear cut bronchioloalveolar adenocarcinoma and adenomatous hyperplasia (AH) are at the ends of the spectrum, whereas atypical AH (AAH) is in the middle with a less clear characterization. Although the World Health Organization defined it as a lesion with mild-to-moderate atypia measuring less than 5 mm, there is still an uncertainty on how to treat AAH. Therefore, an objective marker would be desirable. One of them promises to be X-linked inhibitor of apoptosis protein (XIAP). It belongs to a group of 8 known IAPs. Overexpression in cancer cells renders them resistant to apoptosis-inducing chemotherapeutic agents and radiation. Immunohistochemical studies using XIAP on lung adenocarcinomas and hyperplasias are nonexistent. The small number of cases studied suggests that AAH is not reactive, but preneoplastic. Positive stain for XIAP in borderline lesions may help clinicians to decide on whether or not to remove an AAH lesion even if it is not larger than 5 mm. In fact, the authors support alternate terminology for this type of lesion. They propose naming it alveolar cell dysplasia or alveolar intraepithelial neoplasia.

P. A. Bejarano, MD

Bronchiolitis interstitial pneumonitis: a pathologic study of 31 lung biopsies with features intermediate between bronchiolitis obliterans organizing pneumonia and usual interstitial pneumonitis, with clinical correlation
Mark EJ, Ruangchira-urai R (Massachusetts Gen Hosp and Harvard Med School, Boston)
Ann Diagn Pathol 12:171-180, 2008

Bronchiolitis combined with interstitial pneumonitis generally has been equated with bronchiolitis obliterans organizing pneumonia (BOOP). We describe our experience with lung biopsies that had both bronchiolar and interstitial diseases. We studied 31 patients who had respiratory difficulty leading to open lung biopsy, which showed a combination of both prominent bronchiolitis and prominent interstitial pneumonitis. We compared these cases clinically and pathologically with 6 other pulmonary diseases, namely, bronchiolitis obliterans, BOOP, nonspecific interstitial pneumonitis, usual interstitial pneumonitis, airway-centered interstitial fibrosis, and idiopathic bronchiolocentric interstitial pneumonia, and with 10 cases of cystic fibrosis, an unrelated disease with both bronchiolar and interstitial pathology. The commonality of our cases was a combination of bronchiolitis and interstitial inflammation and fibrosis but little or no intra-alveolar organizing pneumonia. Bronchiolitis obliterans with organizing pneumonia involved less area than the interstitial pneumonitis in each case. All 19 patients for whom we had follow-up received cortico-steroids for their pulmonary diseases. Seven patients had improvement in symptoms and pulmonary function test results and radiographic findings, 5 patients experienced subjective improvement with unchanged results of pulmonary function tests or chest x-ray, 1 patient's condition was unchanged, 6 patients' disease worsened, and 4 of these 6 died. The natural history of these cases, which we have designated bronchiolitis interstitial pneumonitis, seems more sanguine than usual interstitial pneumonitis and worse than BOOP at least in the short term. On the one hand, response to corticosteroids was not as frequent as generally accepted for BOOP. On the other hand, disease did not progress in most patients on corticosteroids.

▶ Nonneoplastic lung diseases became a festival of acronyms. Just the ones mentioned in this article include: BIP, BO, BOOP, NSIP, UIP, ACIF, IBCIP. They stand for bronchiolitis interstitial pneumonitis, bronchiolitis obliterans, non-specific interstitial pneumonitis, usual interstitial pneumonia, airway-centered interstitial fibrosis, and idiopathic bronchiolocentric interstitial pneu-monia, respectively. The latter 2 entities (ACIF, IBCIP) may be the new kids in the block. Of course, there are more acronyms that have been around longer such as DIP, RB-ILD, COP, and AIP. They mean: desquamative interstitial pneumonia, respiratory bronchiolitis associated interstitial lung disease, crypto-genic bronchiolitis, and acute interstitial pneumonia, respectively. This article attempts to explain the patterns of ACIF, IBCIP, and BIP and their distinction from mimickers such as NSIP, UIP, and BOOP. Hypersensitivity pneumonitis should also be included in the differential diagnosis as it is a bronchiolocentric disease with an interstitial component. Until recently, ACIF, BIP, IBCIP, and centrilobular fibrosis, would have been named as unclassifiable interstitial lung disease. Now, we have more entities based on series of small number of cases and with short follow-up. We really need stronger documentation of those entities to immerse them into the every day practice.

P. A. Bejarano, MD

Evidence-Based Pathology and the Pathologic Evaluation of Thymomas: Transcapsular Invasion Is Not a Significant Prognostic Feature
Gupta R, Marchevsky AM, McKenna RJ, et al (Cedars-Sinai Med Ctr, Los Angeles, CA)
Arch Pathol Lab Med 132:926-930, 2008

Context.—Evaluation of transcapsular invasion is currently considered very important in the pathologic examination of thymomas. However, recent studies have questioned the prognostic value of stratifying thymoma patients into stage I and II disease. Evidence-based pathology promotes the use of systematic reviews of literature and metaanalysis of data to synthe-size the results of multiple publications.

Objective.—To analyze the data in the literature regarding the prognostic importance of transcapsular invasion in thymoma stage I and II.

Design.—A systematic review of the English literature was carried out for "thymoma," "stage," and "prognoses." Case reports, case series with fewer than 10 cases, and studies with follow-up periods shorter than 5 years were excluded. Twenty-one retrospective publications reporting the experience with 2451 thymomas were selected for review, including 1419 stage I and 1032 stage II patients. Meta-analysis was performed, and possible publication bias was studied with funnel plots of precision and various statistics.

Results.—Meta-analysis yielded no significant differences in disease-free or overall survival rates in stage I and II thymoma patients. Funnel plots of precision and statistical tests such as the Egger regression intercept test showed no significant publication bias.

Conclusions.—The lack of significant differences in the prognosis of patients with stages I and II thymoma suggests that evaluation of transcapsular invasion is of no clinical value in tumors that lack invasion of neighboring organs or the pleura. The data regarding the prognosis of stage II thymoma patients is somewhat heterogenous, with only some individuals having been treated with radiation therapy, suggesting the need for future randomized controlled trials.

▶ A prospective study is the ideal method to analyze the behavior of tumors. However, those studies require that their series are composed of a large number of cases. Because thymomas are unusual tumors, carrying out meaningful, prospective, randomized, double-blind trials of treated patients in a uniform manner and followed by several decades (Level 1 evidence) is difficult. This is a meta-analysis of the literature of 21 articles showing retrospective characteristics of thymoma patients from 8 countries, thus constituting Level 3 evidence-based pathology. The authors of this study obtained the data stated in the abstracts of the published articles. The abstracts provided limited or no information about details such as surgical procedures used in the treatment of the patients. The Masaoka staging system indicates that Stage I is a completely encapsulated thymoma without microscopic invasion of the capsule. Stage II-1 is macroscopic invasion into surrounding adipose tissue or mediastinal pleura. In Stage II-2, there is microscopic invasion of the capsule. In Stage III there is invasion into adjacent organs. Stage IVa shows dissemination of tumor in the pleura or pericardium. In Stage IVb there is metastasis. Apart from the lack of significant clinical differences between Stages I and II, the inconsistency with which pathologists determine capsular or extracapsular invasion may lend support to the authors' view of simplifying Stages I and II into a single group.

P. Bejarano, MD

Molecular Pathology in the Lungs of Severe Acute Respiratory Syndrome Patients

Ye J, Zhang B, Xu J, et al (Peking Univ Health Science Ctr, Beijing, China; et al)
Am J Pathol 170:538-545, 2007

Severe acute respiratory syndrome (SARS) is a novel infectious disease with disastrous clinical consequences, in which the lungs are the major target organs. Previous studies have described the general pathology in the lungs of SARS patients and have identified some of the cell types infected by SARS coronavirus (SARS-CoV). However, at the time of this writing, there were no comprehensive reports of the cellular distribution of the virus in lung tissue. In this study, we have performed double labeling combining *in situ* hybridization with immunohistochemistry and alternating each of these techniques separately in consecutive sections to evaluate the viral distribution on various cell types in the lungs of seven patients affected with SARS. We found that SARS-CoV was present in bronchial epithelium, type I and II pneumocytes, T lymphocytes, and macrophages/monocytes. For pneumocytes, T lymphocytes, and macrophages, the infection rates were calculated. In addition, our present study is the first to demonstrate infection of endothelial cells and fibroblasts in SARS.

▶ Severe Acute Respiratory Syndrome (SARS) became known to the world in 2004 when an outbreak caused the death of 10% of the infected patients. A coronavirus (CoV) is the responsible agent as it infects pneumocytes, bronchial epithelium, macrophages, and T-lymphocytes. However, the literature has been controversial on what types of cells are indeed infected. The disease manifests as diffuse alveolar damage, pulmonary edema, interstitial lymphocytic infiltrates, and desquamation of pneumocytes into alveolar spaces. Using cRNA probes of SARS-CoV extracted from serum of SARS patients it was confirmed that the virus is present in the cells that have been previously reported. In this study, SARS-CoV was found in a few endothelial cells by in-situ hybridization. The presence of edema, vasculitis, hemorrhage, and thrombosis in this disease in SARS may be explained by the association of direct viral infection of endothelial cells and the production of proinflammatory mediators along with ischemic injury. The disease eventually may lead to fibrosis. The authors also found infection of fibroblasts, thus likely activating them to produce collagen.

P. Bejarano, MD

Cytoplasmic Immunoreactivity of Thyroid Transcription Factor-1 (Clone 8G7G3/1) in Hepatocytes: True Positivity or Cross-Reaction?

Gu K, Shah V, Ma C, et al (Henry Ford Hospital, Detroit, MI)
Am J Clin Pathol 128:382-388, 2007

The nuclear immunoreactivity for thyroid transcription factor-1 (TTF-1) is a useful marker for identification of carcinomas of thyroid and lung origin. Our aim was to determine whether cytoplasmic staining in the liver is a result of cross-reaction of anti–TTF-1 antibody (clone 8G7G3/1, DAKO, Carpinteria, CA) or true positivity resulting from aberrant expression of TTF-1 or products of the alternatively sliced TTF-1 gene. Fresh tissue samples from liver, thyroid, and lung were obtained for H&E-stained sections, TTF-1 immunostaining, and RNA and protein analyses. Western blot revealed an abundant band corresponding to an approximately 160-kd protein from liver but not either thyroid or lung tissue samples. By reverse transcriptase–polymerase chain reaction, messenger RNA of TTF-1 was not detectable in liver tissue. Our study demonstrates that TTF-1 immunoreactivity (clone 8G7G3/1) in the hepatocyte cytoplasm is due to an approximately 160-kd protein; this unique protein is not an alternative splicing product of TTF-1 and neither is it expressed in thyroid and lung tissues.

▶ Thyroid transcription factor-1 (TTF-1) immunohistochemical stain has been a very helpful tool in diagnostic surgical pathology. Its nuclear immunoreactivity suggests that a given tumor is most likely of lung or thyroid origin. However, cytoplasmic staining has been observed in liver tissue. This finding created speculation and controversy regarding the true nature and significance of this pattern of staining. This article adds interesting information about the molecular characterization of the antigen targeted by TTF-1 antibody that shows liver cytoplasmic immunoreactivity. First, it confirms that a particular clone of antibody, 8G7G3/1 manufactured by DAKO produces cytoplasmic staining, which is rarely or not observed using other clones and manufacturers. Western immunoblotting showed a 160-kd protein from liver tissue not present in thyroid or lung tissue when the 8G7G3/1 antibody is used. This protein is not the true protein present in lung and thyroid. The antigen in these 2 organs is a 41-kd protein. So, there is a cross-reaction rather than gene expression of TTF-1 in liver tissue, as there is no mRNA in hepatocytes. It is interesting that the marker, hepatocellular antigen (Hep Par1) antibody, binds a 150-kd mitochondrial liver protein of similar weight to the 160-kd protein detected by 8G7G3/1. This suggests that both TTF1 and Hep Par1 share molecules in the hepatocyte mitochondria. Despite the new knowledge gained, caution is still advised when observing cytoplasmic staining in a tumor of unknown origin because this pattern of staining is not specific for liver origin.

P. Bejarano, MD

7 Cardiovascular

Cardiac Behçet Disease Presenting as Aortic Valvulitis/Aortitis or Right Heart Inflammatory Mass: A Clinicopathologic Study of 12 Cases
Lee I, Park S, Hwang I, et al (Univ of Ulsan College of Medicine, Seoul, Korea)
Am J Surg Pathol 32:390-398, 2008

Behçet disease is an inflammatory disorder of unknown etiology showing diverse clinical presentations. Cardiac involvement is a critical problem that requires a timely diagnosis and management. However, clinicopathologic features have not been characterized clearly. Here, we present clinicopathologic characteristics of this uncommon disease. Patients included 8 males and 4 females, ranging from 24 to 52 years old. They were presented with abrupt heart failure and were mostly diagnosed as having cardiac Behçet disease later in the course. Upon echocardiography, 8 patients showed severe aortic regurgitation with redundant prolapsing aortic cusps and 4 patients showed irregular mass lesions in the right ventricular cavity. No one had both lesions. The aortic root was also involved with aortic valvulitis, showing severe mixed acute and chronic inflammation of various stages. There were frequent microabscess and extensive endothelial loss with fibrinous deposit. The right heart lesions showed similar histopathologic features. Four patients who initially underwent simple aortic valve replacement developed serious postoperative complications requiring reoperations. No serious complications developed after the treatment was changed to a replacement of aortic root with extensive debridement and concomitant immunosuppressive therapy. Cardiac Behçet disease is presented as aortic valvulitis/aortitis or inflammatory mass lesion. Characteristic echocardiographic and pathologic findings seem to be helpful for the timely diagnosis of this critical disease.

▶ This is a multidisciplinary study of Behçet disease affecting the heart. The study includes clinical, echocardiographic, and pathological examination. It is one of the most complete studies of this disease with cardiac manifestations. Cardiovascular involvement by Behçet disease is one of the most serious complications manifesting clinically, as sudden heart failure because of aortic regurgitation. The main findings encountered in this disease are inflammation of the cardiac valves or the aorta, and also a mass in the right heart. Interestingly, both processes did not present simultaneously. It appears that among the initial changes, endotheliitis plays a main role in the pathogenesis of the disease in the heart. Microorganisms were not found. However, an infectious etiology remains a possibility. The cardiac mass is not neoplastic, but inflammatory in nature with the presence of fibrin, neutrophilic infiltrates, blood vessel proliferation, and fibrosis. The authors suggest that echocardiographic findings are valuable as a specific for a tentative diagnosis of Behçet disease.

P. Bejarano, MD

IgG4-positive Plasma Cells in Inflammatory Abdominal Aortic Aneurysm: The Possibility of an Aortic Manifestation of IgG4-related Sclerosing Disease

Sakata N, Tashiro T, Uesugi N, et al (School of Medicine, Fukuoka Univ; Natl Hosp Organization Kyushu Med Ctr, Fukuoka; et al)
Am J Surg Pathol 32:553-559, 2008

Inflammatory abdominal aortic aneurysm (IAA) is associated with autoimmune disease. However, the precise mechanism of IAA remains unclear. There is increasing evidence that IgG4 is involved in the autoimmune mechanism of various idiopathic sclerosing lesions, including sclerosing pancreatitis and retroperitoneal fibrosis. The present study investigated the hypothesis that the IgG4-related autoimmune reaction is involved in the formation of IAA. The study group consisted of 11 cases of IAA (69.2 ± 8.59 y) and 12 age-matched cases of atherosclerotic abdominal aortic aneurysm (AAA, 69.6 ± 5.94 y), which were used in the previous report. A clinicopathologic examination of these lesions was performed, including histology and immunohistochemistry, in relation to the involvement of IgG4-positive plasma cells in the formation of IAA. No difference in the incidence of risk factors for atherosclerosis was observed between the patients with IAA and AAA. Autoimmune diseases were diagnosed in 2 patients with IAA, including rheumatoid arthritis and polyarteritis nodosa. A patient with IAA had pulmonary fibrosis. In contrast, autoimmune diseases were absent in patients with AAA. However, there was no significant difference in the incidence of autoimmune diseases between the patients with IAA and AAA. Lymphocyte and plasma cell infiltration and fibrosis were significantly more intense and extensive in IAA than in AAA. In addition, lymph follicle formation and vasculitis of small veins and arteries were frequently found in the affected lesions of IAA. Immunohistochemically, IAA showed a significant increase in the number of infiltrating IgG4-positive plasma cells and the incidence of a disrupted follicular dendritic cell network in lymph follicles, in comparison with AAA. These findings suggest that IAA may be an aortic lesion reflecting the presence of IgG4-related sclerosing disease, and not a simple inflammatory aneurysm of the aorta.

▶ Atherosclerotic and inflammatory types of aortic aneurysm may share several histologic features. They include lymphocyte and plasma cell infiltration, fibrosis, lymphoid follicle formation, small vein phlebitis, endarteritis and necroinflammation. However, inflammatory abdominal aortic aneurysms (IAAs) show much more prominent lymphoplasmacytic infiltrates, adventitial fibrosis, and lymphoid follicles. This article lends support to the view that IAAs have an autoimmune component as they show a higher number of positive IgG4 plasma cells by immunohistochemistry. Because of this finding it is postulated that IAAs may enter in the group of sclerosing diseases, which includes auto-immune pancreatitis. The prominent lymph follicles are composed of B-cells surrounded by T-cells. Another feature of these follicles is related to the follic-ular dendritic cell network, which is disrupted in the IAA. The patterns are high-lighted using antibodies against CD21/CD35. The normal network of dendritic cells form a well-defined circular meshwork in the lymphoid follicle, whereas the disrupted network shows an irregular and incomplete outline. The point of this article is to highlight the fact that aorta may be affected by the inflamma-tory and sclerosing process driven by IgG4 autoimmune mechanism as observed in other organs.

P. Bejarano, MD

Implications of a congenitally abnormal valve: a study of 1025 consecutively excised aortic valves
Collins MJ, Butany J, Borger MA, et al (Univ Health Network, Toronto, Canada; Univ of Toronto, Canada; et al)
J Clin Pathol 61:530-536, 2008

Background.—An increasing proportion of patients with congenitally abnormal aortic valves (AV) present for AV replacement.

Aims.—To review morphological changes in a large contemporary patient population undergoing AV replacement.

Methods.—A detailed review was conducted for all 1025 patients who underwent AV replacement from 2002 to 2005, including the clinical indi-cation for surgery, the type of native AV disease, the pathological changes observed in each valve and the need for related surgery.

Results.—Tricuspid (TAV), bicuspid (BAV) and unicuspid (UAV) aortic valves were observed in 64.5%, 31.9% and 3.0% of all patients respec-tively. A decreased number of cusps was associated with increasing predi-lection for male gender (83.9%, 73.4%, 59.2% for UAV, BAV, TAV respectively), a younger patient age at surgery (41.6 (14.3), 61.3 (12.8), 67.5 (12.9) years), and an increased occurrence of pathological changes in the cusps, including calcification of both the cusp and the base, ossifica-tion and ulceration. UAV and BAV were also associated with increasing replacement of the ascending aorta due to dilatation and aneurysm forma-tion (54.8, 38.8%, 16.6%). The incidence of infective endocarditis and rheumatic heart disease was 3.8% and 11.2% of all excised valves respec-tively.

Conclusion.—UAV and BAV were increasingly likely to affect men, fail at an earlier age, and show an increasing incidence of pathological changes in the cusps and ascending aorta than TAV. These results suggest that TAV, BAV and UAV may represent a phenotypic continuum of a similar disease process.

▶ The incidence of congenital abnormal aortic valves (AV) in developing countries is increasing in part because infection-driven valvulopathies, in particular rheumatic fever disease, is low. In fact, this study found that 35% of explanted AV were congenitally abnormal. This article offers illustrative photographic material of the gross findings of abnormal valves. In addition, the authors give indirect hints on how to sample these valves for microscopic examination. They took sections of the most severely involved areas. In tricuspid aortic valve (TAV), sections were taken from each cusp and from the fused commissure. In unicuspid aortic valve (UAV) and bicuspid aortic valve (BAV), longitudinal sections were taken from the cusps and transverse sections across the raphe. This is a very detailed morphologic study based on a large number of cases examined by experienced observers of the heart valvular pathology. They found a link between decreased numbers of cusps with incrementally severe valve pathology. It appears that there is chronologic continuum in the damage found in TAV, BAV, and UAV and those may belong to a spectrum of similar diseases.

P. Bejarano, MD

Limited Utility of Endomyocardial Biopsy in the First Year after Heart Transplantation

Hamour IM, Burke MM, Bell AD, et al (Harefield Hosp, Middlesex, UK; et al)
Transplantation 85:969-974, 2008

Background.—Surveillance endomyocardial biopsies (EMBs) are used for the early diagnosis of acute cardiac allograft rejection. Protocols became standardized in an earlier era and their utility with contemporary immunosuppression has not been investigated.

Methods.—We studied 258 patients after orthotopic heart transplantation comparing 135 patients immunosuppressed by mycophenolate mofetil (MMF) with 123 patients treated by azathioprine (AZA); both with cyclosporine and corticosteroids after induction therapy with rabbit antithymocyte globulin. Fifteen EMBs were scheduled in the first year. Additional EMBs were performed for suspected rejection, after treatment, or for inadequate samples. The MMF group had 1875 EMBs vs. 1854 in the AZA group.

Results.—The yield of International Society for Heart and Lung Transplantation (ISHLT) grade≥3A biopsy-proven acute rejection (BPAR) was 1.87% per biopsy (35 of 1875) with MMF vs. 3.13% (58 of 1854) with AZA $P=0.024$. The number of clinically silent BPAR ISHLT grade ≥3A (the true yield of surveillance EMBs) was 1.39% (26 of 1875) of biopsies MMF vs. 2.1% (39 of 1854) AZA, $P=0.48$. There were five serious complications requiring intervention or causing long-term sequelae; 0.13% (5 of 3729) per biopsy and 1.94% (5 of 258) per patient. The incidence of all definite and potential complications was 1.42% (53 of 3729) per biopsy and 20.5% (53 of 258) per patient. There was no biopsy-related mortality.

Conclusion.—The yield of BPAR was low in the AZA group and very low in the MMF group. The incidence of complications was also low, but repeated biopsies led to a higher rate per patient. Routine surveillance EMBs and the frequency of such biopsies should be reevaluated in the light of their low yield with current immunosuppression.

▶ This study shows a very low yield for diagnosis of rejection on routine surveillance endomyocardial biopsies (EMBs). Only 1.8% (65 of 3607) of biopsies showed clinically significant rejection grade 3A. Grade 3A corresponds to 2R (moderate rejection) in the current revised grading system. Historically, the use of routine biopsies was implemented early in the era of transplantation when immunosuppression drugs were less effective. The modern therapies make the probability of rejection a very infrequent diagnosis in the absence of clinical features of rejection. The procedure to obtain an EMB carries serious risks and that is why this article would support the view that less number of biopsies should be performed. If a biopsy shows low-grade rejection (1R) usually treatment is not required. What remains to be seen is if clinically silent rejection grade 2R in the first year after transplantation requires treatment. Replacement of the use of biopsy tissue is not possible at the present time. Other clinical methods are not sensitive or specific for that to happen.

P. A. Bejarano, MD

Aortitis and ascending aortic aneurysm: description of 52 cases and proposal of a histologic classification
Burke AP, Tavora F, Narula N, et al (CVPath Inst, Gaithersburg, MD 20878, USA; Johns Hopkins Univ, Baltimore, MD 21218, USA; Univ of California, Irvine, CA 92623, USA)
Hum Pathol 39:514-526, 2008

Noninfectious aortitis typically involves the ascending aorta and causes aneurysms that result in aortic root repair. Aortitis is clinically categorized into groups that include Takayasu disease, giant cell aortitis, and isolated aortitis. We present a histopathologic classification of 52 patients with aortitis, without reference to clinical findings, which are often unknown to the diagnostic pathologist. The largest group (43 patients) was designated necrotizing aortitis (NA), characterized by zonal medial laminar necrosis, rimmed by giant cells. Healed areas were common and were characterized by extracellular accumulation of proteoglycans imparting the appearance of medial degeneration. NA had a bimodal age distribution with a separation at age 65 (adult NA versus elderly NA). Adult NA (24 patients; 50%

female; age range, 24-60) was generally isolated, but 2 patients had associated autoimmune disease (Crohn disease and lupus erythematosus, respectively). Elderly NA (19 patients; 94% female; age range, 68-80) was likewise usually isolated, but 1 patient had temporal giant cell arteritis and 1 seronegative arthritis. Subsequent complete rheumatologic workup on 17 patients with NA was negative. Adult NA differed significantly from elderly NA (fewer women, $P = .002$; greater adventitial scarring, $P = .007$). The second group of aortitis was designated non-NA (NNA), characterized by the absence of necrosis, with diffuse medial inflammation. The NNA group was composed of 3 men and 6 women, all older than 65 years (mean, 72 ± 6 years). Four had a history of temporal arteritis. NNA patients differed from elderly NA (more frequent temporal arteritis, $P = .03$; less medial destruction and proteoglycan deposits, $P < .01$; increased medial T-lymphocytes, $P = .05$; and more frequent dissection, $P = .002$). We conclude that NA is usually isolated, has distinct histologic features based on age less than or more than 65 years, and is clinicopathologically distinct from NNA. NNA is less often isolated and best classified as giant cell aortitis. Adult NA has histologic features classically associated with Takayasu disease but is limited primarily to the ascending aorta and has no sex predominance.

▶ Currently, classification of aortitis is not based on histologic findings and depends on the patients' clinical presentation. For instance, the term Takayasu syndrome has been applied to any type of aortitis including those occurring in patients under 50 years of age, nonsyphilitic aortitis, with autoimmune etiology, giant cell aortitis, and idiopathic aortitis also. Takayasu syndrome refers to the clinical extension of arteritis disease into branch vessels with peripheral stenoses accompanied by autoimmune diseases such as rheumatoid arthritis and giant cell arteritis in usually young women. The current study classifies aortitis based on the histopathological findings. The authors propose that aortitis should be classified as necrotizing or non-necrotizing variants. Cases of non-necrotizing aortitis are seen in the elderly and are highly suggestive of giant cell aortitis. The necrotizing form of aortitis is usually isolated and infrequently is a manifestation of Takayasu syndrome or other related autoimmune diseases. The photographic material presented in this article is excellent and its viewing is recommended.

P. Bejarano, MD

8 Soft Tissue and Bone

The Controversial Nosology of Benign Nerve Sheath Tumors: Neurofilament Protein Staining Demonstrates Intratumoral Axons in Many Sporadic Schwannomas
Nascimento AF, Fletcher CDM (Brigham and Women's Hosp, Boston, MA; Harvard Med School, Boston, MA)
Am J Surg Pathol 31:1363-1370, 2007

Schwannomas are benign peripheral nerve sheath tumors believed to be composed purely of cells with ultrastructural features of Schwann cells; these tumors are believed to develop eccentrically from the surface of nerves and not to contain axons, other than immediately beneath the capsule. This concept has recently been disputed in cases associated with neurofibromatosis type 2. The usual presence of intratumoral axons in neurofibromas is said to allow easy distinction from schwannomas. Eighty sporadic schwannomas (20 conventional, 20 cellular, 20 ancient, 10 gastric, and 10 plexiform) were retrieved from the authors' files. Hematoxylin-and-eosin stained slides were reviewed, diagnoses were confirmed and all tumors were stained for S-100 protein and neurofilament protein (NFP). The amount (rare, focal, multifocal, and diffuse) and distribution (central and/or peripheral) of axons within the tumors were analyzed. All tumors were strongly and diffusely positive for S-100 protein (nuclear and cytoplasmic staining). NFP-positive axons were identified in 11 of 20 (55%) conventional schwannomas (2 rare, 4 focal, 3 multifocal, and 2 diffuse; 5 central, 4 peripheral, and 2 central and peripheral) and in 15 of 20 (75%) cellular schwannomas (3 rare, 6 focal, and 6 multifocal; 12 central, 1 peripheral, and 2 central and peripheral). Of the 20 ancient schwannomas, 7 cases (35%) showed intratumoral axons, highlighted by NFP immunostaining (1 rare, 4 focal, 1 multifocal, and 1 diffuse; 4 peripheral, 2 central, and 1 central and peripheral). Most cases of gastric schwannoma showed no evidence of intratumoral axons; 9 cases (90%) were negative for NFP and only 1 case (10%) was positive (focal and central). Seven of 10 cases (70%) of plexiform schwannomas were negative for NFP, whereas only 3 cases (30%) showed positive axons (2 multifocal and 1 focal; 3 central). The unexpected but quite frequent presence of intratumoral axons in schwannomas argues against conventional views of these lesions' pathogenesis as an eccentric encapsulated lesion and raises the possibility that a more diverse cell population, perhaps more closely resembling neurofibromas, may constitute these neoplasms. Although NFP-positive axons were most often present in the conventional and cellular variants of schwannoma, their presence was also observed in a minority of ancient, gastric and plexiform schwannomas. Differentiation between neurofibroma and schwannoma in cases with overlapping cytoarchitectural features should not be based solely on the presence or absence of NFP-positive axons within a given tumor.

▶ This article discusses the way schwannomas and neurofibromas are perceived and diagnosed histoligically.

Conventionally, schwannomas are thought to be negative for the neurofilament protein (NFP) because they are made of schwann cells arising eccentrically from the periphery of the nerve, therefore, intratumoral axons are not expected to be present. Although histology alone is most often helpful enough to distinguish these 2 entities, however, there are occasional overlaps of histological features where neurofilament protein (NFP) immunostaining has been helpful to show intratumoral axons in neurofibromas. Distinguishing these 2 entities is important since the neurofibromas have the small potential of malignant transformation.

This article questions the conventional belief about the reliability of neurofilament protein (NFP) staining to distinguish the 2 tumors. Based on this study, NFP immunostain has been found to be positive in conventional and cellular schwannomas as well as few ancient, gastric, and plexiform variants.

The article suggests that schwannomas are composed of mixed population of cells. It further proposes the histology, diffuse staining for S-100, and clinical picture as the criteria to distinguish schwannomas from neurofibromas.

It would be interesting to see if future studies will propose a more reliable immunostain to replace NFP or a more definitive criterion to distinguish these 2 tumors.

For further information on this subject I suggest reading articles by Kawahara et al,[1] Lasota et al,[2] and Weiss et al.[3]

G. Azabdaftari, MD

References

1. Kawahara E, Oda Y, Ooi A, Katsuda S, Nakanishi I, Umeda S. Expression of glial fibrillary acidic protein (GFAP) in peripheral nerve sheath tumors. A comparative study of immunoreactivity of GFAP, vimentin, S-100 protein, and neurofilament in 38 schwannomas and 18 neurofibromas. *Am J Surg Pathol.* 1988;12:115-120.
2. Lasota J, Wasag B, Dansonka-Mieszkowska A, et al. Evaluation of NF2 and NF1 tumor suppressor genes in distinctive gastrointestinal nerve sheath tumors traditionally diagnosed as benign schwannomas: a study of 20 cases. *Lab Invest.* 2003;83:1361-1371.
3. Benign tumors of peripheral nerves. In: Weiss SW, Goldblum JR, eds. *Enzinger and Weiss's Soft Tissue Tumors.* St Louis, MO: Mosby, Inc.; 2001:1111-1208.

An update on plexiform fibrohistiocytic tumor and addition of 66 new cases from the Armed Forces Institute of Pathology, in honor of Franz M. Enzinger, MD

Moosavi C, Jha P, Fanburg-Smith JC (Armed Forces Institute of Pathology, Washington, USA)
Ann Diagn Pathol 11:313-319, 2007

The seminal article of Drs Franz Enzinger and Renyuan Zhang in 1988 defined plexiform fibrohistiocytic tumor (PFHT) as a distinctive entity. They described 65 cases (from 1965 to 1985) in children and young adults, with female and upper extremity predominance. These tumors were morphologically divided into 3 groups: fibroblastic, histiocytic (often with osteoclast-type giant cells), and mixed. Most tumors exhibited a plexiform and infiltrative arrangement of cells at the dermal/subcutaneous junction. Two fibroblastic PFHT had a metaplastic bone formation. Absence of cellular pleomorphism, low mitotic activity, dense hyalinization, hemorrhage, and chronic inflammation were observed. Vascular invasion was present in 1 recurrent, yet nonmetastatic, case. Tumors were negative for S100 protein, desmin, cytokeratin, factor VIIIrag, and lysozyme. Most patients were without disease up to 60 years after excision; 32 (37.5%) cases with follow-up recurred and 2 of those patients had regional lymph node metastasis at 9 and 36 months, respectively, yet there were no systemic metastases. In the interim, there have been additional studies on PFHT. We wanted to update the literature and add 66 new PFHT cases (1986-present) from the Armed Forces Institute of Pathology, since this seminal article, in honor of Dr Franz Enzinger. There were 37 men and 29 women; patient age ranged from 1 to 77 years (median, 20 years; 53% of patients were younger than 20 years). Twenty-eight cases occurred in the upper extremity (mostly forearm), 16 in lower extremity, 11 in trunk, 9 in head and neck, and 2 of unknown site. Although most cases were observed at the dermal/subcutaneous interface, 22 cases were predominantly dermal, and the rest predominantly subcutaneous, with 4 superficially involving skeletal muscle. Except for 12 predominantly dermal cases, most cases had an infiltrative growth pattern. Thirty-four cases were predominantly histiocytic, 16 predominantly fibroblastic, and the remaining 16 mixed. Two fibroblastic cases demonstrated the microfat cells (probably secondary to subcutis infiltration). All cases exhibited a plexiform growth pattern of small- to medium-sized nodules; 41 cases had giant cells, mainly osteoclast type, often the predominantly histiocytic type. The purely fibroblastic often had surrounding inflammation, 2 cases with marked inflammation. Perineural growth was observed in 5 cases, peri-Pacinian corpuscle growth in 2 cases, adnexal trapping in several, and, increased hyalinized collagen in 17 cases. Eight cases demonstrated focal myxoid change. Only 1 case, a histiocytic, had bone formation. Although increased cytologic atypia and mitotic activity were noted in a few cases, an atypical mitosis was only observed in 1 case. No cases demonstrated vascular or lymphatic invasion or necrosis. The tumors were generally positive for CD68 and SMA, occasionally for MSA, and negative for keratin, desmin, HMB45, S100 protein, and CD34. Overall, the findings were very similar to the original observations made by Dr Enzinger and his colleague, with the minor exceptions of roughly equal sex distribution (possibly due to timely referral bias), and additional morphologic features of myxoid change, adnexal sparing, increased inflammation, and microfat similar to recently described lipofibromatosis. The relationship between PFHT and cellular neurothekeoma is also explored.

▶ This article brings together in an organized fashion the results of a study of a large group of the plexiform fibrohistiocytic tumors (PFHT) and builds upon the original seminal article published by Dr Enzinger and Dr Zhang in 1988 where they described this lesion for the first time.

This article is an update of the literature by reviewing 66 cases from archives of Armed Force institute of Pathology (AFIP) from 1986 up to the time of the study took place. These cases were not included in the original study by Dr Enzinger.[1]

This study discusses 3 morphological subclassifications of the PFHT—histiocytic, fibroblastic, and mixed forms. Further observations include a panel of immunohistochemistry studies of the tumor characterizing the lesion as a fibrohistiocytic lesion.

The results of this study are very similar to the original article except that Dr Enzinger and his colleague found this tumor predominantly in female patients. This study states no gender predilection for this entity. There were also additional morphological findings such as increased inflammation, adnexal sparing, microfat, and myxoid changes.

Both this and the original study indicate that the tumor has good prognosis with possible recurrence (low malignant potential). There was no systemic metastasis reported, however, follow-up of 1 patient from the original series showed systemic metastasis.

In addition, this article briefly refers to morphologic and immunophenotypical overlaps between PFHT and cellular neurothekomas exploring the potential relation between these 2 entities.

For further reading on this subject I suggest an article by Hollowood et al.[2]

G. Azabdaftari, MD

References

1. Enzinger FM, Zhang RY. Plexiform fibrohistiocytic tumor presenting in children and young adults An analysis of 65 cases. *Am J Surg Pathol.* 1988;12:818-826.
2. Hollowood K, Holley MP, Fletcher CD. Plexiform fibrohistiocytic tumour: clinicopathological, immunohistochemical and ultrastructural analysis in favour of a myofibroblastic lesion. *Histopathology.* 1991;19:503-513.

Dedifferentiated Liposarcomas With Divergent Myosarcomatous Differentiation Developed in the Internal Trunk: A Study of 27 Cases and Comparison to Conventional Dedifferentiated Liposarcomas and Leiomyosarcomas

Binh MBN, Guillou L, Hostein I, et al (Institut Bergonié and Université Victor Segalen, Bordeaux, France; Univ Inst of Pathology, Lausanne, Switzerland; Institut Bergonié, Bordeaux; et al)
Am J Surg Pathol 31:1557-1566, 2007

Dedifferentiated liposarcoma (DLPS) is one of the most frequent sarcomas of the retroperitoneum and represents most undifferentiated sarcomas of the internal trunk. In about 5% cases, the dedifferentiated component is an heterologous sarcoma such as leiomyosarcoma or rhabdomyosarcoma. We reviewed a series of 65 sarcomas with a myogenic differentiation developed in the internal trunk for which initial diagnoses were leiomyosarcoma (37), rhabdomyosarcoma (6), malignant mesenchymoma (6), and DLPS (16). Immunostainings for MDM2, CDK4, alpha smooth actin, desmin, caldesmon, myogenin, c-kit, and progesterone receptor were performed. In 48 cases, the amplification status of *MDM2* and *CDK4* could be evaluated with quantitative polymerase chain reaction on paraffin-embedded tissues extracted DNAs. After review of the cases, final diagnoses were leiomyosarcoma (35), rhabdomyosarcomatous (20) or leiomyosarcomatous (7) DLPS, probable DLPS (2), and malignant mesenchymoma (1). DLPS were bigger tumors (median: 18.2 cm) than leiomyosarcomas (median: 12 cm). They had a lower 5-year recurrence-free survival than leiomyosarcomas (45% vs. 71%) but a higher 5-year metastasis-free survival (73% vs. 39%). There was no significant difference in overall survival (57% vs. 34%). Outcome of patients with a DLPS with a myosarcomatous component did not differ from conventional DLPS. In conclusion, most sarcomas with a rhabdomyosarcomatous differentiation occurring in the internal trunk of adults are DLPS. Moreover, DLPS with a myogenic component have a low metastatic potential, similar to conventional DLPS and significantly lower to the metastatic potential of leiomyosarcomas.

▶ This is an interesting retrospective study of 65 cases of sarcomas arising in retroperitoneum with myogenic differentiation, composed of rhabdomyosarcoma (6), leiomyosarcoma (LMS) (36), malignant mesenchymoma (6), and dedifferentiated liposarcoma (DLPS) with myogenic differentiation (16). Because DLPS is one of the most common sarcomas of the retroperitoneum and represents most undifferentiated sarcomas of the internal trunk, the authors tried to verify if any of the lesions classified as sarcomas (rhabdomyosarcoma, LMS, and malignant mesenchymoma) were in reality DLPS with myogenic differentiation that lacked atypical lipomatous tumor/well-differentiated liposarcoma (WDL) component. The authors have used immunohistochemistry for MDM2, CDK4, desmin, myogenin, h-caldesmon, progesterone receptors, c-kit, and alpha smooth muscle actin in 65 cases. They have also studied through quantitative polymerase chain reaction (PCR), the amplification status of MDM2 and CDK4 oncogenes in 48 of these cases. Immunohistochemistry and quantitative PCR for MDM2 and CDK4 helped to reclassify 5 malignant mesenchymomas, 1 LMS, and 5 rhabdomysarcomas as DLPS with myogenic component. Clinical follow-up of the patients showed that 5-year metastatic free and local recurrence free of DLPS with myogenic component is similar to the conventional DLPS. Compared with LMS, DLPS with or without myogenic differentiation have higher risk of local recurrence, but the risk of metastasis is low. Although there was no difference in overall survival, the distinction of DLPS from other sarcomas may be helpful in the choice of treatment. Because MDM2 and CDK4 are oncogenes involved in WDL and DLPS, drugs targeting these proteins would be of interest. In the case of the LMS, adjuvant chemotherapy could be considered.

For further reading on this subject I suggest articles by Pilotti et al,[1] Tallini et al,[2] and Evans et al.[3]

G. Azabdaftari, MD

References

1. Pilotti S, Mezzelani A, Vergani B, et al. Morphologic-cytogenetic analysis of dedifferentiated liposarcomas with an extensive misleading leiomyosarcomatous component. *Appl Immunohistochem Mol Morphol.* 2000;8:216-221.
2. Tallini G, Erlandson RA, Brennan MF, Woodruff JM. Divergent myosarcomatous differentiation in retroperitoneal liposarcoma. *Am J Surg Pathol.* 1993;17:546-556.
3. Evans HL, Khurana KK, Kemp BL, Ayala AG. Heterologous elements in the dedifferentiated component of dedifferentiated liposarcoma. *Am J Surg Pathol.* 1994;18:1150-1157.

9 Female Genital Tract

Ovarian Mature Teratomas With Mucinous Epithelial Neoplasms: Morphologic Heterogeneity and Association With Pseudomyxoma Peritonei
McKenney JK, Soslow RA, Longacre TA (Univ of Arkansas for Med Sciences, Little Rock, AR; Sloan-Kettering Cancer Ctr, NY; Stanford Univ School of Medicine, SA)
Am J Surg Pathol 32:645-655, 2008

Mucinous epithelial neoplasms arising in association with mature teratomas are a heterogeneous group of tumors, but with the exception of a single recent study, their full histologic spectrum, detailed immunophenotype, and association with classic pseudomyxoma peritonei (PMP) have not been fully studied. The morphologic, immunohistochemical, and clinical features of 42 patients with mucinous epithelial tumors arising in association with mature ovarian teratomas were evaluated. The patients' ages ranged from 17 to 66 years (mean, 39 y). Tumor size ranged from 5.5 to greater than 200 cm. Most teratoma-associated mucinous tumors were unilateral, although 1 patient harbored bilateral mucinous tumors in association with bilateral teratomas. In all cases, the teratomatous component consisted of mature elements. Using the 2003 World Health Organization criteria for ovarian intestinal type mucinous neoplasms, 17 (40%) were classified as mucinous cystadenoma, 16 (38%) as intestinal-type mucinous epithelial neoplasm of low malignant potential (IM-LMP), 4 (10%) as intraepithelial carcinoma (IEC), and 5 (12%) as invasive mucinous carcinoma. Mucinous cystadenomas had a varied epithelial lining consisting of lower gastroenteric, gastric foveolar, or müllerian appearance. In contrast, the IM-LMP, IEC, and invasive carcinoma cases had a more uniform lower gastroenteric histology. For mucinous cystadenomas, a cytokeratin (CK) 7+/CK20− phenotype (5/13; 38%) was equally as common as a CK7−/CK20+ phenotype (5/13; 38%), with the remaining cases coexpressing both keratins (CK7+/CK20+: 3/13; 23%). In contrast, IM-LMP, IEC, and invasive adenocarcinomas more frequently had a CK7−/CK20+ phenotype (56%, 50%, and 100%, respectively). A CK7+/CK20− phenotype was rare in these later 3 morphologic groups (6%). Of the 42 total cases, 55% had pseudomyxoma ovarii and 24% had classic PMP (1 cystadenoma, 6 IM-LMP, and 3 invasive carcinomas), whereas 5% had more localized accumulations of peritoneal mucin (both IM-LMP). Pathologic evaluation of the peritoneum in these 12 cases revealed 6 with acellular

TABLE 3.—CK20/CK7 Profiles of Teratoma-Associated Mucinous Neoplasms

Epithelium Type	CK20+/CK7−	CK20+/CK7+	CK20−/CK7+	CK20−CK7−
All types combined	17/31 (55%)	7/31 (23%)	6/31 (19%)	1/31 (3%)
Cystadenoma	5/13 (38%)	3/13 (24%)	5/13 (38%)	0/13 (0%)
IM-LMP	5/9 (56%)	3/9 (33%)	1/9 (11%)	0/9 (0%)
IM-LMP with IEC	2/4 (50%)	1/4 (25%)	0/4 (0%)	1/4 (25%)
Invasive carcinoma	5/5 (100%)	0/5 (0%)	0/5 (0%)	0/5 (0%)

(Reprinted from McKenney JK, Soslow RA, Longacre TA. Ovarian mature teratomas with mucinous epithelial neoplasms: morphologic heterogeneity and association with pseudomyxoma peritonei. *Am J Surg Pathol.* 2008;32:645-655.)

mucin alone, 3 with low-grade mucinous epithelium (all 3 with ovarian IM-LMP), and 3 with high-grade mucinous carcinomatosis (all 3 with ovarian mucinous adenocarcinoma). No appendiceal lesions were identified. Follow-up was available in 48% of patients (mean, 61 mo). The only adverse outcomes occurred in the 3 patients with ovarian carcinoma and associated peritoneal carcinomatosis. We report that a significant proportion of mucinous tumors associated with mature ovarian teratomas present with clinical PMP, which in most cases is associated with IM-LMP. PMP in this setting may harbor microscopic intra-abdominal low-grade mucinous epithelium that is histologically and immunophenotypically similar to that typically seen in appendiceal-related PMP. Pseudomyxoma ovarii is common in this setting, particularly in tumors with IM-LMP histology, but pseudomyxoma ovarii is not predictive of PMP. Ovarian teratoma-associated benign and IM-LMP mucinous neoplasms with microscopic peritoneal low-grade mucinous epithelium do not seem to be at significant risk for intra-abdominal recurrence, but numbers are few and follow-up is limited. In contrast, teratomas with an invasive carcinomatous component and microscopic peritoneal carcinomatosis follow an aggressive clinical course (Table 3).

▶ This study addresses an important and less understood area of gynecological pathology, which is the relationship between mucinous tumors associated with mature teratomas and mucinous tumors of the gastrointestinal tract. Studies have shown that these tumors display a spectrum of histological and immuno-histochemical characteristics. This is a large series of cases (n = 42) of ovarian neoplasms that contain a mixture of mature teratoma and a mucinous epithelial neoplasm. The study also addresses the concurrent presence of pseudomyxoma peritonei in these cases. The authors have combined the review of clinicopathological features with the clinical follow-up on these cases.

The results of this study are very interesting and show that a large proportion of the ovarian mucinous tumors associated with a mature teratoma present with clinical pseudomyxoma peritonei (24% in the current series). This study confirms the previous observations that most of these types of tumors resemble tumors and share the same immunoprofile as those arising in the lower gastrointestinal tract, particularly the intestinal-type mucinous epithelial neoplasms of low malignant potential (IM-LMP) and the carcinomas (Table 3).

Interestingly, the cystadenoma group in this study, in multiple cases, displayed a more "non-enteric" immunoprofile. These findings are important for the surgical pathologist because when they are evaluating an ovarian tumor where the teratomatous component is not identified because of undersampling and the tumor otherwise resembles a lower gastrointestinal tumor, the latter may be misclassified as metastatic tumor to the ovary. This misclassification may be more in cases where there is an association with pseudomyxoma peritonei (one-fourth of the cases in this series).

For further reading on this subject I suggest articles by Vang et al[1] and Ronnett et al.[2]

A. V. Parwani, MD

References

1. Vang R, Gown AM, Zhao C, et al. Ovarian mucinous tumors associated with mature cystic teratomas: morphologic and immunohistochemical analysis identifies a subset of potential teratomatous origin that shares features of lower gastrointestinal tract mucinous tumors more commonly encountered as secondary tumors in the ovary. *Am J Surg Pathol.* 2007;31:854-869.
2. Ronnett BM, Yan H, Kurman RJ, Shmookler BM, Wu L, Sugarbaker PH. Patients with pseudomyxoma peritonei associated with disseminated peritoneal adenomucinosis have a significantly more favorable prognosis than patients with peritoneal mucinous carcinomatosis. *Cancer.* 2001;92:85-91.

Vascular "Pseudo Invasion" in Laparoscopic Hysterectomy Specimens: A Diagnostic Pitfall

Logani S, Herdman AV, Little JV, et al (Emory Univ Hosp; Crawford Long Hosp, Atlanta, GA; et al)
Am J Surg Pathol 32:560-565, 2008

Total laparoscopic hysterectomy has been shown to be an equally effective and safe technique when compared with conventional abdominal surgery for endometrial carcinoma. The procedure, as performed at our institution, involves the use of a uterine balloon manipulator (RUMI manipulator and Koh Colpotomizer system) for optimal surgical control. The fallopian tubes are cauterized to prevent transtubal spread of the tumor. The balloon manipulator thus creates a positive closed pressure system within the uterine cavity. After observing extensive displacement of tumor into small and large blood vessels in 1 case of grade 1, stage 1b endometrial carcinoma, we reviewed slides from 37 hysterectomy specimens (7 for endometrial carcinoma or atypical hyperplasia and 30 for benign conditions) performed laparoscopically between August 2004 and March 2006 at Emory University and Crawford Long Hospitals. We reviewed all slides for the presence or absence of endometrial tumor/tissue in vascular spaces. Patients with endometrial carcinoma/atypical complex hyperplasia included 6 FIGO grade I endometrioid carcinomas (3 stages 1A; 3 stages 1B) and 1 patient with atypical complex hyperplasia. Tumor within blood vessels was noted in 5 of 7 (71%) cases. In 3 cases, including the case of atypical complex hyperplasia, the number of vessels containing tumor were too numerous to count small and large caliber blood vessels. In the remainder, 1 case had 2 small vessels involved and in the other 7 small vessels showed tumor within vascular lumina. Benign endometrial glands and stromal tissue were noted within vascular spaces in 4 of 30 (13%) hysterectomy specimens removed for benign conditions. We describe a hitherto unreported artifact of vascular pseudo invasion in hysterectomy specimens obtained using the technique of total laparoscopic abdominal hysterectomy. We postulate that the creation of a closed pressure system generated as part of the operative technique is likely responsible for this phenomenon. Pathologists need to be aware of this artifact to avoid misinterpretation of vascular invasion in these cases with its associated therapeutic and prognostic implications.

▶ This article illustrates a potential artifact of the surgical procedure employed for laparoscopic hysterectomy that results in displacement of tissue into small and larger vessels, resulting in a false appearance of vascular invasion to the pathologist who is reviewing the slides.

The procedure, as performed at our institution, involves the use of a uterine balloon manipulator for optimal surgical control. The balloon manipulator thus creates a positive closed pressure system within the uterine cavity. The authors discovered this artifact when they were reviewing pathology slides for a case of grade 1, stage 1b endometrial carcinoma. Extensive vascular invasion was noted in their review. This prompted a pathology review of 37 additional cases of laparoscopic hysterectomy, 7 malignant, and 30 for benign conditions. The results were surprising and showed that in 5/7 cases of malignant conditions, "pseudovascular invasion" was identified. Similarly, tumor displacement or "pseudoinvasion" was seen in 4/30 cases where the same procedure was done for benign conditions.

The findings in this study are important because they highlight the occurrence of this tumor displacement artifact associated with the use of a balloon manipulator. This is an important observation because it will alert pathologists not to "overcall" vascular invasion, particularly in lower stage, lower grade tumor cases, or more importantly in cases where there is atypical complex hyperplasia. A combination of observing tumors in the vessels and identifying the atypical complex hyperplasia may result in a diagnosis of endometrial carcinoma because the tumor displacement was misinterpreted as true vascular invasion. This will alert the pathologist to also seek out and communicate with the surgeon about the particular technique used for the hysterectomy in the hospital that they practice so such a diagnostic pitfall may be avoided.

For further reading on this subject I suggest articles by Koh[1] and Sivridis et al.[2]

A. V. Parwani, MD

References

1. Koh CH. A new technique and system for simplifying total laparoscopic hysterectomy. *J Am Assoc Gynecol Laparosc.* 1998;5:187-192.
2. Sivridis E, Buckley CH, Fox H. The prognostic significance of lymphatic vascular space invasion in endometrial adenocarcinoma. *Br J Obstet Gynaecol.* 1987;94:991-994.

Expression of Glypican 3 in Ovarian and Extragonadal Germ Cell Tumors
Zynger DL, Everton MJ, Dimov ND, et al (Northwestern Univ, Chicago, IL; et al)
Am J Clin Pathol 130:224-230, 2008

Germ cell tumors (GCTs), rare malignancies that occur in a wide range of locations and display variable histologic patterns, may pose diagnostic challenges. Glypican 3 (GPC3), a membrane-bound heparan sulfate proteoglycan, has been shown to be a novel diagnostic marker in testicular GCT. However, GPC3 expression in ovarian and extragonadal GCT has not been reported. We evaluated GPC3 immunoreactivity in GCTs from 63 patients (57 children and 6 adults), including 14 ovarian and 20 extragonadal primary GCTs and 8 metastases along with 21 primary testicular GCTs for comparison. All 33 yolk sac tumors (YSTs) and both choriocarcinomas were immunoreactive for GPC3. In contrast, a minority of immature (4/10) and mature (4/35) teratomas were positive. No positivity was seen in 6 embryonal carcinomas or 5 germinomas. GPC3 is differentially expressed in ovarian and extragonadal GCTs, with expression predominantly observed in YSTs and choriocarcinoma (Image 1).

▶ This is an important study that reviews the expression of glypican 3, a membrane-bound heparan sulfate proteoglycan, for utilization as a diagnostic marker for subclassification of ovarian and extragonadal germ cell tumors. Germ cell tumors are subtyped into germinomas, yolk sac tumors, embryonal carcinomas, choriocarcinomas, or teratomas. Each of the subtypes displays a wide spectrum of histological appearances with overlaps considerably within subtypes. These overlapping morphological appearances can often pose diagnostic difficulties for the surgical pathologist. A recognition and accurate classification and quantification of each of the components within a mixed germ cell tumor become important because of different prognostic and therapeutic implications. In addition, the classification may become more challenging when evaluating extragonadal germ cell tumors.

Glypican 3 expression, as validated in this study, is a useful diagnostic immunohistochemical marker that is preferentially expressed in yolk sac tumors and choriocarcinomas and in a minority of teratomas (Image 1). More importantly, this marker is negative in embryonal carcinomas and germinomas. The predominant expression of glypican 3 in yolk sac tumors is an important diagnostic aid

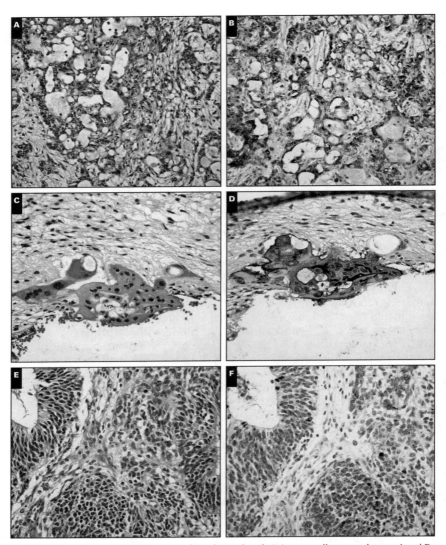

IMAGE 1.—Glypican 3 (GPC3) immunohistochemical analysis in germ cell tumor subtypes. **A** and **B**, Yolk sac tumor. Strong and diffuse reactivity (**A**, H&E, ×20; **B**, GPC3 immunostain, ×20). **C** and **D**, Choriocarcinoma. Strong positivity within syncytiotrophoblasts (**C**, H&E, ×40; **D**, GPC3 immunostain, ×40). **E** and **F**, Immature teratoma. Weak reactivity within primitive neural elements (**E**, H&E, ×20; **F**, GPC3 immunostain, ×20). (Reprinted from Zynger DL, Everton MJ, Dimov ND, et al. Expression of glypican 3 in ovarian and extragonadal germ cell tumors. *Am J Clin Pathol.* 2008;130:224-230, with permission from the American Society for Clinical Pathology.)

for the surgical pathologist because these tumors have a more complex and wider spectrum of histological appearances, are more difficult to identify, and are often misclassified or underclassified. In addition, there are specific growth and architectural patterns such as the papillary growth pattern of yolk sac tumors, which can be confused with an embryonal carcinoma with predominant papillary architecture. This type of distinction is particularly important because studies have shown that a higher proportion of embryonal carcinoma may have a worse prognosis.

Similar overlaps in the histology occur between other germ cell tumors, highlighting the importance of accurate diagnosis of the different components of germ cell tumors by the surgical pathologist to aid in appropriate patient management. In these situations, glypican 3 serves as a useful marker. Because the total numbers of this study were small (n = 63) with only 2 cases of choriocarcinomas, additional larger studies may be helpful to further validate the use of glypican 3 as a diagnostic marker for germ cell tumors.

For further reading on this subject I suggest articles by McKenney et al[1] and Ulbright.[2]

A. V. Parwani, MD

References

1. McKenney JK, Heerema-McKenney A, Rouse RV. Extragonadal germ cell tumors: a review with emphasis on pathologic features, clinical prognostic variables, and differential diagnostic considerations. *Adv Anat Pathol.* 2007;4:69-92.
2. Ulbright TM. Germ cell tumors of the gonads: a selective review emphasizing problems in differential diagnosis, newly appreciated, and controversial issues. *Mod Pathol.* 2005;8:S61-S79.

Granulosa Cell Tumors of the Ovary With a Pseudopapillary Pattern: A Study of 14 Cases of an Unusual Morphologic Variant Emphasizing Their Distinction From Transitional Cell Neoplasms and Other Papillary Ovarian Tumors

Irving JA, Young RH (Royal Jubilee Hosp, Victoria, Canada; Univ of British Columbia, Vancouver, Canada; et al)
Am J Surg Pathol 32:581-586, 2008

Granulosa cell tumors of the ovary with a pseudopapillary pattern have received only passing mention in the literature. We have reviewed the clinicopathologic features of 10 cases of juvenile granulosa cell tumor and 4 cases of adult granulosa cell tumor with a pseudopapillary pattern. Twelve cases were received in consultation; the referring pathologist favored a diagnosis of a transitional cell neoplasm in 3 of these cases, and a retiform Sertoli-Leydig cell tumor in 2 cases; in most of the remainder, the diagnosis of granulosa cell tumor was considered but uncertainty expressed because of the unusual papillarylike pattern. All 14 tumors were unilateral, and the majority were predominantly cystic, 3 unilocular, and 6 multilocular. Multiple papillary projections lining the cyst wall were noted grossly in 10 cases; these ranged in size from 0.1 to 1.5 cm and were typically soft, edematous, fleshy, or rubbery. Microscopically, pseudopapillae were formed by intracystic cellular projections with surrounding necrotic debris and/or undulating folds of neoplastic cells in the absence of appreciable necrosis. In all tumors, thorough sampling revealed areas with architectural patterns and cytomorphology typical of granulosa cell tumor. Granulosa cell tumors of adult and juvenile type may have a pseudopapillary pattern that can be confused with other ovarian tumors with a papillary architecture. Identification of areas that are more characteristic of granulosa cell tumor resolves most cases, although immunohistochemistry can be used in more problematic tumors. This phenomenon seems to be related to the cystic change that is a feature of many granulosa cell tumors.

▶ This is an interesting article that describes a series of 14 cases of granulosa cell tumors of the ovary with a pseudopapillary pattern. This is a unique morphology that can cause diagnostic dilemma for surgical pathologists. Most of these cases in this series were sent for a second opinion because of this unique papillary-like pattern. Interestingly, in most cases, on gross examination, numerous papillary-like projections were identified.

These projections were lining the cyst wall and had a consistency which was described as soft, edematous, fleshy, or rubbery. The interesting finding was the microscopic identification of pseudopapillae, which were projecting into the cystic cavity. These pseudopapillae lack true stromal cores. A recognition of this pattern in graulosa tumors is important for pathologists because other ovarian tumors may have a papillary architecture. Furthermore, this appearance of a papillary-like architecture may be confused with transitional cell carcinomas, as was the case in 3 of the cases in this series. This study highlights the importance of recognizing this morphologic variant of graulosa cell tumors, so a misinterpretation may be avoided by the surgical pathologist.

For further reading on this subject I suggest an article by Young et al.[1]

A. V. Parwani, MD

Reference

1. Young RH, Scully RE. Differential diagnosis of ovarian tumors based primarily on their patterns and cell types. *Semin Diagn Pathol.* 2001;18:161-235.

Adenocarcinoma of the uterine cervix: prognostic significance of clinicopathologic parameters, flow cytometry analysis and HPV infection
Dabić MM, Nola M, Tomičić I, et al (Clinical Hosp Ctr Zagreb, Croatia)
Acta Obstet Gynecol Scand 87:366-372, 2008

Background.—This study was designed to determine the possible impact of status of human papillomavirus (HPV) infection (no infection, single, multiple infections) on the survival of patients with cervical adenocarcinoma, to correlate the HPV status with other clinicopathologic parameters, and to examine clinical, histological and flow cytometric parameters as predictors of survival in cervical adenocarcinoma.

Methods.—The clinical data of 51 patients with adenocarcinoma of the cervix who were treated at the Department of Gynecology and Obstetrics, Zagreb University School of Medicine, from 1978 to 2004 were analysed: age at presentation, menstrual status, clinical stage, relapse, survival. Exact histologic subtype, architectural grade and nuclear grade were determined. DNA flow cytometry was performed to determine DNA ploidy and proliferative index. Polymerase chain reaction (SPF primers), followed by reverse hybridisation for genotyping, was used to determine the HPV status.

Results.—The status of HPV infection had no impact on patient survival, and could not be correlated with any of the analysed clinicopathologic parameters. Univariate analysis showed significant association between patient survival and clinical stage ($p = 0.002$) and architectural grade ($p = 0.033$). Multivariate analysis confirmed both parameters as significantly associated with survival. Menstrual status, nuclear grade, DNA ploidy and proliferative activity had no impact on patient survival.

Conclusion.—Clinical stage and architectural grade are significant predictors for survival of patients with cervical adenocarcinoma. Status of HPV infection, flow cytometric parameters, nuclear grade and menstrual status do not predict patient survival.

▶ Several studies have shown that human papillomavirus (HPV) is found in a large majority of adenocarcinomas. Types 16, 18, and 45 are most frequently seen. The sensitivity of HPV detection assays has improved significantly in recent years and there are increasing reports of multiple HPV infections. However, there is limited information on this and its role in cervical cancer progression.

This study investigates the potential impact of the status of HPV infection (no infection, single infection, or multiple infections) on patient survival and other clinicopathological parameters in 51 cases of cervical adenocarcinoma from a single institute. This is an important study area in gynecological pathology because there is limited or conflicting information available for the impact of HPV infections and outcome. Only 1 previous study has addressed the impact of multiple HPV infections. A previous study by Bachiatry et al[1] had shown that there was a correlation of multiple HPV infections with poor response and reduced survival.

The results from this study are interesting and show that clinical stage and architectural grade are significant predictors for survival of patients with cervical adenocarcinomas. More importantly, and contrary to the study by Bachiatry et al, in this study the status of HPV infections had no impact on survival of patients with cervical adenocarcinomas. There is a need for a larger study with more cases to confirm these findings and compare them with earlier studies.

A. V. Parwani, MD

Reference

1. Bachtiary B, Obermair A, Dreier B, et al. Impact of multiple HPV infection on response to treatment and survival in patients receiving radical radiotherapy for cervical cancer. *Int J Cancer.* 2002;102:237-243.

Oncofetal Protein Glypican-3 Distinguishes Yolk Sac Tumor From Clear Cell Carcinoma of the Ovary

Esheba GE, Pate LL, Longacre TA (Stanford Univ, CA)
Am J Surg Pathol 32:600-607, 2008

Clear cell carcinoma (CCC) of the ovary is the surface epithelial neoplasm most often confused with primitive germ cell tumors, particularly yolk sac tumor (YST) and dysgerminoma. OCT3/4 has proven to be a sensitive and relatively specific marker for the latter entity, but existing markers for YST are limited. Recent studies suggest that glypican-3 (GPC3), an oncofetal protein expressed in fetal liver and malignant tumors of hepatocytic lineage, is also expressed in germ cell tumors, particularly YST. To investigate whether GPC3 is useful in distinguishing YST from ovarian CCC, we studied the expression of GPC3 in a large series of ovarian neoplasms and compared it to the expression profiles of CK7 and alpha-fetoprotein. Tissue microarrays containing over 400 benign and malignant ovarian neoplasms, including 34 CCCs were stained with monoclonal GPC3 (clone 1G12, Biomosaics, Burlington, VT). These arrays contained a wide assortment of ovarian surface epithelial neoplasms and sex cord stromal neoplasms, as well as germ cell tumors. Full paraffin tissue sections from 32 YSTs and 10 CCCs were also assessed. All but one YST (97%), including those associated with mixed germ cell tumor were positive for GPC3, whereas all teratomas and embryonal carcinomas were negative. Both cytoplasmic and membrane staining were present in the positive cases, with no background staining. The syncytiotrophoblastic cells in the germ cell tumors and placental villi included in the arrays were also positive for GPC3. Most CCCs (83%) were completely negative for GPC3, as were 99% serous, 94% endometrioid, and 100% mucinous tumors. Five CCCs exhibited focal, moderate to strong GPC3 expression and in 2 the expression was focal and weak. All other tissues, including normal ovary were negative for GPC3. GPC3 seems to be a promising diagnostic marker for differentiating YST from ovarian CCC ($P < 0.0001$). Because GPC3 may be associated with alpha-fetoprotein expression, further studies are required to determine the utility of GPC3 in differentiating YST from CCC with hepatoid differentiation.

▶ Glypican-3 (GPC3) is a cell surface heparan sulfate proteoglycan, which binds to the cell membrane via glycosylphosphatidylinositol anchors. GPC3 is normally expressed in fetal tissues and trophoblastic cells with little or no expression in adult tissues.

This is an important article because it describes the use of GPC3 for yolk sac tumor (YST) of the ovary from a clear cell carcinoma (CCC) of the ovary. These 2 entities share morphological appearance and often pose a diagnostic challenge for the surgical pathologist to distinguish one from the other. This is particularly challenging when one encounters a glandular and papillary YST. The histological features overlap significantly with a CCC.

Often the pathologist employs a combination of CD15, alpha-fetoprotein (AFP) and CK7 to distinguish YSTs from the CCCs. However, both CD15 and AFP have poor sensitivity and specificity, and CK7 may only show patchy or focal positivity for CK7, necessitating a more reliable immunohistochemical marker to distinguish the 2 entities.

In this study, 97% of the YSTs were positive for GPC3, whereas 83% of the CCCs were negative. Only 5 cases of CCCs showed focal, moderate to strong GPC3 staining. Furthermore, most of the ovarian neoplasm were negative for GPC3 including serous (99% negative), endometrioid (94% negative), and mucinous tumors (100% were negative). The latter results confirm the results previously described in the literature for testicular germ cell tumors. The current study shows that the GPC3 is a useful marker that can reliably distinguish between YSTs and CCCs.

For further reading on this subject, I suggest articles by Ulbright,[1] and Zynger et al.[2]

A. V. Parwani, MD

References

1. Ulbright TM. Germ cell tumors of the gonads: a selective review emphasizing problems in differential diagnosis, newly appreciated, and controversial issues. *Mod Pathol.* 2005;18:S61-S79.
2. Zynger DL, Dimov ND, Luan C, Teh BT, Yang XJ. Glypican 3: a novel marker in testicular germ cell tumors. *Am J Surg Pathol.* 2006;30:1570-1575.

Stage IA Vulvar Squamous Cell Carcinoma: An Analysis of Tumor Invasive Characteristics and Risk
Yoder BJ, Rufforny I, Massoll NA, et al (Univ of Florida College of Medicine, Gainesville, FL)
Am J Surg Pathol 32:765-772, 2008

Early invasive vulvar squamous cell carcinoma (SCC) with less than 1.0 mm of invasion (FIGO stage IA) has been shown to have a minimal risk of lymph node metastasis and is associated with an excellent prognosis. The prognostic significance of other histologic parameters other than depth of invasion, however, remains controversial. Seventy-eight consecutive cases of vulvar SCC having a depth of invasion of 5.0 mm or less were reviewed and the clinical outcome compared with the type

TABLE 3.—Risk of SCC Disease Recurrence

Factor	Univariate Analysis Hazard Ratio (95% CI)	P	Multivariate Analysis Hazard Ratio (95% CI)	P
Depth	1.51 (1.06-2.16)	0.023	1.84 (1.22-2.77)	0.003
Grade	—	0.018	—	0.003
2 from 1	2.35 (0.69-8.02)	0.174	2.75 (0.79-9.64)	0.113
3 from 1	6.72 (1.77-25.4)	0.005	13.20 (2.96-59.1)	0.001
2 from 3	0.35 (0.11-1.11)	0.075	0.21 (0.06-0.72)	0.013
SCC margin	11.5 (2.47-53.9)	0.020	6.32 (1.19-33.5)	0.030

(Reprinted from Yoder BJ, Rufforny I, Massoll NA, et al. Stage IA vulvar squamous cell carcinoma: An analysis of tumor invasive characteristics and risk. *Am J Surg Pathol.* 2008;32:765-772.)

of surgical excision, the presence of concurrent lymph node metastases, the depth of tumor invasion, the tumor thickness, the tumor horizontal spread, the estimated tumor volume, tumor histologic subtype, tumor histologic grade, tumor pattern of invasion, tumor multifocality, presence of perineural invasion, presence of angiolymphatic invasion and the presence of precursor lesions, including the type of vulvar intraepithelial neoplasia and presence of lichen sclerosus. The only histologic feature for predicting concurrent lymph node metastasis was tumor depth of invasion. The 3 most important features of stage IA tumors in predicting tumor recurrence were the depth of invasion, presence of SCC at the surgical margins, and the histologic grade (Table 3).

▶ This article examines cases of vulvar squamous cell carcinoma, International Federation of Gynecology and Obstetrics (FIGO) stage 1A (with less than 1.0 mm of invasion) for a better understanding of the prognostic significance of other histological parameters such as the pattern of growth, histological differentiation, tumor volume, perineural invasion, vascular invasion, multifocality of disease, and the concurrent presence of precursor lesions including vulvar intraepithelial neoplasia (VIN) and lichen sclerosus (LS). The current stage IA definition includes horizontal spread and tumor depth of invasion only. There is only limited and often conflicting information available about all the other features listed above.

The study included 78 patients with vulvar squamous cell carcinoma with a tumor depth of invasion, which was 5.0 mm or less. The clinical outcome of these patients was compared with the various clinicopathological features such as the type of surgical excision and the concurrent presence of lymph node metastases. The results were very interesting and demonstrated that the only histological feature that was predictive of concurrent lymph node metastasis was the tumor depth of invasion. Forty patients in this series had inguinal lymph node dissections, and of those only 5 had lymph node metastases. None of the cases with a depth of invasion less than 1.0 mm had positive lymph nodes, 5 of the cases had positive nodes, 2 had a depth of invasion between 1 mm and 3 mm, and 3 had a depth of invasion between 3 mm and 5 mm.

Another important conclusion from the study was that the 3 most important features that were predictive of tumor recurrence were the depth of invasion, presence of carcinoma at the margin, and the histological grade of the tumor (Table 3). These findings have important therapeutic implications and highlight the importance of an accurate measurement of the depth of invasion of the tumor to stratify patients into appropriate stage. This data also support the general clinical opinion that the treatment of patients with a stage IA vulvar squamous cell carcinoma with only a wide local excision, without an inguinal-femoral lymphadenectomy (Table 3).

For further reading on this subject I suggest articles by Wilkinson.[1,2]

A. V. Parwani, MD

References

1. Wilkinson EJ. Protocol for the examination of specimens from patients with carcinomas and malignant melanomas of the vulva: a basis for checklist. Cancer Committee of the American College of Pathologists. *Arch Pathol Lab Med.* 2000;124:51-56.
2. Wilkinson EJ. Premalignant and malignant tumors of the vulva. In: Kurman RJ, ed. *Blaustein's Pathology of the Female Genital Tract.* New York, NY: Springer-NewVerlag; 2002:99-149.

Serous papillary adenocarcinoma of the female genital organs and invasive micropapillary carcinoma of the breast. Are WT1, CA125, and GCDFP-15 useful in differential diagnosis?
Moritani S, Ichihara S, Hasegawa M, et al (Nagoya Med Ctr, Aichi, Japan; et al)
Hum Pathol 39:666-671, 2008

Serous papillary adenocarcinoma of the female genital organs and invasive micropapillary carcinoma of the breast have close histologic similarities. Thus, when these cancers occur synchronously or metachronously in the same patient, it is difficult to determine the primary site. We examined 23 serous papillary adenocarcinomas (16 ovarian, 5 endometrial, and 2 peritoneal) and 37 invasive micropapillary carcinomas of the breast (12 pure and 25 mixed types) on immunohistochemical expression of Wilm's tumor antigen-1 (WT1), CA125, and gross cystic disease fluid protein-15 (GCDFP-15), which have been reported to be useful in the differential diagnosis of primary ovarian carcinomas versus metastatic breast cancer to the ovary. The positive rates of WT1, CA125, and GCDFP-15 in serous papillary adenocarcinomas were 78%, 78%, and 0%, respectively, and the corresponding rates in invasive micropapillary carcinomas were 3%, 40%, and 38%. The CA125-positive rate of invasive micropapillary carcinoma was higher than the rate reported for other types of breast carcinomas. We consider CA125 to be not always useful in the differential diagnosis of serous papillary adenocarcinoma and invasive micropapillary carcinoma. Although the positive rate of

WT1 was significantly higher in serous papillary adenocarcinoma than in invasive micropapillary carcinoma, WT1 expression in endometrial serous papillary adenocarcinoma was infrequent (20%). WT1 and GCDFP-15 could be useful markers for the differential diagnosis of ovarian and peritoneal serous papillary adenocarcinoma versus breast invasive micropapillary adenocarcinoma. However, the availability of GCDFP-15 is limited because of the low positive rate of GCDFP-15 in invasive micropapillary carcinomas.

▶ There is a significant histological overlap between papillary serous adenocarcinoma of the female genital tract and invasive micropapillary carcinoma of the breast such that reliably distinguishing the 2 entities may lead to diagnostic difficulties for the surgical pathologist, particularly in the setting when the patient has a history of both the neoplasms. The latter may occur when there is synchronous or metachronous occurrence of both these tumors in the same patient. In addition to histological similarities between breast and ovarian carcinomas, many immunohistochemical stains are positive in both breast and ovarian tumors. These include estrogen and progesterone receptors, Her2/Neu, p53, MUC1, and MUC2 as well the expression patterns of CK7 and CK20.

This study examines a large series of both papillary serous adenocarcinoma of the female genital tract and invasive micropapillary carcinoma of the breast and uses a panel of immunohistochemical markers such as WT-1, GCDFP-15, and CA125. The latter immunohistochemistry panel has been previously proposed to be useful in differentiating primary ovarian carcinomas from metastatic breast carcinoma to the ovary. However, there are no reports of immunohistochemical comparison with matched histological subtypes such as the papillary serous carcinomas and the micropapillary carcinomas of the breast.

The results showed that CA125 had limited use in distinguishing papillary serous adenocarcinoma and invasive micropapillary carcinoma of the breast. WT-1 immunostaining was more helpful in this study with a positive rate that was significantly higher in serous papillary adenocarcinoma than in invasive micropapillary carcinoma. However, WT-1 had some limitations as well because WT-1 expression in endometrial serous papillary carcinoma was very low (only 20% in this study). Overall, this panel has limited use in the differential diagnosis of serous adenocarcinoma and invasive micropapillary carcinoma and should be used with caution. Additional newer and more sensitive and specific immunostains are needed for a more accurate diagnosis of morphologically challenging entities.

For further reading on this subject I suggest articles by Tornos et al[1] and Goldstein et al.[2]

A. V. Parwani, MD

References

1. Tornos C, Soslow R, Chen S, et al. Expression of WT1, CA 125, and GCDFP-15 as useful markers in the differential diagnosis of primary ovarian carcinomas versus metastatic breast cancer to the ovary. *Am J Surg Pathol.* 2005;29:1482-1489.

2. Goldstein NS, Uzieblo A. WT1 immunohistochemistry in uterine papillary serous carcinoma is different from ovarian serous carcinomas. *Am J Clin Pathol.* 2002; 117:541-545.

Tumor cell type can be reproducibly diagnosed and is of independent prognostic significance in patients with maximally debulked ovarian carcinoma

Gilks CB, Ionescu DN, Kalloger SE, et al (Genetic Pathology Evaluation Centre of the Res Centre, Vancouver, BC)
Hum Pathol 39:1239-1251, 2008

Ovarian surface epithelial carcinomas are routinely subclassified by pathologists based on tumor cell type and grade. It is controversial whether cell type or grade is superior in predicting patient response to treatment or survival, in patients stratified by stage of disease. The aim of this study was to uniformly apply updated criteria for cell-type and grade assignment to a series of 575 cases of ovarian surface epithelial carcinoma. All patients were optimally surgically debulked, with no macroscopic residual disease after primary surgery. Slides from these cases were reviewed by a single pathologist, who was blinded to patient outcomes. In 50 cases, 2 additional pathologists reviewed the slides independently to determine interobserver variation in assessment of cell type and grade. The distribution of tumor stage was as follows: stage I—233 cases, stage II—246 cases, stage III—96 cases. The most common cell type encountered was serous carcinoma (229/575, 40%), followed by clear cell (149/575, 26%), endometrioid (139/575, 24%), and mucinous (36/575, 6%). Serous carcinomas were significantly more likely to present with advanced stage disease (76/229 [33.2%] were stage III, and 82% of all stage III tumors were serous), whereas all nonserous cell types were stage I or II at diagnosis in greater than 90% of cases. Both FIGO grade and Silverberg grade stratified patients into groups with significantly different risks of relapse and survival, but the Silverberg grading system was a more powerful prognosticator. In multivariate analysis, stage was the most powerful prognostic indicator ($P < .0001$), followed by tumor cell type ($P = .015$), but grade was not of independent significance. Interobserver variation in assignment of cell type was very good ($\kappa = 0.77$) with moderate reproducibility in assignment of Silverberg grade ($\kappa = 0.40$) and minimal reproducibility in assignment of FIGO grade ($\kappa = 0.27$). Thus, in this series of cases of ovarian surface epithelial carcinomas with no macroscopic residual disease after primary debulking surgery, assignment of tumor cell type was both more reproducible and provided superior prognostic information compared with assignment of tumor grade. As tumor cell type also correlates with underlying molecular abnormalities and may predict response to chemotherapy, this suggests

TABLE 5.—Interobserver Reproducibility of Assessment of Histopathologic Features

	κ statistic
Architectural score	0.45
Nuclear score	0.34
Mitotic activity	0.62
Silverberg grade	0.40
FIGO grade	0.26
Tumor cell type	0.77

(Reprinted from Gilks CB, Ionescu DN, Kalloger SE, et al. Tumor cell type can be reproducibly diagnosed and is of independent prognostic significance in patients with maximally debulked ovarian carcinoma. *Hum Pathol* 2008;39:1239-1251, with permission from Elsevier.)

that tumor cell type could be used to guide treatment decisions for patients with ovarian surface epithelial carcinoma (Table 5).

▶ Recent studies on ovarian carcinomas have shown that tumor cell type correlates with epidemiological risk factors, BRCA1 or 2 mutation status, differences in gene expression profile and genetic events during oncogenesis, and response to treatment. Therefore, a correct diagnosis of tumor cell type by the pathologist has important prognostic and therapeutic implications. The reproducibility between pathologists in assessing tumor cell types is of critical importance because this has the potential to guide the therapy of patients with ovarian carcinomas. This study illustrates the importance of an accurate diagnosis of the tumor cell type in the overall pathological evaluation of ovarian surface epithelial carcinomas from patients with no macroscopic residual disease after primary debulking surgery. The authors have examined the histology of a large number of cases (n = 575) of ovarian surface epithelial carcinomas and applied the updated criteria for cell type and grade assignment to these tumors. The grading and assessment were done by 1 pathologist for all the cases and a subset of the cases (n = 50) were also evaluated by 2 additional pathologists.

The results were striking and showed that serous carcinomas were significantly more likely to present with advanced stage disease (33.2% of the cases) as compared with nonserous cell types. In this study, the nonserous cell types were stage I or II in greater than 90% of the cases. There was good overall interobserver variation in assignment of cell types between the study pathologists (κ = 0.77) (Table 5).

The results of this study are significant because the authors have shown that assignment of the tumor cell type in ovarian surface epithelial carcinomas from patients with no macroscopic residual disease after primary debulking surgery had superior reproducibility. Secondly, this approach of assessing the tumor cell type provided useful prognostic information as compared with the assignment of tumor grade. The stratification of patients into different groups on the basis of the tumor cell type may be of value in the future to administer more appropriate and customized adjuvant therapies.

For further reading on this subject I suggest articles by Schwartz et al[1] and Risch et al.[2]

A. V. Parwani, MD

References

1. Schwartz DR, Kardia SL, Shedden KA, et al. Gene expression in ovarian cancer reflects both morphology and biological behavior, distinguishing clear cell from other poor-prognosis ovarian carcinomas. *Cancer Res.* 2002;62:4722-4729.
2. Risch HA, McLaughlin JR, Cole DE, et al. Prevalence and penetrance of germline BRCA1 and BRCA2 mutations in a population series of 649 women with ovarian cancer. *Am J Hum Genet.* 2001;68:700-710.

The Use of p16 in Enhancing the Histologic Classification of Uterine Smooth Muscle Tumors
Atkins KA, Arronte N, Darus CJ, et al (Univ of Virginia, Charlottesville, VA)
Am J Surg Pathol 32:98-102, 2008

Background.—Uterine smooth muscle tumors can usually be divided histologically into leiomyoma (L) and leiomyosarcoma (LMS). Occasionally, the histologic features are indeterminate and classified as smooth muscle tumor of uncertain malignant potential (STUMP). Recent gene expression studies have found p16 overexpressed in LMS when compared with normal myometrium. This study evaluated the protein expression of p16 by immunohistochemistry in LMS, L, and normal myometrium. Additionally, 8 tumors originally classified as STUMP were evaluated for p16 expression and correlated to their clinical outcome.

Methods.—A tissue microarray was constructed and composed of 15 LMS, 8 STUMPs, 22 L, and 10 samples of normal myometrium. p16 expression was correlated with clinical outcome and histologic features.

Results.—Twelve of the 15 LMS strongly and diffusely expressed p16, 3 of the L had focal p16 staining, and none of the normal myometria were p16 positive. Three of the tumors originally classified as STUMP developed metastatic disease and 2 of these tumors had strong, diffuse p16 positivity. Histologically, these 2 cases were characterized by coagulative tumor cell necrosis and only mild cytologic atypia.

Conclusions.—p16 is preferentially expressed in LMS with only rare L showing positivity. Histologically, tumors with coagulative tumor cell necrosis alone were clinically LMS. In those cases in which the type of necrosis is uncertain (coagulative tumor cell vs. hyalinized), the addition of p16 may aid in discerning a subset of STUMP that should be classified as LMS.

▶ The histological classification of uterine smooth muscle tumors into leiomyomas (L) and leiomyosarcomas (LMS) are based on mitotic activity, cytological activity, and necrosis. In the current study, the investigators explored the use of

P16 immunostaining in further refining the classification of uterine smooth muscle tumors including L and LMS as well as a small subset of smooth muscle tumors referred to as smooth muscle tumor of uncertain malignant potential (STUMP). The latter has indeterminate histological features and is not easily classifiable as either L or LMS. In addition, there is a lack of clinical experience with STUMPs making the optimal clinical management of these patients more challenging.

Recent gene expression studies have shown that there is an overexpression of p16 in LMS when compared with normal myometrium. The authors have used a tissue microarray with 15 cases of LMS, 8 STUMPs, 22 leiomyoma, and 10 samples of normal myometrium. The case number is small but the data are interesting and shows a definite trend. A majority of the LMS (12 out of 15 cases) expressed p16, a small number of L (only 3 of the 22 cases had focal p16 staining). More importantly, none of the normal myometria had any p16 expression. Interestingly, 2 of 3 of the STUMP cases with metastatic disease had strong p16 expression.

Although the number of STUMP cases were very few, this study provides support of using p16 for refining the diagnosis of uterine smooth muscle tumors, particularly when encountering cases which fall under the STUMP category or have some atypical features but are otherwise histologically consistent with L.

For further reading on this subject, I suggest articles by Skubitz et al,[1] and Bodner et al.[2]

A. V. Parwani, MD

References

1. Skubitz KM, Skubitz AP. Differential gene expression in leiomyosarcoma. *Cancer.* 2003;98:1029-1038.
2. Bodner K, Bodner-Adler B, Czerwenka K, Kimberger O, Leodolter S, Mayerhofer K. Expression of p16 protein in patients with uterine smooth muscle tumors: an immunohistochemical analysis. *Gynecol Oncol.* 2005;96:62-66.

Expression of gonadotrophin releasing hormone receptor I is a favorable prognostic factor in epithelial ovarian cancer

Wilkinson SJ, Kucukmetin A, Cross P, et al (Newcastle Univ, Newcastle, UK; Queen Elizabeth Hosp, Gateshead, UK)
Hum Pathol 39:1197-1204, 2008

The majority of epithelial ovarian cancers originate in the ovarian surface epithelium. The ovarian surface epithelium is a hormonally responsive tissue, and hormones are thought to play a key role in the development of this type of cancer. Gonadotrophin releasing hormone II is one of 2 isoforms which are thought to act through gonadotrophin releasing hormone receptor I, and gonadotrophin releasing hormone II has been shown to cause growth inhibition of cultured ovarian surface epithelium. The aim of this study was to investigate the expression levels and prognostic significance of gonadotrophin releasing hormone II and the gonadotrophin releasing hormone receptor I in epithelial ovarian cancer. Gonadotrophin releasing hormone II and gonadotrophin releasing hormone receptor I messenger RNA expression was examined in 23 cancers and 7 normal ovarian surface epithelium samples by quantitative real time polymerase chain reaction. An ovarian cancer tissue microarray containing 139 cases was constructed and immunohistochemical analysis of gonadotrophin releasing hormone II and gonadotrophin releasing hormone receptor I protein expression was performed and correlated with clinical outcome data. Gonadotrophin releasing hormone II messenger RNA expression was lower in cancer samples compared to normal ovarian surface epithelium samples ($P < .05$). Gonadotrophin releasing hormone II protein expression correlated with histologic subtype (25% serous versus 45% nonserous, $P < .05$) but not with overall survival. Gonadotrophin releasing hormone receptor I messenger RNA expression was highest in serous tumors when compared to non serous ($P < .05$) and normal tissue ($P < .001$). Expression of the gonadotrophin releasing hormone receptor I protein was also found to correlate with patient survival ($P < .05$). We have demonstrated gonadotrophin releasing hormone II and its receptor, gonadotrophin releasing hormone receptor I, are present in clinical ovarian samples, and that gonadotrophin releasing hormone receptor I protein expression is a favorable prognostic factor, suggesting these proteins play an important role in the development of epithelial ovarian cancer (Fig 3).

▶ This article examines the levels of 2 isotypes of gonadotrophin releasing hormone, GnRH-I and GnRH-II. These investigations are important because

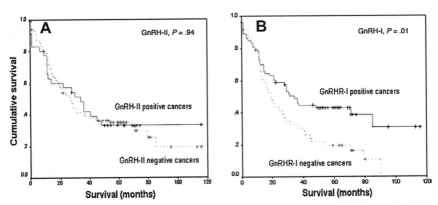

FIGURE 3.—Kaplan-Meier curves demonstrating relationship between GnRH-II and GnRHR-I expression and patient survival. Protein expression was measured using immunohistochemistry on 139 samples of epithelial ovarian cancer and correlated with survival. Staining was categorized as negative, weak, moderate, or strong and, for the purpose of analysis, further categorized as negative (negative/weak) or positive (moderate/strong). A, Correlation between GnRH-II expression and survival was not statistically significant ($P = .94$). B, Survival was greater in patients whose tumor expressed GnRHR-I protein ($P < .01$). (Reprinted from Wilkinson SJ, Kucukmetin A, Cross P, et al. Expression of gonadotrophin releasing hormone receptor I is a favorable prognostic factor in epithelial ovarian cancer. *Hum Pathol.* 2008;39:1197-1204, with permission from Elsevier.)

of some recent data about these hormones and their receptors and the potential mechanisms of action. Recent studies have shown that when GnRH-II is administered to ovarian cancer cells, there is a decrease in cell proliferation. Also, studies have suggested that in ovarian cancer cells, the effects of GnRH-II are mediated through the GnRH receptor I and the protein kinase C pathway, and not the type 2 receptor.

The authors constructed an ovarian carcinoma tissue microarray, which had 139 cases of epithelial ovarian cancer. The immunohistochemical expression of gonadotrophin releasing hormone II and the gonadotrophin releasing hormone receptor I in these cases of epithelial ovarian cancer was quantitated to evaluate for prognostic significance.

The results were very interesting and revealed that expression of the gonadotrophin releasing hormone receptor I protein correlated with patient survival ($P < .05$), with the patients whose tumors have expressed the type I receptor having an overall greater survival (Fig 3). Overall, it was also seen that GnRH-II was down-regulated in cancers when compared with normal tissue. The investigators also found that gonadotrophin releasing hormone receptor I messenger RNA expression was highest in serous tumors when compared with nonserous ($P > .05$) and normal tissue ($P > .001$). Also, it was found that the serous tumors expressed the lowest levels of GnRH-II protein. The findings of this study highlight the importance of GnRH-II and its receptor in ovarian epithelial neoplasia.

For further reading on this subject I suggest articles by Kim et al,[1] and Chien et al.[2]

A. V. Parwani, MD

References

1. Kim KY, Choi KC, Auersperg N, Leung PC. Mechanism of gonadotropin-releasing hormone (GnRH)-I and -II-induced cell growth inhibition in ovarian cancer cells: role of the GnRH-I receptor and protein kinase C pathway. *Endocr Relat Cancer.* 2006;13:211-220.
2. Chien CH, Chen CH, Lee CY, Chang TC, Chen RJ, Chow SN. Detection of gonadotropin-releasing hormone receptor and its mRNA in primary human epithelial ovarian cancers. *Int J Gynecol Cancer.* 2004;14:451-458.

Role of Immunohistochemical Overexpression of Matrix Metalloproteinases MMP-2 and MMP-11 in the Prognosis of Death by Ovarian Cancer

Périgny M, Bairati I, Harvey I, et al (Ctr Hospitalier Universitaire de Québec, l'Hôtel-Dieu de Québec, Canada, et al)
Am J Clin Pathol 129:226-231, 2008

Matrix metalloproteinases (MMPs) are enzymes thought to be involved in tumor invasion. We hypothesized that MMP-2 and MMP-11 overexpression was associated with the aggressiveness of ovarian carcinoma.

This study was performed on samples from 100 patients with stage III ovarian carcinomas treated surgically between 1990 and 2000. Immuno-histochemical staining was performed on ovarian tumors and peritoneal implants using monoclonal antibodies. Overexpression was defined as more than 10% of cells expressing the marker. Multivariate analyses showed that only MMP-2 overexpression by cancer cells in peritoneal implants was associated with a significant risk of death by disease (hazard ratio, 2.65; 95% confidence interval, 1.41-4.97; $P = .003$). MMP-11 over-expression was not predictive of survival. These results suggest that MMP-2 overexpression by cancer cells in peritoneal implants and not in the primary ovarian cancer is predictive of ovarian cancer prognosis and more likely reflects the presence of particularly aggressive clones of cancer cells (Fig 1).

▶ The investigators in this study were interested in assessing if the overexpression of matrix metalloproteinases (MMP-2 and MMP-11) were associated with poor prognosis of ovarian carcinomas. Many recent studies, including studies on breast and prostate carcinoma, have shown that matrix metalloproteinases, members of a family of zinc-dependent endopeptidases, are involved in tumor growth, invasion, and metastasis. Immunohistochemical staining was performed on ovarian tumors and peritoneal implants using monoclonal antibodies specific for MMP-2 and MMP-11.

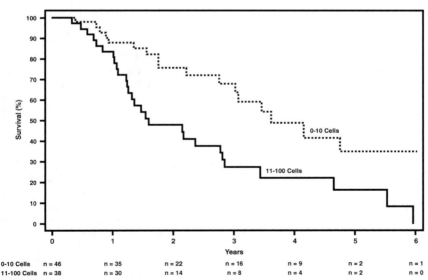

FIGURE 1.—Kaplan-Meier survival curves for time to death according to matrix metalloproteinase-2 expression by epithelial cells in peritoneal implants. For 0-10 cells, median survival was 3.6 years and for 11-100 cells, 1.6 years. $P = .0021$; log-rank test. (Reprinted from Périgny M, Bairati I, Harvey I, et al. Role of immunohistochemical overexpression of matrix metalloproteinases MMP-2 and MMP-11 in the prognosis of death by ovarian cancer. *Am J Clin Pathol.* 2008;129:226-231, with permission from the American Society of Clinical Pathology.)

Although the study only used 100 cases of stage III ovarian carcinomas, both primary and in peritoneal implants, the results were very interesting. On the basis of multivariate analysis, it was shown in this study that only the MMP-2 overexpression by cancer cells and only in peritoneal implants, there was a significant risk of death by disease (Fig 1). Another interesting finding in this study is the observation that MMP-2 overexpression in peritoneal implants and not ovarian tumors is associated with tumor aggressiveness.

Interestingly, MMP-11 overexpression in this study was not associated with survival. This is in contrast to prostate and breast carcinomas, where both MMP-2 and MMP-11 overexpression was found to be associated with poor prognosis. This observation needs to be confirmed with a larger number of cases of ovarian carcinomas, particularly in peritoneal implants. The validation of these findings has therapeutic implications including the use of synthetic MMP inhibitors.

For further reading on this subject I suggest articles by Overall et al[1] and Trudel et al.[2]

A. V. Parwani, MD

References

1. Overall CM, Kleifeld O. Tumour microenvironment: opinion: validating matrix metalloproteinases as drug targets and anti-targets for cancer therapy. *Nat Rev Cancer.* 2006;6:227-239.
2. Trudel D, Fradet Y, Meyer F, Harel T, Têtu B. Significance of MMP-2 expression in prostate cancer: an immunohistochemical study. *Cancer Res.* 2003;63:8511-8515.

Human Papillomavirus (HPV) Profiles of Vulvar Lesions: Possible Implications for the Classification of Vulvar Squamous Cell Carcinoma Precursors and for the Efficacy of Prophylactic HPV Vaccination
Skapa P, Zamecnik J, Hamsikova E, et al (Charles Univ, Prague, Czech Republic; Inst of Hematology and Blood Transfusion, Prague, Czech Republic)
Am J Surg Pathol 31:1834-1843, 2007

The term vulvar intraepithelial neoplasia (VIN) introduced in 1986 incorporates 3 grades of usual VIN (u-VIN I-III) and the differentiated VIN (d-VIN). Although u-VIN is etiologically associated with the human papillomavirus (HPV) infection, d-VIN represents an alternative HPV negative pathway of vulvar carcinogenesis. In 2004, the u-VIN I category was abandoned and u-VIN II and III were merged. Further, an alternative Bethesda-like terminology scheme presenting the term vulvar intraepithelial lesion was proposed recently. To analyze the impact of HPV profiles of vulvar precancerous lesions for their classification and to assess the presumable efficacy of the prophylactic HPV vaccination, 269 vulvar excisions representing lichen sclerosus, lichen simplex chronicus, condylomata acuminata, d-VIN, all grades of u-VIN and squamous cell carcinomas were subjected to the HPV typing by use of GP5+/6+

polymerase chain reaction and reverse line blot hybridization. The results showed different HPV profiles, and also differing frequency of multiple-type HPV infection and the age structure in patients with u-VIN II and III. The biologic heterogeneity within the u-VIN II category was also demonstrated. u-VIN I was distinguished as a rare disorder associated with high-risk HPV infection. We conclude that the original VIN terminology proposed in 1986 seems to be appropriate for the classification of vulvar squamous dysplastic lesions. The spectrum of HPV types found in vulvar squamous cell carcinomas indicates that the efficacy of HPV vaccination in preventing vulvar cancer might be diminished in the studied population, because the recently developed prophylactic vaccines are targeted against a limited number of HPV types.

▶ This is an important article because it highlights the human papillomavirus (HPV) profiles of vulvar lesions, information that is very valuable as it relates to the assessment of the efficacy of the recently developed prophylactic HPV vaccine. Several studies have demonstrated that squamous preneoplastic lesions and invasive squamous cell carcinoma of the lower female genital tract are linked to HPV infection, particularly the cervix. However, this is not the case for most of the vulvar squamous cell carcinomas, which are HPV-negative.

In 2004, the Vulvar Oncology Subcommittee of the International Society for the Study of Vulvar Diseases (ISSVD) developed the classification system for vulvar intraepithelial neoplasia (VIN), which is classified into 2 main groups as follows: (1) VIN, usual type (VINu), which includes the warty type VIN, basaloid type VIN, and mixed type VIN, and (2) the differentiated VIN, VINd (Table 1 in the original article).

Many studies have focused on vulvar squamous cell carcinoma (SCC) and have shown the vulvar SCC develops from 2 different pathways. In HPV-negative lesions, vulvar SCC can develop in a background of lichen sclerosus (LS), differentiated vulvar intraepithelial neoplasia (VINd), or both. The second pathway, which results in vulvar SCC, is the one that is associated with HPV. The HPV-associated preneoplastic condition is VINu.

The authors have performed a correlation study between the histological appearance and the HPV profile of vulvar non-neoplastic, preneoplastic, and neoplastic squamous cell lesions. The lesions included in this study (n = 269 cases) represented cases of lichen sclerosus, lichen simplex chronicus, condylomata acuminata, VINd, all grades of VINu, and squamous cell carcinomas.

The results of this study are striking. The authors have shown that there is variability in the HPV profiles between vulvar and cervical preneoplastic and neoplastic squamous cell lesions. Furthermore, there was geographical variability in the distribution of HPV subtypes in the vulvar lesions. Among vulvar lesions, the authors found an increased prevalence of HPV type 33, whereas there was a decreased prevalence of HPV 16 and HPV 18 types. This finding has important epidemiological implications for the potential lack of the HPV vaccine against vulvar lesions because the vaccine's primary target is HPV 16 and HPV 18.

For further reading on this subject I suggest articles by Chiesa-Vottero et al[1] and Clifford et al.[2]

A. V. Parwani, MD

References

1. Chiesa-Vottero A, Dvoretsky PM, Hart WR. Histopathologic study of thin vulvar squamous cell carcinomas and associated cutaneous lesions: a correlative study of 48 tumors in 44 patients with analysis of adjacent vulvar intraepithelial neoplasia types and lichen sclerosus. *Am J Surg Pathol.* 2006;30:310-318.
2. Clifford G, Franceschi S, Diaz M, Muñoz N, Villa LL. Chapter 3: HPV-type distribution in women with and without cervical neoplastic diseases. *Vaccine.* 2006;24: 26-34.

10 Urinary Bladder and Male Genital Tract

Malignant germ cell tumours in the elderly: a histopathological review of 50 cases in men aged 60 years or over
Berney DM, Warren AY, Verma M, et al (St Bartholomew's Hosp, West Smithfield, London; Addenbrooke's Hosp, Cambridge)
Mod Pathol 21:54-59, 2008

Malignant testicular germ cell tumours in the elderly are extremely rare with anecdotal accounts of their aggressive behaviour. Fifty cases of germ cell tumour, diagnosed at the age of 60 years or above, were pathologically reviewed. The oldest patient was 86 years of age, with 78% of cases presenting in men in their 60s. Forty-one (82%) of the tumours were seminomas with only nine cases (18%) of mixed or non-seminomatous germ cell tumour. However, all non-seminomatous types of tumour were represented in the series. The macroscopic tumour size was significantly larger (median = 6 cm, range = 2–11 cm) than comparable series in younger men. They were also of higher stage with more frequent vascular invasion and rete testis invasion than is typically seen in a younger population. The tumours were less associated with intratubular germ cell neoplasia than in younger men as it was present in only 47% of assessable cases. We conclude that germ cell tumours, in man aged 60 years or above, present at a later stage than in younger men, and although most are seminomas, non-seminomatous tumours may occur with a wide spectrum of morphology.

▶ Testicular malignant germ cell tumors are typically seen in young males. The vast majority of these tumors are diagnosed in the third and fourth decade of life. Rare reports of prepubescent malignant germ cell tumors are there, but they have a very different histopathologic profile and behavior. The incidence of malignant germ cell tumors declines markedly after the age of 50. Malignant germ cell tumors in patients above the age of 60 are extremely rare. Spermatocytic seminomas are an entirely separate lesion from the remainder of the germ cell tumors. They are well reported in the elderly and have a distinct morphology and immunophenotype. This study documents the existence of 50 cases seen in the age group > 60 years. Eighty-two percent of the tumors were seminomas. The mixed tumors present had all the different morphologic types represented. This study is important, establishing the prevalence of malignant germ cell tumors in older males. Testicular malignant germ cell tumors should, therefore, be considered in the differential when the microscopic features suggest this diagnosis in older males.

R. Dhir, MD

Is the utility of prostate–specific antigen velocity for prostate cancer detection affected by age?
Loeb S, Roehl KA, Catalona WJ, et al (Johns Hopkins School of Medicine, Baltimore, MD; Univ School of Medicine, St. Louis, MO; Northwestern Feinberg School of Medicine, Chicago, IL)
BJU Int 101:817-821, 2008

Objective.—To determine whether prostate-specific antigen velocity (PSAV) is useful for prostate cancer detection in men from different age groups, and whether the same PSAV thresholds can reasonably be applied to all men aged ≥40 years.

Patients and Methods.—From a large prostate cancer screening study, 13 615 men had data on age and a calculable PSAV. We used statistical analysis to examine the ability of PSAV to predict prostate cancer risk in each age decade.

Results.—For men of all ages, the median PSAV was 0.6–0.7 ng/mL/year in men with prostate cancer, and 0–0.1 ng/mL/year in men with no prostate cancer ($P < 0.005$ for all). On receiver operating characteristic (ROC) analysis, the area under the curve was 0.800, 0.697, 0.693, and 0.668 for predicting prostate cancer risk using PSAV for men aged 40–49, 50–59, 60–69 and ≥70 years, respectively. In the multivariate model controlling for race, family history, and the total PSA level, both PSA and PSAV were significant independent predictors of prostate cancer risk in men of all ages.

Conclusions.—The PSAV is significantly higher in men of all ages with prostate cancer compared with men with no prostate cancer; although on ROC analysis it performed the best in young men. Interestingly, the median PSAV in men with prostate cancer was <0.75 ng/mL/year regardless of age, suggesting that this threshold may be too high. Overall, this data confirms that PSAV is a useful tool for prostate cancer detection for men aged ≥40 years.

▶ Serum prostate-specific antigen (PSA) screening is very common. Prostate-specific antigen velocity (PSAV) measures the rate at which PSA is increasing and is considered a useful adjunct to serum PSA values. This study evaluates whether age affects the use of PSAV in prostate cancer detection in men from different age groups, and whether the same PSAV thresholds can reasonably be applied to all men aged ≥40 years. This study used data from a large prostate cancer screening study that had enrolled 13 615 men with information regarding age and a calculable PSAV. Statistical analysis ascertained ability of

PSAV to predict prostate cancer risk in each age decade. PSAV is significantly higher in men of all ages with prostate cancer compared with men with no prostate cancer. PSAV showed best results in the 40 to 49 age group with the best receiver operating characteristic (ROC) results. The median PSAV in men with prostate cancer was 0.75 ng/mL/year as compared with 0 to 0.1 in the men without prostate cancer. This particular study reinforces the value of PSAV in prostate cancer screening. It also highlights the fact that age really is no barrier to using either PSA or PSAV and is useful across the younger and older age ranges. In fact, the PSAV increases were most dramatic in the youngest age group evaluated (40-49 years).

R. Dhir, MD

Value of multicolour fluorescence in situ hybridisation (UroVysion) in the differential diagnosis of flat urothelial lesions
Schwarz S, Rechenmacher M, Filbeck T, et al (Univ of Regensburg, Germany; Hosp Eichstaett, Germany, et al)
J Clin Pathol 61:272-277, 2008

Aims.—During the past 10 years, multitarget fluorescence in situ hybridisation has been established as a valuable adjunct in the cytological diagnosis of precancerous and malignant lesions of the urinary tract. The aim of the present study was to define its value in detecting chromosomal imbalances in patients with various flat urothelial lesions in routine paraffin-embedded bladder biopsy samples. In addition, the HER2 gene amplification and HER2 expression pattern were examined, since alterations of the HER2 expression patterns have been demonstrated in invasive bladder cancer.

Methods.—29 samples of normal urothelium and 86 flat urothelial lesions (hyperplasia, reactive atypia, dysplasia and carcinoma in situ (CIS)) from 73 patients were analysed patients using tissue microarrays and centromeric probes for chromosomes 3, 7 and 17, and gene-specific probes for 9p21/P16 and HER2 (UroVysion, PathVysion). The expression of HER2 was studied by immunohistochemistry.

Results.—Polysomy of at least one of the chromosomes was found in about half of the dysplastic cells, and in more than 90% of cells in CIS or cells in invasive bladder tumours. Polysomic cells were found in only 17% of urothelial hyperplasia, reactive atypia and normal urothelium of healthy patients, whereas about 30% of non-neoplastic lesions in patients with concomitant urothelial carcinoma showed polysomy of at least one chromosome. These alterations indicate a field effect and are associated with synchronous development of dysplastic lesions of a higher grade. Deletion of the P16 locus was most frequently observed in aneuploid lesions, whereas overexpression of HER2 was found in 10–20% of invasive urothelial carcinomas, and only occasionally in CIS (5%). An altered HER2 expression pattern was present in non-neoplastic lesions (25%).

Conclusions.—UroVysion fluorescence in situ hybridisation is a valuable tool for the detection of genetically unstable flat urothelial lesions, and can help to resolve difficult cases, particularly the differential diagnosis of reactive atypia and dysplasia.

▶ Histological diagnosis of flat urothelial lesions can sometimes be challenging. Although urothelial carcinoma in situ (CIS) usually has distinctive atypia, it might occasionally be challenging when dealing with severe reactive atypia/urothelial dysplasia. Similar issues may be faced with noninvasive papillary tumor and papillary cystitis with atypia. Polysomy of at least one of the chromosomes was found in about half of the dysplastic cells, and in more than 90% of cells in CIS or cells in invasive bladder tumors. The nonneoplastic cases (urothelial hyperplasia/reactive atypia/normal urothelium) showed polysomic cells in only 17% of cases. Evidence of field effect is also seen with 30% of nonneoplastic lesions in patients with concomitant urothelial carcinoma showing polysomy of at least 1 chromosome. Use of UroVysion fluorescence in situ hybridization (FISH) should be considered as an ancillary tool for the detection of genetically unstable flat urothelial lesions. This FISH test can help resolve difficult morphologic issues especially the differential diagnosis of reactive atypia, dysplasia, and CIS.

R. Dhir, MD

D2-40 is a sensitive and specific marker in differentiating primary adrenal cortical tumours from both metastatic clear cell renal cell carcinoma and phaeochromocytoma
Browning L, Bailey D, Parker A (Wycombe Hospital, High Wycombe; The John Radcliffe Hospital, Oxford)
J Clin Pathol 61:293-296, 2008

Background.—The morphological similarities between the cells of clear cell renal cell carcinoma (CCRCC) and those of the adrenal cortex impose diagnostic difficulties, for example in the context of a solitary nodule in the adrenal gland in a patient with renal cell carcinoma (RCC). This problem is confounded by the variable and patchy staining seen with the established panel of antibodies utilised in this context, namely EMA, cytokeratins, vimentin, inhibin, melan-A, and RCC marker; particularly on biopsy material. D2-40, an antibody commonly used to highlight lymphatic endothelial cells, is consistently positive in the normal adrenal cortex.

Aims.—To investigate the utility of D2-40 in distinguishing neoplastic and non-neoplastic adrenal cortical cells from those of CCRCC, and from phaeochromocytoma.

Methods.—D2-40 antibody was applied to tissue sections from 10 normal adrenal glands, 15 renal carcinomas (13 clear cell, 2 papillary variants), 1 metastatic CCRCC in the adrenal gland, 6 adrenal cortical hyperplasias, 5 adrenal cortical adenomas, 3 adrenal cortical carcinomas, and 4 phaeochromocytomas.

Results.—D2-40 was strongly and diffusely positive in the cells of the neoplastic and non-neoplastic adrenal cortex, but negative in the cells of the CCRCC, both primary and metastatic, in 100% of the cases. The cells of the adrenal medulla, and those of the phaeochromocytomas, were negative for D2-40.

Conclusions.—D2-40 may be a useful marker for distinguishing primary adrenal cortical neoplasms from both metastatic CCRCC and phaeochromocytoma.

▶ Discriminating clear cell renal cell carcinoma (CCRCC) from neoplasms of the adrenal cortex may be difficult. This discrimination is important especially in the context of possible metastasis from a CCRCC to the adrenal. Coexistence of solitary nodules in the adrenal gland in a patient with RCC is also seen. The current established panel of antibodies have issues and may show variable and patchy staining. There is a need for a definitive marker that highlights renal cortical tissue/neoplasms. This article describes the use of D2-40, an antibody commonly used to highlight lymphatic endothelial cells. D2-40 is consistently positive in the normal adrenal cortex as well as in adrenal cortical hyperplasias, adrenal cortical adenomas, and adrenal cortical carcinomas. It was consistently negative in renal carcinomas (clear cell and papillary variants) and a CCRCC metastatic to the adrenal gland. In addition, adrenal medulla and phaeochromo-cytomas were negative. D2-40 should be considered when discriminating between a metastasis from a CCRCC and adrenal tissue/lesion.

R. Dhir, MD

Aberrant Diffuse Expression of p63 in Adenocarcinoma of the Prostate on Needle Biopsy and Radical Prostatectomy: Report of 21 Cases
Osunkoya AO, Hansel DE, Sun X, et al (The Johns Hopkins Hosp, Baltimore, MD; The Cleveland Clinic Foundation, OH; Lakewood Pathology Associates, NJ)
Am J Surg Pathol 32:461-467, 2008

Aberrant diffuse expression of p63 in prostate carcinoma cells is a rare and poorly understood phenomenon. We studied 19 cases of prostate cancer with aberrant diffuse expression of p63 on needle biopsy and reviewed the subsequent radical prostatectomies in 6 cases. In 19/21 cases, 100% of the cancer nuclei stained intensely for p63, with 70% staining in the remaining 2 cases. Two additional radical prostatectomies with aberrant p63 staining with no needle biopsies available for review were also analyzed. On the hematoxylin and eosin-stained slides, 19/21 cases (90.5%) showed a distinctive morphology composed predominantly of glands, nests, and cords with atrophic cytoplasm, hyperchromatic nuclei, and visible nucleoli. Needle biopsy cases ranged from Gleason patterns 3 to 5 with tumor identified on one or more cores, ranging from a minute focus to 80% of the core. In all 8 radical prostatectomies p63 positive cancer was present, with in 2/8 cases both p63 positive cancer and usual p63 negative acinar prostate cancer. In all 8 cases, the tumors were organ confined with negative margins and there was no seminal vesicle involvement or lymph node metastasis. The presence of p63 positive atypical glands with an infiltrative pattern and perineural invasion on radical prostatectomy confirmed the needle biopsy diagnosis of carcinoma. Rarely, prostate cancer can aberrantly express diffuse p63 staining in a non-basal cell distribution leading to the erroneous diagnosis of atrophy or atypical basal cell proliferation. The diagnosis of prostate cancer is based on the morphology and confirmed by the absence of high molecular weight cytokeratin staining and positivity for α-methylacyl-CoA racemase in the atypical glands. Pathologists need to be aware of this rare and unusual phenomenon, which is a potential pitfall in prostate cancer diagnosis.

▶ Confirmation of light microscopic impression of prostate cancer typically uses a panel of immunohistochemical stains. The most commonly used stains label basal cells of benign prostate glands and are negative in prostate cancer. The stains used are p63 (a nuclear stain) and HWCK/CK903 (cytoplasmic stain). The prostate cancer cells typically express racemase. There are reports of sporadic HWCK positivity in prostate cancer cells. This study describes a rare phenomenon of diffuse p63 positive prostate cancers. These tumors have an atrophic morphology and can be confused with atrophy/atypical atrophy. Pathologists need to be aware of this variant of prostate cancer because it can be a source of misdiagnosis. It is also important to realize the need for using both basal cell markers in this situation. These tumors with aberrant p63 expression express prostate-specific antigen (PSA) (confirms prostate origin) and racemase and are negative for HWCK. On a related note, there are no prostate cancers described with diffuse HWCK positivity, nor are there prostate cancers described with focal positivity for both basal cell markers p63 and HWCK.

R. Dhir, MD

Whole genome SNP arrays as a potential diagnostic tool for the detection of characteristic chromosomal aberrations in renal epithelial tumors
Monzon FA, Hagenkord JM, Lyons-Weiler MA, et al (Univ of Pittsburgh, PA)
Mod Pathol 21:599-608, 2008

Renal tumors with complex or unusual morphology require extensive workup for accurate classification. Chromosomal aberrations that define subtypes of renal epithelial neoplasms have been reported. We explored if whole-genome chromosome copy number and loss-of-heterozygosity analysis with single nucleotide polymorphism (SNP) arrays can be used to identify these aberrations and classify renal epithelial tumors. We analyzed 20 paraffin-embedded tissues representing clear cell, papillary renal and chromophobe renal cell carcinoma, as well as oncocytoma with Affymetrix GeneChip 10K 2.0 Mapping arrays. SNP array results were in concordance with known genetic aberrations for each renal tumor subtype. Additional chromosomal aberrations were detected in all renal cell tumor types. The unique patterns allowed 19 out of 20 tumors to be readily categorized by their chromosomal copy number aberrations. One papillary renal cell carcinoma type 2 did not show the characteristic 7/17 trisomies. Clustering using the median copy number of each chromosomal arm correlated with histological class when using a restricted set of chromosomes. In addition, three morphologically challenging tumors were analyzed to explore the potential clinical utility of this method. In these cases, the SNP array-based copy number evaluation yielded information with potential clinical value. These results show that SNP arrays can detect characteristic chromosomal aberrations in paraffin-embedded renal tumors, and thus offer a high-resolution, genome-wide method that can be used as an ancillary study for classification and potentially for prognostic stratification of these tumors.

▶ There has been a surge in the incidence of renal cell carcinomas, especially over the last decade. This is presumed to be partly because of earlier detection with more sophisticated radiologic methods. Although there exist definite criteria and panels of immunohistochemical stains, morphologically complex tumors can represent a diagnostic challenge, especially in classification of exact histologic type. Use of single nucleotide polymorphism (SNP) chips represents a high-throughput effort to profile the chromosomal changes (loss-of-heterozygosity[-LOH]/mutations/amplifications). This data set demonstrates consistent SNP patterns in different morphologic subtypes. This approach will have value in the future as these techniques become reimbursable and more commonly available.

R. Dhir, MD

Polypoid/Papillary Cystitis: A Series of 41 Cases Misdiagnosed as Papillary Urothelial Neoplasia
Lane Z, Epstein JI (The Johns Hopkins Hosp, Baltimore, MD)
Am J Surg Pathol 32:758-764, 2008

Polypoid cystitis and its more chronic phase papillary cystitis, which results as a reaction to injury to the bladder mucosa, is a benign lesion mimicking various papillary urothelial neoplasms. Analogous lesions occur throughout the urothelial tract and are referred to as polypoid urethritis, polypoid ureteritis, and polypoid pyelitis when present in the urethra, ureter, and renal pelvis, respectively. For simplicity, these lesions in different sites and papillary cystitis will typically be referred to as polypoid cystitis in this manuscript. A search of the consultation files from our institution from January 2000 to July 2007 was performed. Of 155 cases diagnosed as polypoid cystitis, we identified 41 cases that were diagnosed as papillary urothelial neoplasms by contributing pathologists and only sent to us, typically at the request of the urologist after the case had be signed out. For cases where information was available, clinical symptoms included bladder obstruction (n = 7), gross hematuria (n = 6), colovesicular fistula (n = 4), follow-up status posttreatment of bladder and ureter carcinoma (n = 4), bladder/urethral stones (n = 2), benign prostate hyperplasia (n = 2), follow-up after radiation for prostate cancer (n = 2), long-standing urinary stents (n = 2), and voiding dysfunction (n = 1). Original diagnoses included noninvasive low grade papillary urothelial carcinoma (n = 23), noninvasive high grade papillary urothelial carcinoma (n = 6), papillary urothelial neoplasm of low malignant potential (n = 5), papilloma (n = 3), urothelial neoplasia (n = 2), carcinoma in situ (n = 1), and squamous carcinoma (n = 1). The mean age at diagnosis was 63 years (range, 19 to 93 y; median 63 y). Male to female ratio was 3.1 to 1. Clinical symptoms varied with the most common manifestations, including gross hematuria, bladder/urethral stones, history of prostate cancer treated with radiation, follow-up after bladder/ureter carcinoma treatment, long-term urinary stents, and colovesicular fistulas. At cystoscopy, lesions were variably described as polypoid, trabeculations, bullous polyps, and diffuse erythema and edema. The locations of polypoid cystitis were bladder (n = 34), ureteral orifice (n = 2), urethra (n = 2), renal pelvis (n = 2), and undesignated (n = 1). Architecturally, 31 cases had isolated papillary fronds with in 1 case branching papillary structures. The base of the papillary stalks were characterized as both broad and narrow (n = 24), only broad (n = 9), and only narrow (n = 3). The overlying urothelium of polypoid cystitis was diffusely and focally thickened in 8 cases and 5 cases, respectively. Umbrella cells were identified in 32 cases. Acute and chronic inflammation was present in 28 cases, moderate in 15, and mild in 13 cases. Eleven cases showed chronic inflammation, mild in 10, and moderate in 1 case. Reactive urothelial atypia was noted in 26 cases with mitotic figures present in 22 cases, frequent in 3 and rare in 19 cases. Stroma edema was seen in 32 cases with fibrosis within the polypoid stalks seen in 16 cases. The key to correctly diagnosing polypoid/papillary cystitis is to recognize at low magnification the reactive nature of the process with an inflamed background that is edematous or densely fibrous with predominantly simple, non-branching, broad-based fronds of relatively normal thickness urothelium, and not focus at higher power on the exceptional frond that may more closely resemble a urothelial neoplasm either architecturally or cytologically. In cases where the diagnosis of papillary neoplasia is not straightforward and there is a question of polypoid cystitis, pathologists should seek clinical history that might suggest a reactive process. Because the urologist can more often better recognize the inflammatory nature of the lesion than the pathologist, the pathologist should hesitate diagnosing urothelial neoplasia when the cystoscopic impression is that of an inflammatory lesion.

▶ Distinguishing papillary neoplasms of the urinary bladder from benign mimickers can be difficult. This is further compounded by the fact that inflammatory lesions may have associated atypia and occasional mitoses. The key to correctly diagnosing polypoid/papillary cystitis is to recognize at low magnification the reactive nature of the process. Typically, the lesion will have an inflamed background with edema/fibrosis. The epithelial architecture is of predominant simple, nonbranching, broad-based fronds of relatively normal thickness urothelium. The misleading feature can be the exceptional frond resembling an urothelial neoplasm either architecturally or cytologically. Pathologists should seek clinical history in cases where the diagnosis of papillary neoplasia is not straightforward and there is a question of polypoid cystitis. The history might indicate a reactive process. It is also important to correlate with the cystoscopic picture because the urologist can more often better recognize the inflammatory nature of the lesion than the pathologist. One should be conservative in diagnosing urothelial neoplasia when the cystoscopic impression is that of an inflammatory lesion.

R. Dhir, MD

Development of a Multiplexed Urine Assay for Prostate Cancer Diagnosis
Vener T, Derecho C, Baden J, et al (Veridex LLC, Johnson & Johnson Company, Warren, NJ; et al)
Clin Chem 54:874-882, 2008

Background.—Several studies have demonstrated the value of DNA methylation in urine-based assays for prostate cancer diagnosis. However, a multicenter validation with a clinical prototype has not been published.

Methods.—We developed a multiplexed, quantitative methylation-specific polymerase chain reaction (MSP) assay consisting of 3 methylation markers, *GSTP1*, *RARB*, and *APC*, and an endogenous control, *ACTB*, in a closed-tube, homogeneous assay format. We tested this format with urine samples collected after digital rectal examination from 234 patients with prostatespecific antigen (PSA) concentrations ≥2.5 µg/L in 2 independent patient cohorts from 9 clinical sites.

Results.—In the first cohort of 121 patients, we demonstrated 55% sensitivity and 80% specificity, with area under the curve (AUC) 0.69. In the second independent cohort of 113 patients, we found a comparable sensitivity of 53% and specificity of 76% (AUC 0.65). In the first cohort, as well as in a combined cohort, the MSP assay in conjunction with total PSA, digital rectal examination status, and age improved the AUC without MSP, although the difference was not statistically significant. Importantly, the *GSTP1* cycle threshold value demonstrated a good correlation (R = 0.84) with the number of cores found to contain prostate cancer or premalignant lesions on biopsy. Moreover, samples that exhibited methylation for either *GSTP1* or *RARB* typically contained higher tumor volumes at prostatectomy than those samples that did not exhibit methylation.

Conclusions.—These data confirm and extend previously reported studies and demonstrate the performance of a clinical prototype assay that should aid urologists in identifying men who should undergo biopsy.

▶ Screening for prostate cancer relies heavily on prostate-specific antigen (PSA) screening. This modality has its associated challenges related to false positive and false negative issues. One of the issues is that clinical guidance by PSA does result in unnecessary biopsy procedures. There is the need to have ancillary tests that can increase performance of positive biopsy procedures without unnecessary negative procedures. There has been a push to develop molecular panels associated with malignancy. One of these areas relate to methylated markers. This study has evaluated a methylation-specific polymerase chain reaction (MSP) assay consisting of 3 methylation markers—glutathione-S-transferase pi (*GSTP1*), retinoic acid receptor β (*RARB*), and adenomatous polyposis coli (*APC*). This study demonstrates respectable specificity. The sensitivity is relatively low and needs improvement. These results were reproducible and, therefore, represent testing initiative that could have clinical relevance. Another interesting feature was that the increased values of *GSTP1* (*GSTP1* cycle threshold value) demonstrated a good correlation with the number of cores with prostate cancer. Also, identification of methylation for either *GSTP1* or *RARB* correlated with higher tumor volumes at prostatectomy compared with those samples that did not exhibit methylation. Although these types of tests have issues that need to be resolved, they represent progress in developing molecular test panels.

R. Dhir, MD

Stat3 Promotes Metastatic Progression of Prostate Cancer
Abdulghani J, Gu L, Dagvadorj A, et al (Kimmel Cancer Ctr, Thomas Jefferson Univ, Philadelphia, PA; et al)
Am J Pathol 172:1717-1728, 2008

There are currently no effective therapies for metastatic prostate cancer because the molecular mechanisms that underlie the metastatic spread of primary prostate cancer are unclear. Transcription factor Stat3 is constitutively active in malignant prostate epithelium, and its activation is associated with high histological grade and advanced cancer stage. In this work, we hypothesized that Stat3 stimulates metastatic progression of prostate cancer. We show that Stat3 is active in 77% of lymph node and 67% of bone metastases of clinical human prostate cancers. Importantly, adenoviral gene delivery of wild-type Stat3 (AdWTStat3) to DU145 human prostate cancer cells increased the number of lung metastases by 33-fold in an experimental metastasis assay compared with controls. Using various methods to inhibit Stat3, we demonstrated that Stat3 promotes human prostate cancer cell migration. Stat3 induced the formation of lamellipodia in both DU145 and PC-3 cells, further supporting the concept that Stat3 promotes a migratory phenotype of human prostate cancer cells. Moreover, Stat3 caused the rearrangement of cytoplasmic actin stress fibers and microtubules in both DU145 and PC-3 cells. Finally, inhibition of the Jak2 tyrosine kinase decreased both activation of Stat3 and prostate cancer cell motility. Collectively, these data indicate that transcription factor Stat3 is involved in metastatic behavior of human prostate cancer cells and may provide a therapeutic target to prevent metastatic spread of primary prostate cancer.

▶ There has been a significant push in the past few years in the evaluation of phosphorylated antigens. Many factors important in neoplastic pathways are activated by the process of phosphorylation. Detection of phosphorylated molecules reflects their activation status and is more meaningful than detection of just the molecule. A major reason for the increasing importance of the study of these phosphorylated molecules is the presence of therapeutic tools that can target or prevent phosphorylation, thereby inactivating these molecules. This study evaluates the role of phosphorylated Stat3 (pStat3) in prostate cancer. Although preliminary, the data indicates a role of pStat3 in prostate cancer. The data shows that transcription factor Stat3 is involved in metastatic behavior of human prostate cancer cells and may provide a therapeutic target to prevent metastatic spread of primary prostate cancer.

R. Dhir, MD

MUC2 **expression in primary mucinous and nonmucinous adenocarcinoma of the prostate: an analysis of 50 cases on radical prostatectomy**
Osunkoya AO, Adsay NV, Cohen C, et al (Emory Univ School of Medicine, Atlanta, GA; et al)
Mod Pathol 21:789-794, 2008

The expression of mucin (*MUC2*) in prostate cancer has not been well studied previously and may be of prognostic and pathobiologic significance. It is, however, well known that *MUC2* expression in mucinous pancreatic and breast cancer represents an indolent pathway since these tumors have a significantly better outcome than their conventional counterparts. Twenty-five cases each of Gleason pattern 3 and 4 mucinous adenocarcinoma of the prostate defined by greater than 25% mucinous component and nonmucinous adenocarcinoma of the prostate were obtained from the surgical pathology files of the Johns Hopkins Hospital and Emory University Hospital. Immunohistochemical stains were performed for *MUC2* on all 50 cases. Mean patient age was 60 years (range 44–72 years). *MUC2* was expressed in all 25 cases (100%) of mucinous adenocarcinoma of the prostate, irrespective of the Gleason pattern. The nonmucinous component of these cases was negative for *MUC2*. In contrast, *MUC2* expression was significantly lower in nonmucinous adenocarcinoma of the prostate, detected in only 6/25 cases as a focal finding, while 19/25 (76%) of nonmucinous adenocarcinoma of the prostate were completely negative for *MUC2* (*P*<0.01). In six cases that showed focal positivity, *MUC2* was expressed in areas with Gleason pattern 3 cancer with extensive mucinous fibroplasia (one case) and prominent intraluminal mucin (five cases). Other areas of these tumors were negative for *MUC2*. Mucinous adenocarcinoma of the prostate shows diffuse expression of

MUC2, a known tumor suppressor, which is not present in either normal prostate or the majority of conventional adenocarcinomas of this organ. This indicates that mucinous adenocarcinoma of the prostate is indeed of the 'colloid type' akin to those in other exocrine organs. It is highly conceivable that this *de novo* expression of *MUC2* has a role, not only in the mucinous differentiation of these tumors and their colloid pattern, but also in their relatively indolent behavior that has been recently elucidated.

▶ Current experience indicates that certain mucinous tumors, notably mucinous carcinomas of the pancreas and breast, behave in an indolent manner. Studies have delineated a strong association of indolent behavior and better outcome and the expression of MUC2, a known tumor suppressor. This study evaluated MUC2 expression in conventional and mucinous carcinomas of the prostate. One hundred percent of the mucinous carcinoma of the prostate expressed MUC2, irrespective of the Gleason pattern. The nonmucinous areas were MUC2 negative. In contrast, MUC2 expression was significantly lower in nonmucinous adenocarcinoma and was seen in less than 25% of cases. When seen, the expression was focal. It was also observed that MUC2 expression was not present in normal prostate. MUC2 may, therefore, have a role not only in the mucinous differentiation of these tumors, but also in their relatively indolent behavior.

R. Dhir, MD

Evaluation of whole slide image immunohistochemistry interpretation in challenging prostate needle biopsies
Fine JL, Grzybicki DM, Silowash R, et al (Univ of Pittsburgh School of Medicine, PA)
Hum Pathol 39:564-572, 2008

Whole slide images (WSIs), also known as virtual slides, can support electronic distribution of immunohistochemistry (IHC) stains to pathologists that rely on remote sites for these services. This may lead to improvement in turnaround times, reduction of courier costs, fewer errors in slide distribution, and automated image analyses. Although this approach is practiced de facto today in some large laboratories, there are no clinical validation studies on this approach. Our retrospective study evaluated the interpretation of IHC stains performed in difficult prostate biopsies using WSIs. The study included 30 foci with IHC stains identified by the original pathologist as both difficult and pivotal to the final diagnosis. WSIs were created from the glass slides using a scanning robot (T2, Aperio Technologies, Vista, CA). An evaluation form was designed to capture data in 2 phases: (1) interpretation of WSIs and (2) interpretation of glass slides. Data included stain interpretations, diagnoses, and other parameters such as time required to diagnose and image/slide quality. Data were also collected from an expert prostate pathologist, consensus meetings, and a poststudy focus group. WSI diagnostic validity (intraobserver pairwise κ statistics) was "almost perfect" for 1 pathologist, "substantial" for 3 pathologists, and "moderate" for 1 pathologist. Diagnostic agreement between the final/ consensus diagnoses of the group and those of the domain expert was "almost perfect" (κ = 0.817). Except for one instance, WSI technology was not felt to be the cause of disagreements. These results are encouraging and compare favorably with other efforts to quantify diagnostic variability in surgical pathology. With thorough training, careful validation of specific applications, and regular postsignout review of glass IHC slides (eg, quality assurance review), WSI technology can be used for IHC stain interpretation.

▶ Emerging technologies are playing an increasingly important role in medicine. Pathology is no exception to this evolution. Whole slide images (WSIs) are also known as virtual slides. WSI are digital facsimiles of entire histopathologic sections originally mounted on glass microscope slides. WSI images are viewed using software termed "virtual microscopy software." This software allows the user to adjust magnification and navigate to any portion of the image. WSI has primarily been limited to education and proficiency testing. However, it is now being used for quality assurance (QA) activities as well. The clinical effectiveness of WSI, using static and dynamic digital imaging telepathology, is well documented. This study evaluated the role of WSI in the interpretation of immunohistochemistry (IHC). The results indicate that WSI technology is mature for its adoption as a means of IHC interpretation. This has wide ranging significance because it will allow pathologists in relatively remote locations to rapidly access stains performed for them in reference laboratories. This process will be facilitated further by the availability of free/cheap viewing software.

R. Dhir, MD

Assessing the Value of Reflex Fluorescence In Situ Hybridization Testing in the Diagnosis of Bladder Cancer When Routine Urine Cytological Examination is Equivocal
Kipp BR, Halling KC, Campion MB, et al (Mayo Clinic and Foundation, Rochester, MN)
J Urol 179:1296-1301, 2008

Purpose.—We evaluated the usefulness of fluorescence in situ hybridization in the treatment of patients with equivocal cytology.
Materials and Methods.—Fluorescence in situ hybridization was performed in residual urine from 124 patients with a cytological diagnosis of cell clusters (22), atypical findings (46) and suspicious findings (56) who had a same day cystoscopy result and bladder biopsy within 6 months of the cytology diagnosis. Urologists and fluorescence in situ hybridization

technologists were blinded to the matching fluorescence in situ hybridization and cystoscopy results, respectively.

Results.—In conjunction with cystoscopy fluorescence in situ hybridization was significantly more sensitive than cystoscopy alone for detecting cancer (87% vs 67%, p <0.001) and muscle invasive cancer (94% vs 56%, p = 0.031). Of the 124 equivocal cytology specimens 58 (47%) were positive by fluorescence in situ hybridization. Of these patients 53 (91%) had subsequent evidence of carcinoma, including Ta tumors in 17, Tis in 13, T1 in 8 and T2 or greater in 15, on the first followup biopsy. Three of the 5 remaining patients with a positive fluorescence in situ hybridization result and negative first followup biopsy had evidence of cancer at a later date, including TxN+ disease in 2 and Tis in 1. A total of 66 specimens were diagnosed as negative by fluorescence in situ hybridization. Of these patients 34 (52%) had negative biopsy results, whereas the remaining 32 (48%) demonstrated bladder cancer, including Ta disease in 20, Tis in 8, T1 in 2 and T2+ in 2. Cystoscopy detected 21 of the 32 tumors (66%) not detected by fluorescence in situ hybridization, while fluorescence in situ hybridization detected 17 of the 28 (61%) not detected by cystoscopy.

Conclusions.—Our data suggest that fluorescence in situ hybridization with cystoscopy can aid clinicians in the diagnosis of bladder cancer in patients with equivocal cytology.

▶ Detection and surveillance of patients with urothelial carcinoma (UC) relies heavily on urine cytology and cystoscopy. Urine cytology is widely used as it is noninvasive, inexpensive, and has good specificity. However, cytology has relatively low sensitivity for detecting low-grade UC. An equivocal cytology result creates a clinical conundrum. Data suggest that fewer than 50% of patients with an equivocal cytology result have cancer on follow-up. Ancillary testing that provides additional insight into this problem would be of great value. UroVysion fluorescence in situ hybridization (FISH) testing has become an accepted mechanism for screening and surveillance for UC. In this study, 91% of the FISH-positive equivocal cytology specimens had subsequent evidence of carcinoma on the first follow-up biopsy. The negative predictive value of FISH was not that good because 48% demonstrated bladder cancer. This is an evolving methodology and can have use in specific clinical situations.

R. Dhir, MD

Change in Prostate Specific Antigen Following Androgen Stimulation is an Independent Predictor of Prostate Cancer Diagnosis
Svatek RS, Shulman MJ, Benaim EA, et al (Univ of Texas Southwestern Med Ctr at Dallas, TX)
J Urol 179:2192-2196, 2008

Purpose.—We tested the hypothesis that a single exogenous androgen injection in men with low prostate specific antigen would provoke a differential prostate specific antigen response that would correlate with the presence and volume of cancer at biopsy.

Materials and Methods.—Following institutional review board approval 40 men with prostate specific antigen between 2.5 and 4.0 ng/ml were given 1 intramuscular injection of 400 mg testosterone cypionate at the start of the study. Prostate specific antigen and early morning serum testosterone were measured at baseline, 48 hours, and weeks 1, 2 and 4. All men underwent 12-core transrectal ultrasound guided biopsy at week 4.

Results.—Of the 40 men 18 (45%) were diagnosed with prostate cancer. The mean change in prostate specific antigen from baseline to 4 weeks was 3.1 to 3.4 ng/ml (9.7%) in men found to have benign findings on biopsy compared to a mean increase of 2.9 to 3.8 ng/ml (29%) in those with prostate cancer ($p = 0.006$). The change in prostate specific antigen following androgen stimulation was significantly associated with the percent of tissue involved with cancer and it was an independent predictor of cancer diagnosis on univariate and multivariate analysis.

Conclusions.—An increase in prostate specific antigen following androgen stimulation in men with prostate specific antigen between 2.5 and 4.0 ng/ml was highly predictive of the subsequent diagnosis of prostate cancer and it correlated with disease volume. If these findings are corroborated, prostate specific antigen provocation may become an important strategy to identify men at risk for harboring prostate cancer and minimize the number undergoing unnecessary biopsies.

▶ Prostate-specific antigen (PSA) screening is a traditional approach for prostate cancer. A total PSA threshold of 4.0 ng/mL has been the traditional trigger point for a biopsy. However, studies have shown that a lower threshold may be indicated because approximately 20% to 25% of men with PSA 2.5 to 4.0 ng/mL are found to have clinically and pathologically significant prostate cancer. Unfortunately, the diagnostic performance characteristics of PSA are particularly poor in the less than 4.0 ng/mL range. Lowering PSA threshold for a biopsy trigger event could significantly increase the number of unnecessary biopsies. This article describes a new strategy to help identify prostate cancer while avoiding unnecessary biopsies. The approach of androgen stimulation and assessment of PSA levels seem to provide a mechanism to stratify patients with PSA level less than 4. Individuals showing a 10% or higher PSA increase had pure red cell aplasia (PRCA) in 36% of cases as compared with only 8% who demonstrated PSA increase of less than 10%. This approach needs to be validated with a larger patient cohort. In addition, it also will need to be assessed for possible side effects of exogenous testosterone administration in individuals with a hormone sensitive tumor.

R. Dhir, MD

Hypoxia-inducible factor-1α expression correlates with focal macrophage infiltration, angiogenesis and unfavourable prognosis in urothelial carcinoma

Chai C-Y, Chen W-T, Hung W-C, et al (Kaohsiung Med Univ, Taiwan; Kaohsiung Med Univ Chung-Ho Memorial Hosp, Taiwan; Natl Sun Yat-Sen Univ, Kaohsiung, Taiwan)
J Clin Pathol 61:658-664, 2008

Background.—Hypoxia inducible factor (HIF)-1α is a critical regulatory protein of cellular response to hypoxia and is closely related to angiogenic process.

Aims.—To explore the potential role and the prognostic value of HIF-1α in urothelial carcinoma (UC).

Methods.—Clinicopathological and follow-up data on 99 UC cases were reviewed and immunostained for HIF-1α, CD68, vascular endothelial growth factor (VEGF) and CD34 antigen. Tumour-associated macrophage (TAM) counts and HIF-1α expression were compared with clinicopathologic characteristics, overall survival (OS) and disease-free survival rates (DFS).

Results.—High expression of HIF-1α was detected in 55 of 99 (55.6%) tumours. HIF-1α expression was correlated with tumour size, histological grade, tumour invasiveness and recurrence. VEGF and microvessel density (MVD) demonstrated their positive correlation with HIF-1α overexpression, supporting the correlation of HIF-1α upregulation with tumour angiogenesis. Higher TAM infiltration was identified in high expression of HIF-1α cases rather than HIF-1α low expression cases (p = 0.002). Kaplan-Meier analysis found that HIF-1α overexpression and high TAM count was only associated with worse DFS (p = 0.009, p = 0.023) but was not associated with OS (p = 0.696, p = 0.141). Multivariate analyses indicated only tumour size (p = 0.038) to be an independently significant prognostic factor for OS, in addition, HIF-1α expression (p = 0.011), as well as histological grade (p = 0.038), and MVD (p = 0.004), to be independently significant prognostic factors for DFS.

Conclusions.—Our results indicate that HIF-1α is a key regulator of the angiogenic cascade. We show that HIF-1α is an independent prognostic factor for disease-free survival.

▶ There is a need for identifying markers that can provide prognostic information in urothelial carcinomas. One approach is to evaluate markers associated with angiogenesis. Angiogenesis is essential for the growth, invasion, and metastasis of tumors. Absence of angiogenesis limits tumor growth. In addition, it is documented that regions of hypoxia may contribute to resistance to chemotherapy and radiotherapy, poor prognosis, and progression of disease (local and distant). Hypoxia inducible factor-1 (HIF-1) is a major regulator of cell adaptation to hypoxic stress, and plays a critical role in tumorigenesis and angiogenesis. High expression of HIF-1α was seen and correlated with tumor size, grade, invasiveness, and recurrence. Vascular endothelial growth factor (VEGF) and microvessel density (MVD) also correlated with HIF-1α overexpression.

HIF-1α is an independently significant prognostic factor for disease-free survival. Assessment of this marker could be of value in urothelial carcinoma assessment.

R. Dhir, MD

Comparison of Prostate Specific Antigen Velocity in Screened Versus Referred Patients With Prostate Cancer

Meeks JJ, Thaxton CS, Loeb S, et al (Northwestern Feinberg School of Medicine, Chicago, IL; The Johns Hopkins School of Medicine, Baltimore, MD; et al)
J Urol 179:1340-1343, 2008

Purpose.—Despite the tremendous stage migration associated with prostate cancer screening to our knowledge it remains unproven whether prostate specific antigen based screening decreases prostate cancer specific mortality. Recent studies have shown that prostate specific antigen velocity more than 2 ng/ml per year in the year before diagnosis is associated with a significantly greater risk of prostate cancer specific mortality after treatment. This may serve as a surrogate marker for prostate cancer outcomes. We compared the prostate specific antigen velocity profile between patients with prostate cancer in whom the tumor was detected in a formal screening study and those who were referred for treatment.

Materials and Methods.—We evaluated prostate specific antigen velocity in 1,101 men from a prostate cancer screening study and in 368 not enrolled in a screening study who were referred for treatment. All patients underwent radical prostatectomy for clinically localized disease and had multiple preoperative prostate specific antigen measurements to calculate prostate specific antigen velocity.

Results.—Median prostate specific antigen velocity before diagnosis was significantly higher in referred vs screened men (1.35 vs 0.68 ng/ml per year, p <0.0001). In addition, a significantly greater proportion of referred patients had prostate specific antigen velocity more than 2 ng/ml per year (38% vs 17%, p <0.0001). On multivariate analysis using prostate specific antigen, clinical stage and biopsy Gleason score screened vs referred status was a significant independent predictor of prostate specific antigen velocity more than 2 ng/ml per year (p <0.0004).

Conclusions.—Prostate specific antigen velocity more than 2 ng/ml per year has been linked to a significantly greater risk of prostate cancer specific mortality. Patients who underwent serial screening had a more favorable prostate specific antigen velocity profile at diagnosis, suggesting that screen detected prostate cancer may be more likely to be cured with definitive therapy.

▶ It is well documented that prostate cancer (PCa) screening is associated with a significant stage migration as the cancers are detected earlier. However, it has not been evaluated whether prostate-specific antigen (PSA)-based screening decreases PCa specific mortality. It has also been documented that PSA velocity

(PSAV) of > 2 ng/mL per year in the year before diagnosis is associated with a significantly greater risk of PCa specific mortality after treatment. This study compared PSAV profile and outcomes between patients with PCa in a formal screening study versus those referred for treatment (nonscreened). The nonscreened group had a significantly higher PSAV versus the screened group (median 1.35 vs 0.68 ng/mL/y). In addition, a significantly greater proportion of nonscreened patients had PSAV > 2 ng/mL per year (38% vs 17%). The data suggest that patients who underwent serial screening had a more favorable PSAV profile at diagnosis, suggesting that screen-detected PCa may be more likely to be cured with definitive therapy.

R. Dhir, MD

Tertiary Gleason Pattern 5 in Gleason 7 Prostate Cancer Predicts Pathological Stage and Biochemical Recurrence
Sim HG, Telesca D, Culp SH (Univ of Washington, Seattle, WA; et al)
J Urol 179:1775-1779, 2008

Purpose.—Gleason sum 7 prostate cancers are a heterogeneous group with diverse tumor behaviors and disease outcomes. Tertiary Gleason patterns are reported with increasing frequency, particularly in prostatectomy pathology reports. We studied the pathological and biochemical outcome following radical prostatectomy in men with Gleason sum 7 and tertiary Gleason pattern 5.

Materials and Methods.—We reviewed 1,110 cases of clinically localized prostate cancer treated with primary radical prostatectomy between January 1998 and August 2006 through a prospectively collected prostate cancer database. Patients who underwent neoadjuvant or adjuvant hormonal deprivation, radiation or systemic chemotherapy were excluded.

Results.—Of the 1,110 patients 509 had Gleason sum 7 cancer. Tertiary Gleason pattern was present in 66 of 509 cases (13%) and it was absent in 443 (87%). On multivariate analysis tertiary Gleason pattern 5 was associated with higher pT stage (OR 2.55, 95% CI 1.40–4.65) and biochemical recurrence (HR 1.78, 95% CI 1.00–3.17). On subgroup analysis when patients with Gleason sum 3 + 4 + 5 and 4 + 3 + 5 were compared to their respective referent groups without the tertiary Gleason pattern, the 2 groups showed a trend toward higher pathological stage and prostate specific antigen progression. Patients with Gleason sum 3 + 4 with no tertiary pattern had higher PSA recurrence-free probability than those with Gleason sum 3 + 4 + 5 or 4 + 3 and patients with Gleason sum 4 + 3 + 5 had the lowest PSA recurrence-free probability.

Conclusions.—In patients with Gleason sum 7 prostate cancer tertiary Gleason grade 5 is significantly associated with higher pT stage and biochemical recurrence. Larger studies are needed to assess the predictive value of tertiary grade compared to other established parameters in predicting the long-term oncological outcome after radical prostatectomy.

▶ The Gleason system is the most commonly used system worldwide for grading prostate cancer. Histological grade is divided into primary and secondary patterns based on glandular differentiation at low magnification. The sum of the assigned primary and secondary patterns is called the Gleason score and has been shown to correlate with pathological stage and biochemical recurrence. There may exist smaller areas with tumor patterns of a higher grade compared with the primary and secondary patterns; so called tertiary patterns. Limited studies have examined the usefulness of reporting the tertiary Gleason patterns and found association with higher pathological stage and probable worse prostate-specific antigen (PSA) progression. This study looked at the specific issue of pathological and biochemical outcome after radical prostatectomy in men with Gleason sum 7 and tertiary Gleason pattern 5. Not surprisingly Gleason 7 tumors with tertiary pattern 5 were significantly associated with a higher pT stage and biochemical recurrence. It is therefore important to recognize and report a tertiary 5 pattern in the RP.

R. Dhir, MD

PCA3 Molecular Urine Assay Correlates With Prostate Cancer Tumor Volume: Implication in Selecting Candidates for Active Surveillance

Nakanishi H, Groskopf J, Fritsche HA, et al (The Univ of Texas M. D. Anderson Cancer Ctr, Houston, TX; Gen-Probe Incorporated, San Diego, California)
J Urol 179:1804-1810, 2008

Purpose.—Prostate cancer gene 3 (PCA3) has shown promise as a molecular marker in prostate cancer detection. We assessed the association of urinary PCA3 score with prostatectomy tumor volume and other clinical and pathological features.

Materials and Methods.—Urine specimens were collected after digital rectal examination from 59 men scheduled for prostate biopsy and 83 men scheduled for radical prostatectomy. Prostatectomy findings were evaluable for 96 men. PCA3 and prostate specific antigen mRNAs were quantified with Gen-Probe DTS® 400 System. The PCA3 score was defined as the ratio of PCA3 mRNA/prostate specific antigen mRNA $\times 10^3$.

Results.—The PCA3 score in men with negative biopsies (30) and positive biopsies (29) were significantly different (median 21.1 and 31.0, respectively, p = 0.029). The PCA3 score was significantly correlated with total tumor volume in prostatectomy specimens (r = 0.269, p = 0.008), and was also associated with prostatectomy Gleason score (6 vs 7 or greater, p = 0.005) but not with other clinical and pathological features. The PCA3 score was significantly different when comparing low volume/low grade cancer (dominant tumor volume less than 0.5 cc, Gleason score 6) and significant cancer (p = 0.007). On multivariate analysis PCA3 was the best predictor of total tumor volume in prostatectomy (p = 0.001). Receiver operating characteristic curve analysis showed that the PCA3 score could discriminate low volume cancer (total tumor volume less than 0.5 cc) well with area under the curve of 0.757.

Conclusions.—The PCA3 score appears to stratify men based on prostatectomy tumor volume and Gleason score, and may have clinical applicability in selecting men who have low volume/low grade cancer.

▶ Molecular methods for prostate cancer (PCa) detection are now commercially available. One such method uses the prostate cancer gene 3 (PCA3). PCA3 was first described in 1999 and is a noncoding, prostate-specific messenger RNA (mRNA) highly overexpressed in PCa tissue compared with benign prostatic tissue. PCA3 diagnostic testing is available as a urinary assay as a PCa marker, measuring relative overexpression of PCA3 mRNA compared with PSA mRNA. The test generates a PCA3 score. Recent studies have shown that the PCA3 test could improve diagnostic accuracy of PCa detection, especially in the PSA gray zone. This study assessed association of urinary PCA3 score with prostatectomy tumor volume and other clinical and pathological features. PCA3 discriminated the cancer versus noncancer patients. In addition, the PCA3 score stratified men based on prostatectomy tumor volume and Gleason score. It may therefore have clinical applicability in selecting men who have low volume/low grade cancer for possible conservative nonsurgical approaches like watchful waiting.

R. Dhir, MD

[-2]Proenzyme Prostate Specific Antigen for Prostate Cancer Detection: A National Cancer Institute Early Detection Research Network Validation Study

Sokoll LJ, Wang Y, Feng Z, et al (Johns Hopkins Med Institutions, Baltimore, MD; Fred Hutchinson Cancer Res Ctr, Seattle, WA; et al)
J Urol 180:539-543, 2008

Purpose.—This study evaluated the [-2]proenzyme prostate specific antigen serum marker using a blinded reference specimen set from 3 National Cancer Institute Early Detection Research Network centers from men with an indication for prostate biopsy.

Materials and Methods.—Serum was collected before biopsy from 123 men with no prior biopsy or prostate cancer history. Specimens (cancer cases 51%, noncancer controls 49%) were selected equally from the 3 sites, and analyzed for prostate specific antigen, free prostate specific antigen, [-2]proenzyme prostate specific antigen, benign prostate specific antigen and testosterone (Beckman Coulter ACCESS® analyzer).

Results.—There was no difference in total prostate specific antigen concentrations (noncancer 6.80 ± 5.20 ng/ml, cancer 6.94 ± 5.12 ng/ml) among the groups. Overall %[-2]proenzyme prostate specific antigen had the greatest area under the curve (AUC 0.69) followed by percent free prostate specific antigen (AUC 0.61). For %[-2]proenzyme prostate specific antigen maximal sensitivity was 60% and specificity was 70%. A logistic regression model combining prostate specific antigen, benign prostate specific antigen, percent free prostate specific antigen, %[-2]proenzyme prostate specific antigen, [-2]proenzyme prostate specific antigen/benign prostate specific antigen and testosterone had an AUC of 0.73. In the 2 to 10 ng/ml prostate specific antigen range %[-2]proenzyme prostate specific antigen and the model had the largest AUC (0.73). The AUC for percent free prostate specific antigen was 0.53. Specificities for %[-2]proenzyme prostate specific antigen, the logistic regression model and percent free prostate specific antigen at 90% sensitivity were 41%, 32% and 18%, and at 95% sensitivity were 31%, 26% and 16%, respectively.

Conclusions.—%[-2]proenzyme prostate specific antigen was the best predictor of prostate cancer detection compared to percent free prostate specific antigen, particularly in the 2 to 10 ng/ml total prostate specific antigen range. These findings provide a rationale for broader validation studies to determine whether %[-2]proenzyme prostate specific antigen alone can replace other molecular prostate specific antigen assays (such as percent free prostate specific antigen) for improving the accuracy of prostate cancer early detection. These findings also support the usefulness of well characterized, carefully collected reference sets to evaluate new biomarkers.

▶ Prostate-specific antigen (PSA) is used for screening for prostate cancer (PCa). There are issues with the sensitivity and specificity associated with use of PSA. It is known that PSA has various disease-specific isoforms. Use of these may improve some of the current limitations of PSA in the early detection of PCa. [-2]proPSA is the most prevalent form in tumor extracts and is a promising biomarker. This article presents the experience of the National Cancer Institute Early Detection Research Network (NCI EDRN) evaluating new prostate biomarkers using a common, retrospective, archival, blinded reference set of serum samples collected from men with an indication for prostate biopsy at 3 EDRN sites. Percent[-2]proenzyme PSA was the best predictor of PCa detection compared with percent-free PSA, particularly in the 2 to 10 ng/mL total PSA range. Larger validation studies are needed before this marker can become part of the clinical diagnostic algorithm.

R. Dhir, MD

The Impact of the 2005 International Society of Urological Pathology Consensus Conference on Standard Gleason Grading of Prostatic Carcinoma in Needle Biopsies
Billis A, Guimaraes MS, Freitas LLL, et al (State Univ of Campinas (Unicamp), Brazil)
J Urol 180:548-553, 2008

Purpose.—At an International Society of Urological Pathology consensus conference in 2005 the Gleason grading system for prostatic carcinoma underwent its first major revision. We compared the concordance of pattern and change of prognostic groups for the conventional and the modified Gleason grading, and checked the discriminative power of the modified Gleason grading.

Materials and Methods.—The grading was based on 172 prostatic needle biopsies of patients subsequently undergoing radical prostatectomy. Four prognostic Gleason grading groups were considered, divided into scores of 2–4, 5–6, 7 and 8–10. To check the discriminative power of the modified Gleason grading we compared the time of biochemical (prostate specific antigen) progression-free outcome according to prognostic groups between standard and revised grading.

Results.—The greatest impact of the International Society of Urological Pathology consensus recommendations for Gleason grading was seen on the secondary pattern which had the lowest percentage of concordance and was reflected in a change toward higher Gleason prognostic groups. Of 172 patients in whom the Gleason prognostic group was changed (to higher grades) based solely on the consensus criteria, 46 (26.7%) had higher preoperative prostate specific antigen, more extensive tumors and positive surgical margins, and higher pathological stage. The revised Gleason grading identified in this series a higher number of patients in the aggressive prognostic group Gleason score 8–10 who had a significantly shorter time to biochemical progression-free outcome after radical prostatectomy (log rank $p = 0.011$).

Conclusions.—The findings of this study indicate that the recommendations of the International Society of Urological Pathology are a valuable refinement of the standard Gleason grading system.

▶ The 2005 International Society of Urological Pathology (ISUP) consensus conference modified the Gleason grading system for prostatic carcinoma. This study compares the concordance of patterns and change of prognostic groups for the conventional and modified Gleason grading on needle prostatic biopsies of patients subsequently undergoing radical prostatectomy (RP). It evaluates the discriminative power of modified Gleason grading on the time of biochemical prostate-specific antigen (PSA) progression-free outcome according to prognostic groups between the standard and revised grading. The greatest impact of the modified grading was on the secondary pattern and resulted in a shift toward the higher Gleason groups. These patients demonstrated an aggressive behavior with a significantly shorter time to biochemical recurrence after RP. The findings of this study validate the modified Gleason scoring schema recommended by the ISUP.

R. Dhir, MD

11 Kidney

Loss of chromosome 9p is an independent prognostic factor in patients with clear cell renal cell carcinoma
Brunelli M, Eccher A, Gobbo S, et al (Univ of Verona, Italy; et al)
Mod Pathol 21:1-6, 2008

Loss of chromosome 9p has been implicated in the progression of renal cell carcinoma. We evaluated the clinical utility of fluorescence *in situ* hybridization analysis of loss of chromosome 9p in 73 patients with clear cell renal cell carcinomas with varied stage, size, grade, necrosis (SSIGN) scores. Loss of chromosome 9p was observed in 13 tumors (18%). The 5-year cancer-specific survival of patients without loss of chromosome 9p was 88% and was 43% in those with loss of chromosome 9p ($P < 0.001$). Local extension of the primary tumor according to the 2002 TNM staging system, lymph node involvement, the presence of distant metastases, and the SSIGN score were the other variables that predicted cancer-specific survival in univariate analysis. Loss of chromosome 9p was an independent prognostic factor in multivariate analysis. Our data indicate that the detection of chromosome 9p loss by fluorescence *in situ* hybridization analysis of clear cell renal cell carcinoma adds prognostic information beyond the pathological factors included in the current predictive models for renal cell carcinoma, such as SSIGN score.

▶ There are no definite prognostic markers available for renal tumors. The most frequent historical parameter used is the Fuhrman nuclear grade. A higher Fuhrman grade is associated with a poorer outcome. This article highlights loss of chromosome 9p as an independent prognostic marker in patients with clear cell renal cell carcinomas. Of the 73 cases analyzed, loss of chromosome 9p was observed in 13 tumors (18%). This loss had a significant association with 5-year cancer-specific survival. Patients without loss of chromosome 9p had a cancer-specific survival of 88% versus 43% in those with loss of chromosome 9p. Loss of chromosome 9p was an independent prognostic factor in multivariate analysis. It seems to be of value to assess chromosome 9p loss by fluorescence in situ hybridization (FISH) because it provides definite prognostic information.

R. Dhir, MD

Identification of Pro-MMP-7 as a Serum Marker for Renal Cell Carcinoma by Use of Proteomic Analysis

Sarkissian G, Fergelot P, Lamy P-J, et al (Cezanne SAS, Parc Scientifique Georges Besse, Nimes; Univ Hosp Ctr-Pontchaillou Hosp, Rennes; Val d'Aurelle-Paul Lamarque Cancer Inst, Montpellier, et al)
Clin Chem 54:574-581, 2008

Background.—No validated renal cell carcinoma (RCC) marker is known for detection of asymptomatic disease in selected populations or for prognostic purposes or treatment monitoring. We identified immunogenic proteins as tumor markers for RCC by combining conventional proteome analysis with serological screening, and we investigated the diagnostic clinical value of such markers in serum.

Methods.—We studied the immunogenic protein expression profile of CAL 54, a human RCC cell line, by 2-dimensional electrophoresis combined with immunoblotting using sera from healthy donors compared with RCC patients. We developed a homogeneous, fluorescent, dual-monoclonal immunoassay for metalloproteinase 7 (MMP-7) and used it to measure MMP-7 in sera from 30 healthy donors, 30 RCC patients, and 40 control patients.

Results.—Pro-MMP-7 (29 kDa; pI 7.7) in the CAL 54 cell line secretome was an immunogenic protein reactive with RCC patient sera but not with control sera. The concentrations of pro-MMP-7 were increased (P <0.0001) in sera of RCC patients (median 7.56 µg/L; range 3.12–30.5 µg/L) compared with healthy controls (median 2.13 µg/L; range 0.17–3.5 µg/ L). Serum pro-MMP-7 had a sensitivity of 93% (95% CI 78%–99%) at a specificity of 75% (59%–87%) for RCC in the samples tested.

Conclusion.—Proteomics technology combined with serology led to the identification of serum pro-MMP-7 as a marker of RCC and represents a powerful tool in searching for candidate proteins as biomarkers.

▶ The identification of renal cell carcinomas (RCCs) is dependent primarily on either radiology or investigation of clinical symptoms (mass/hematuria/flank pain). There currently is no validated RCC marker for detection of asymptomatic disease. This particular study is provocative and provides interesting data. The design used immunogenic protein profile of a cell line using 2-dimensional electrophoresis and combined it with immunoblotting using sera from healthy donors combined with patients with RCC. This novel approach resulted in identification of metalloproteinase 7 (MMP-7) as a potential marker for screening for RCC. This marker has a high sensitivity and is fairly specific. This approach could have diagnostic value as a screening serum marker for RCC. In addition, this approach could also lead to identification of other novel markers.

R. Dhir, MD

Renal medullary carcinoma: rhabdoid features and the absence of INI1 expression as markers of aggressive behavior
Cheng JX, Tretiakova M, Gong C, et al (Univ of Chicago, IL)
Mod Pathol 21:647-652, 2008

Renal medullary carcinoma is a rare, well-recognized highly aggressive tumor of varied histopathology, which occurs in young patients with sickle cell trait or disease. Rhabdoid elements, occasionally seen in high-grade renal tumors including renal medullary carcinoma, possibly represent a pathologic marker of aggressive behavior. INI1 (hSNF5/SMARCB1/BAF47) is a highly conserved factor in the ATP-dependent chromatin-modifying complex. Loss of this factor in mice results in aggressive rhabdoid tumors or lymphomas. In humans, the loss of INI1 expression has been reported in pediatric renal rhabdoid tumors, central nervous system atypical teratoid/rhabdoid tumors and epithelioid sarcomas, a possible primary soft tissue rhabdoid tumor. This study compares five renal medullary carcinomas with 10 high-grade renal cell carcinomas (five with rhabdoid features), two urothelial carcinomas and two pediatric renal rhabdoid tumors. All five renal medullary carcinomas, irrespective of histopathology, showed complete loss of INI1 expression similar to that seen in pediatric renal rhabdoid tumors. In contrast, all renal cell carcinomas or urothelial carcinomas, including those with histological rhabdoid features, expressed INI1. Clinically, all five of the patients with renal medullary carcinoma and the two patients with rhabdoid tumors presented with extra-renal metastases at the time of diagnosis. This study demonstrates that renal medullary carcinoma and renal rhabdoid tumor share a common molecular/genetic alteration, which is closely linked to their aggressive biological behavior. However, the absence of INI1 expression is not necessarily predictive of rhabdoid histopathology but remains associated with aggressive behavior in renal medullary carcinoma.

▶ Young patients with sickle cell trait or disease can rarely present with a highly aggressive tumor of varied histopathology, called renal medullary carcinomas. Some of the medullary carcinomas may show rhabdoid features and could be difficult to differentiate from the more frequent conventional renal cell carcinomas with rhabdoid features. Discrimination is facilitated by the presence of definitive conventional tumor; however, sometimes this might not be the case as there might be predominant rhabdoid tumor. This article describes a mechanism to discriminate between the medullary carcinomas with rhabdoid features versus the rhabdoid tumors from the conventional renal carcinomas. INI1 (hSNF5/SMARCB1/BAF47) is a highly conserved factor in the ATP-dependent chromatin-modifying complex and is of value in addressing this issue. In humans, the loss of INI1 expression has been reported in pediatric renal rhabdoid tumors, central nervous system atypical teratoid/rhabdoid tumors, and epithelioid sarcomas. This study shows complete loss of INI1 expression in all 5 renal medullary carcinomas. In contrast, all renal cell carcinomas or urothelial carcinomas, including those with histological rhabdoid features, expressed INI1. Immunohistochemical staining for INI1 is therefore of great value in discriminating rhabdoid medullary carcinomas from rhabdoid renal cell carcinoma (RCC) (clear/papillary/chromophobe).

R. Dhir, MD

Differential expression of prognostic markers in histological subtypes of papillary renal cell carcinoma
Perret AG, Clemencon A, Li G, et al (North Hosp, CHU Saint-Etienne, France)
BJU Int 102:183-187, 2008

Objective.—To assess the expression of the tumour markers stromelysin 3, MUC1, p53 and cytokeratin-7 in papillary renal cell carcinoma (pRCC, for which two histological subtypes are distinguished, i.e. type 1 and type 2, the latter appearing to be associated with a poorer prognosis) and to determine whether any of these markers might be of prognostic value.

Patients and Methods.—In a retrospective study of 50 patients, the type and nuclear grade of tumours was determined by histological analyses, the presence of microvascular emboli detected, and the markers assessed by immunohistochemical analysis using anti-stromelysin 3, anti-MUC1, anti-p53 and anti-cytokeratin-7 antibodies.

Results.—Twenty-five patients each had a type 1 or type 2 tumour. MUC1 and cytokeratin-7 were principally expressed in type 1 tumours, being detected in 76% and 84%, respectively. By contrast, p53 accumulated principally in type 2 tumours (36%); the accumulation of p53 was also associated with poorer survival. In patients with type 2 tumours with a more unfavourable development, stromelysin-3 expression was associated with a more advanced stage and a higher risk of metastases.

Conclusion.—Subtyping pRCC according to the recommended morphological criteria appears to be worthwhile, and can be reinforced by immunohistochemical tests capable of detecting cytokeratin-7 and MUC1 expression. Immunohistochemical detection of p53 is of prognostic value, as accumulation of this factor is associated with poorer survival.

▶ The subclassification of papillary carcinomas is a relatively recent phenomenon. This subclassification does have prognostic bearing because the Type 2 renal cell carcinomas demonstrate a poorer outcome. This study evaluates a panel of markers of potential value in discriminating Type 1 from Type 2 carcinomas. Based on the data presented, Muc-1 and cytokeratin 7 are principally expressed in Type 1 RCC. p53 accumulation was more frequent in the Type 2 RCC. In addition, stromelysin-3 expression was associated with more aggressive disease in the Type 2 RCC. This panel is of potential value in evaluating papillary RCC. Because CK7 and Muc1 positivity is seen very frequently with

RCC Type 1 and not in Type 2, this panel provides diagnostic value. Expression of p53 and stromelysin-3 provides prognostic information.

R. Dhir, MD

A Comparison of Urinary Albumin–Total Protein Ratio to Phase-Contrast Microscopic Examination of Urine Sediment for Differentiating Glomerular and Nonglomerular Bleeding

Ohisa N, Yoshida K, Matsuki R, et al (Kumamoto Univ; Tohoku Univ Hosp, Sendai, Japan; et al)
Am J Kidney Dis 52:235-241, 2008

Background.—Hematuria can be classified as either glomerular or non-glomerular, depending on the bleeding source. We recently reported that urinary albumin–total protein ratio is potentially useful for identifying the source of hematuria.

Study Design.—Diagnostic test study.

Setting & Participants.—579 fresh urine specimens with microhematuria (≥ 5 red blood cells/high-power field) collected from patients with the source of the hematuria confirmed on histopathologic and/or imaging studies and clinical criteria assessed.

Index Test.—Each urine specimen was evaluated morphologically by using phase-contrast microscopy and biochemically by using urinary albumin–total protein ratio, albumin-creatinine ratio, and total protein–creatinine ratio.

Reference Test.—Each patient had a definitive clinical diagnosis established by means of biopsy (64.4%), imaging studies (21.2%), and routine optimal microscopic examination of urine sediment (14.3%).

Results.—Of 579 specimens, 329 were obtained from patients with glomerular disease and 250 were obtained from patients with nonglomerular disease. Mean urinary albumin–total protein, albumin-creatinine, and total protein–creatinine ratios for those with glomerular versus nonglomerular diseases were 0.73 ± 0.11 versus 0.41 ± 0.14 mg/mg ($P < 0.001$), $1,110 \pm 1,850$ versus 220 ± 560 mg/g ($P < 0.001$), and $1,600 \pm 3,010$ versus $480 \pm 1,160$ mg/g ($P < 0.001$), respectively. The percentage of patients with greater than 3% glomerular red cells was 83.3% versus 24.8% ($P < 0.001$). Receiver operating characteristic curve analysis showed that areas under the curve for albumin–total protein ratio, albumin-creatinine ratio, and total protein–creatinine ratio were 0.992, 0.781, and 0.688, respectively ($P < 0.001$, albumin–total protein versus albumin-creatinine; $P < 0.001$, albumin–total protein versus total protein–creatinine). At cutoff values of 0.59 mg/mg, 71 mg/g, and 265 mg/g, albumin–total protein ratio, albumin-creatinine ratio, and total protein–creatinine ratio had sensitivities and specificities of 97.3% and 100%, 78.9% and 61.1%, and 68.8% and 62.0% for detecting glomerular disease, respectively. Phase-contrast microscopy had sensitivity of 83.3% and specificity of 75.2% for detecting glomerular disease.

Limitations.—Albumin–total protein ratio cannot be used in patients with urinary total protein less than 5 mg/dL (<0.05 g/L). Use of only 1 sample from 1 patient may not be sufficient to obtain definitive results.

Conclusions.—Urinary albumin–total protein ratio is much more useful than phase-contrast microscopy for differentiating between glomerular and nonglomerular disease in patients with microscopic hematuria.

▶ Hematuria is a common diagnostic problem in clinical practice. It is of clinical importance to distinguish glomerular and Nonglomerular bleeding, with impact on the diagnostic and therapeutic approach. Currently, one of the mechanisms is to use phase contrast microscopy. Dysmorphic erythrocytes are suggestive of glomerular bleeding. Isomorphic erythrocytes are suggestive of bleeding from the pelvis, ureter, or bladder. However, studies indicate that the diagnostic value of urinary dysmorphic red blood cells may be limited. This study evaluates urinary albumin to total protein ration as a new mechanism to address this issue. Using appropriate cutoffs, this approach has a sensitivity of 97.3% and specificity of 100%. The urinary protein has to be > 5 mg/dL. It is also recommended to evaluate multiple samples, as use of only 1 sample might not provide definitive results.

R. Dhir, MD

12 Head and Neck

Histopathologic Characterization of Radioactive Iodine-refractory Fluorodeoxyglucose-Positron Emission Tomography-positive Thyroid Carcinoma

Rivera M, Ghossein RA, Schoder H, et al (Mem Sloan-Kettering Cancer Ctr, NY)
Cancer 113:48-56, 2008

Background.—Radioactive iodine-refractory (RAIR) 18F-fluorodeoxyglucose (FDG)-positron emission tomography (PET) positive thyroid carcinomas represent the major cause of deaths from thyroid carcinomas (TC) and are therefore the main focus of novel target therapies. However, to the authors' knowledge, the histology of FDG-PET-positive RAIR metastatic thyroid carcinoma has not been described to date.

Methods.—Metastatic tissue from RAIR PET-positive patients identified between 1996 and 2003 at the study institution were selected for histologic examination. The biopsied metastatic site corresponded to a FDG-PET positive lesion sampled within 2 years (87% of which were sampled within 1 year) of the PET scan. Detailed microscopic examination was performed on the metastatic deposit and the available primary tumors. Poorly differentiated thyroid carcinomas (PDTC) were defined on the basis of high mitotic activity (≥ 5 mitoses/10 high-power fields) and/or tumor necrosis. Other types of carcinomas were defined by conventional criteria. The histology of the metastases and primary were analyzed, with disease-specific survival (DSS) as the endpoint.

Results.—A total of 70 patients satisfied the selection criteria, 43 of whom had primary tumors available for review. Histologic characterization of the metastasis/recurrence in 70 patients revealed that 47.1% (n = 33 patients) had PDTC, 20% (n = 14 patients) had the tall cell variant (TCV) of papillary thyroid carcinoma, 22.9% (n = 16 patients) had well-differentiated papillary thyroid carcinoma (WDPTC), 8.6% (n = 6 patients) had Hurthle cell carcinoma (HCC), and 1.4% (n = 1 patient) had anaplastic carcinomas. The histopathologic distribution of the tumor in the primaries was: PDTC, 51%; TCV, 19%; WDPTC, 23%; and widely invasive HCC, 7%. A differing histology between the primary tumor and metastasis was observed in 37% of cases (n = 16 patients). In the majority of instances (63%; 10 of 16 patients) this was noted as transformation to a higher grade. Of the primary tumors classified as PTC, 70% progressed to more aggressive histotypes in the metastasis. Tumor necrosis and extensive extrathyroid extension in the primary tumor were found to be independent predictors of poorer DSS in this group of patients

($P = .015$). Approximately 68% of the PDTC primary tumors were initially classified by the primary pathologist as better-differentiated tumors on the basis of the presence of papillary and/or follicular architecture or the presence of typical PTC nuclear features.

Conclusions.—Several observations can be made based on the results of the current study. The majority of metastases in patients with RAIR PET-positive metastases are of a histologically aggressive subtype. However, well-differentiated RAIR metastatic disease is observable. Poorly differentiated disease is underrecognized in many cases if defined by architectural and nuclear features alone. The presence of tumor necrosis was found to be a strong predictor of aggressive behavior, even within this group of clinically aggressive tumors. Finally, there is a significant amount of histologic plasticity between primary tumors and metastases that may reflect the genetic instability of these tumors.

▶ Generally, follicular-derived thyroid carcinomas have an excellent prognosis with long-term cure being the norm. However, a small percentage will recur and may progress histologically or biologically, leading to patient morbidity and mortality. This more aggressive group is often clinically characterized radioactive iodine resistance (RAIR) and FDG-PET avidity. This study is one of the few that attempts to correlate histologic subtype with RAIR/PET positivity in both primary tumors and their metastases. As expected, RAIR/PET-positive cases had aggressive primary histology (poorly differentiated carcinomas), and even in the well-differentiated carcinomas with this metabolic profile, most metastases showed evidence of histologic progression. However, this is the first large series to confirm this. An ancillary finding is that poorly differentiated carcinoma has been initially underdiagnosed, and that using previously validated criteria of mitotic count and necrosis alone, rather than also requiring a solid/trabecular/insular growth pattern (as in the Turin proposal), more RAIR/PET-positive cases were identified as poorly differentiated. It is still important to note that almost one-fourth of RAIR/PET-positive cases were well differentiated. In the future, perhaps a more relevant problem is to address the molecular differences between the well-differentiated tumors that progress to a RAIR/PET-positive status and those that do not.

For further reading on this subject I suggest articles by Are et al[1] and Hiltzik et al.[2]

R. Seethala, MD

References

1. Are C, Hsu JF, Ghossein RA. Histological aggressiveness of fluorodeoxyglucose positron-emission tomogram (FDG-PET)-detected incidental thyroid carcinomas. *Ann Surg Oncol.* 2007;14:3210-3215. Epub 2007 Aug 23.
2. Hiltzik D, Carlson DL, Tuttle RM, et al. Poorly differentiated thyroid carcinomas defined on the basis of mitosis and necrosis: a clinicopathologic study of 58 patients. *Cancer.* 2006;106:1286-1295.

Array comparative genomic hybridization analysis of olfactory neuroblastoma

Guled M, Myllykangas S, Frierson HF Jr, et al (Univ of Helsinki, Finland; Univ of Virginia Health System, Charlottesville, VA)
Mod Pathol 21:770-778, 2008

Olfactory neuroblastoma is an unusual neuroectodermal malignancy, which is thought to arise at the olfactory membrane of the sinonasal tract. Due to its rarity, little is understood regarding its molecular and cytogenetic abnormalities. The aim of the current study is to identify specific DNA copy number changes in olfactory neuroblastoma. Thirteen dissected tissue samples were analyzed using array comparative genomic hybridization. Our results show that gene copy number profiles of olfactory neuroblastoma samples are complex. The most frequent changes included gains at 7q11.22– q21.11, 9p13.3, 13q, 20p/q, and Xp/q, and losses at 2q31.1, 2q33.3, 2q37.1, 6q16.3, 6q21.33, 6q22.1, 22q11.23, 22q12.1, and Xp/q. Gains were more frequent than losses, and high-stage tumors showed more alterations than low-stage olfactory neuroblastoma. Frequent changes in high-stage tumors were gains at 13q14.2–q14.3, 13q31.1, and 20q11.21–q11.23, and loss of Xp21.1 (in 66% of cases). Gains at 5q35, 13q, and 20q, and losses at

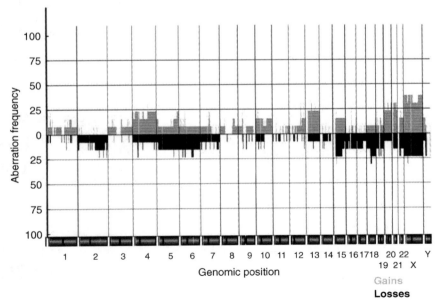

FIGURE 2.—Frequency profile of copy number aberrations in 13 olfactory neuroblastoma samples. CGH explorer software and piecewise Constant Fit algorithm were used to determine copy number aberrations in olfactory neuroblastoma samples. The chromosomal alterations are shown in each probe position as incidence bar. Gains of genomic material are indicated in gray on the upper side of the middle line (at 0). Losses are indicated in black on the bottom side of the middle line. Genomic positions of the aCGH probes are marked on the *x* axis. (Reprinted from Guled M, Myllykangas S, Frierson HF Jr, et al. Array comparative genomic hybridization analysis of olfactory neuroblastoma. *Mod Pathol.* 2008:21:770-778, with permission from USCAP, Inc.)

2q31.1, 2q33.3, and 6q16–q22, were present in 50% of cases. The identified regions of gene copy number change have been implicated in a variety of tumors, especially carcinomas. In addition, our results indicate that gains in 20q and 13q may be important in the progression of this cancer, and that these regions possibly harbor genes with functional relevance in olfactory neuroblastoma (Fig 2).

▶ Olfactory neuroblastoma is a rare neuroendocrine tumor presumed to arise from the olfactory epithelium. A combined multimodal approach has improved 5-year survival to about 70%. The underlying molecular pathogenesis of this tumor is poorly understood. Recently, assessment for chromosomal gains and losses by comparative genomic hybridization (CGH) has become more accessible to investigators. Here, the authors use array CGH to characterize 13 olfactory neuroblastomas. Before this study, these tumors had only been investigated using metaphase CGH. Here the authors find some previously reported chromosomal gains and losses, as well as some novel alterations (Fig 2). Notably, gains in 13q and 20q appear to correlate with higher-stage, more aggressive tumors, and are worth further investigation. Array CGH, particularly the Agilent platform used here, has improved resolution as compared with metaphase CGH. In this study, the authors used formalin-fixed, paraffin-embedded tissue, which may not be ideal for array CGH, though high concordance between frozen and paraffin tissues has been reported. Although frozen tissues for this tumor type are difficult to obtain, it would have been ideal if at least 1 or 2 tumors were validated using corresponding frozen tissue. Another method of validation, which would have been feasible, is confirmation of select gains and losses by fluorescent in-situ hybridization. Overall, this study adds to the expanding literature on chromosomal alterations in olfactory neuroblastoma and may help to localize biologically important genes in future studies.

For further reading on this subject, I suggest important articles by Bockmühl et al,[1] and another article by Holland et al.[2]

R. Seethala, MD

References

1. Bockmühl U, You X, Pacyna-Gengelbach M, Arps H, Draf W, Petersen I. CGH pattern of esthesioneuroblastoma and their metastases. *Brain Pathol.* 2004;14: 158-163.
2. Holland H, Koschny R, Krupp W, et al. Comprehensive cytogenetic characterization of an esthesioneuroblastoma. *Cancer Genet Cytogenet.* 2007;173:89-96.

Prognostic Significance of Somatic *RET* Oncogene Mutations in Sporadic Medullary Thyroid Cancer: A 10-Year Follow-Up Study
Elisei R, Cosci B, Romei C, et al (Univ of Pisa, Italy; et al)
J Clin Endocrinol Metab 93:682-687, 2008

Background.—Medullary thyroid carcinoma (MTC) is a well-differentiated thyroid tumor that maintains the typical features of C cells. An advanced stage and the presence of lymph node metastases at diagnosis have been demonstrated to be the most important bad prognostic factors. Somatic *RET* mutations have been found in 40–50% of MTCs. Although a relationship between somatic mutations and bad prognosis has been described, data are controversial and have been performed in small series with short-term follow ups. The aim of this study was to verify the prognostic value of somatic *RET* mutations in a large series of MTCs with a long follow up.

Methods.—We studied 100 sporadic MTC patients with a 10.2 yr mean follow-up. *RET* gene exons 10–11 and 13–16 were analyzed. The correlation between the presence/absence of a somatic *RET* mutation, clinical/pathological features, and outcome of MTC patients was evaluated.

Results.—A somatic *RET* mutation was found in 43 of 100 (43%) sporadic MTCs. The most frequent mutation (34 of 43, 79%) was M918T. *RET* mutation occurrence was more frequent in larger tumors ($P = 0.03$), and in MTC with node and distant metastases ($P < 0.0001$ and $P = 0.02$, respectively), thus, a significant correlation was found with a more advanced stage at diagnosis ($P = 0.004$). A worse outcome was also significantly correlated with the presence of a somatic *RET* mutation ($P = 0.002$). Among all prognostic factors found to be correlated with a worse outcome, at multivariate analysis only the advanced stage at diagnosis and the presence of a *RET* mutation showed an independent correlation ($P < 0.0001$ and $P = 0.01$, respectively). Finally, the survival curves of MTC patients showed a significantly lower percentage of surviving patients in the group with *RET* mutations ($P = 0.006$).

Conclusions.—We demonstrated that the presence of a somatic *RET* mutation correlates with a worse outcome of MTC patients, not only for the highest probability to have persistence of the disease, but also for a lower survival rate in a long-term follow up. More interestingly, the presence of a somatic *RET* mutation correlates with the presence of lymph node metastases at diagnosis, which is a known bad prognostic factor for the definitive cure of MTC patients.

▶ The outcome in sporadic medullary thyroid carcinoma (MTC) is generally determined by stage. However, it has been known for several years that even sporadic MTC may have mutations in the *RET* proto-oncogene. There has been some evidence to suggest that the mutational status is also a prognosticator. However, most series were too small and did not have a sufficient length of follow-up to support this with conviction. This study is one of the more recent attempts to answer this question in a large cohort of 100 patients with a median follow-up of over 10 years. In this series, *RET* mutations correlated with nodal status and outcome as an independent prognosticator in multivariate analysis. The prevalence was in keeping with previously published literature as was the high frequency of mutations at codon 918. Even though some tumors tested were paraffin embedded, whereas others were snap frozen, the methodology as previously described appears to be fairly robust, making this somewhat of a nonissue. Of note, it appears that the codon 918 mutations (as suggested by other reports) had a higher percentage of lymph node metastases as compared with other mutations. This may simply be a function of its high prevalence, but interestingly, germline mutations here are associated with MEN-2B, which is a familial multiple endocrine neoplasia syndrome characterized by more aggressive MTC. A subgroup analysis of the different RET mutants within a similarly large series with extended follow-up would be of interest in the future.

For further reading on this subject I suggest articles by Nikiforov[1] and Zedenius.[2]

R. Seethala, MD

References

1. Nikiforov YE. Thyroid carcinoma: molecular pathways and therapeutic targets. *Mod Pathol*. 2008;2:S37-S43.
2. Zedenius J. Is somatic RET mutation a prognostic factor for sporadic medullary thyroid carcinoma? *Nat Clin Pract Endocrinol Metab*. 2008; 2008 [Epub ahead of print].

NUT Rearrangement in Undifferentiated Carcinomas of the Upper Aerodigestive Tract

Stelow EB, Bellizzi AM, Taneja K, et al (Univ of Virginia, Charlottesville, VA; Brigham and Women's Hosp Boston, MA)
Am J Surg Pathol 32:828-834, 2008

Background.—Undifferentiated carcinomas of the upper aerodigestive tract (UCUAT) occur most frequently within the nasopharynx and are most often associated with infection by Epstein-Barr virus (EBV) (WHO undifferentiated nonkeratinizing squamous cell carcinoma). An unusual group of aggressive carcinomas are characterized by translocations that involve Nuclear Protein in Testis (*NUT*), a novel gene on chromosome 15. In about two-thirds of cases, *NUT* is fused to *BRD4* on chromosome 19. These tumors, here termed NUT midline carcinomas (NMCs), are undifferentiated, may have focal squamous differentiation, and are reported to occur in children and young adults. This study investigates the prevalence of *NUT* rearrangement and the diagnostic significance of NUT expression in a series of upper aerodigestive tract undifferentiated carcinomas. The histologic features of these tumors are described in detail.

Methods.—All UCUAT not associated with EBV infection seen at the University of Virginia (UVA) over a 16-year period were reviewed. Clinical and histologic features were noted. Additional material was submitted for fluorescent in situ hybridization (FISH) using split-apart probes to the *NUT* and *BRD4* genes. Immunohistochemistry (IHC) was performed on all cases using a polyclonal antibody to NUT, and on select cases with antibody to p63.

Results.—Thirty-one UCUAT were identified. Twenty-five tumors had originally been diagnosed as sinonasal undifferentiated carcinomas. Five of 28 cases (2 males, 3 females; average age 47; range 31 to 78) with interpretable results showed rearrangements of the *NUT* and *BRD4* genes by FISH. Three of these 5 cases showed diffuse (>90%) nuclear staining for NUT by IHC; 22 of 23 other tumors showed at most focal (<50%) nuclear staining. Undifferentiated carcinomas with *NUT* gene rearrangement had focal abrupt squamous differentiation in 2 cases, and intense and diffuse immunoreactivity with antibody to p63 in 4 cases.

Conclusions.—Approximately, 20% of UCUAT not associated with EBV infection were found to have rearrangements of *NUT* by FISH. Although previous reports suggest that NMCs afflict only children and young adults, 4 of 5 of the patients described are mature adults older than any heretofore reported, suggesting that previous reports may have been biased in their case selections. Furthermore, because these tumors are indistinguishable from other poorly differentiated carcinomas, IHC using NUT antibody may be a useful method for the identification of these tumors. Despite the lack of overt squamous differentiation in most cases, their p63 immunoreactivity suggests that NMCs may generally be of squamous lineage.

▶ NUT gene rearrangements have been recently described in midline carcinomas with poorly to undifferentiated histology with a predilection for a young age group. This series examines the prevalence of NUT rearrangements in sinonasal tumors with poorly to undifferentiated histology in all age groups, including entities that would be placed in the sinonasal undifferentiated carcinoma category (SNUC). Results are interesting, in that the rearrangement does not appear to be restricted to the pediatric age group here. Additionally, focal abrupt keratinization within a diffuse proliferation of undifferentiated cells and p63 immunoreactivity were common characteristic findings in tumors with NUT rearrangements. From a taxonomic standpoint, the question of how much differentiation is allowed in a SNUC is raised because the presence of focal squamous differentiation correlates (albeit based on small numbers) with NUT rearrangement. Immunohistochemistry for the NUT protein may be a useful surrogate, though it does not appear to be entirely sensitive or specific for at least the known NUT rearrangements. In future studies, the impact of the rearrangement status on outcome and possible targeted therapy will likely be addressed.

For further reading on this subject I suggest articles by French et al.[1,2]

R. Seethala, MD

References

1. French CA, Kutok JL, Faquin WC, et al. Midline carcinoma of children and young adults with NUT rearrangement. *J Clin Oncol.* 2004;22:4135-4139.
2. French CA. Molecular pathology of NUT midline carcinomas. *J Clin Pathol.* 2008; 2008 [Epub ahead of print].

Poorly Differentiated Thyroid Carcinoma: The Turin Proposal for the Use of Uniform Diagnostic Criteria and an Algorithmic Diagnostic Approach
Volante M, Collini P, Nikiforov YE, et al (University of Turin, Orbassano; Pathology Istituto Nazionale Tumori, Milan, Italy; Pittsburgh School of Medicine; et al)
Am J Surg Pathol 31:1256-1264, 2007

Poorly differentiated (PD) thyroid carcinomas lie both morphologically and behaviorally between well-differentiated and undifferentiated (anaplastic) carcinomas. Following the original description of this entity, different diagnostic criteria have been employed, resulting in wide discrepancies and confusion among pathologists and clinicians worldwide. To compare lesions occurring in different geographic areas and the diagnostic criteria applied in those countries, we designed a study with a panel of internationally recognized thyroid pathologists to develop consensus diagnostic criteria for PD carcinomas. Eighty-three cases were collected from Europe, Japan, and the United States, and circulated among 12 thyroid pathologists. Diagnoses were made without any knowledge of the clinical parameters, which were subsequently used for survival analysis. A consensus meeting was then held in Turin, Italy, where an agreement was reached concerning the diagnostic criteria for PD carcinoma. These include (1) presence of a solid/trabecular/insular pattern of growth, (2) absence of the conventional nuclear features of papillary carcinoma, and (3) presence of at least one of the following features: convoluted nuclei; mitotic activity $\geq 3 \times 10$ HPF; and tumor necrosis. An algorithmic approach was devised for practical use in the diagnosis of this tumor.

▶ Poorly differentiated thyroid carcinoma is a nebulous entity that is a presumed biologic intermediate between well-differentiated carcinomas and undifferentiated (anaplastic) carcinoma. This article attempts to standardize the criteria to define this entity. This was a consensus conference between thyroid experts worldwide who used a test set of tumors that were essentially "handpicked" from the files of some of the authors. The conclusions and criteria used to define poorly differentiated carcinoma in general are valid. However, it is evident even in this series that mitotic rate and necrosis are the prevailing determinants of behavior. One previous highly clinically annotated large single institution study demonstrated that this holds even in tumors without the solid-trabecular-insular growth pattern or those with obvious nuclear features of papillary carcinoma. This raises the question as to why follicular or papillary patterned tumors, or solid tumors with overt nuclear features of papillary carcinoma, should not be considered poorly differentiated as well if they have a high mitotic rate or necrosis. Additionally, the definition of "convoluted nuclei" is insufficient for a general audience. Overall, although this consensus report has merit as a guideline and does attempt to provide an outcome-based approach to this problem, it is not the best study on this subject and is influenced to some extent by "expert opinion" instead of concrete evidence.

For further reading on this subject I suggest articles by Hiltzik et al[1] and Carcangiu et al.[2]

R. Seethala, MD

References

1. Hiltzik D, Carlson DL, Tuttle RM, et al. Poorly differentiated thyroid carcinomas defined on the basis of mitosis and necrosis: a clinicopathologic study of 58 patients. *Cancer.* 2006;106:1286-1295.
2. Carcangiu ML, Zampi G, Rosai J. Poorly differentiated ("insular") thyroid carcinoma. a reinterpretation of Langhans' "wuchernde Struma." *Am J Surg Pathol.* 1984;8:655-668.

Expression of Parafibromin in Distant Metastatic Parathyroid Tumors in Patients with Advanced Secondary Hyperparathyroidism Due to Chronic Kidney Disease

Tominaga Y, Tsuzuki T, Matsuoka S, et al (Nagoya Second Red Cross Hosp, Showa-ku, Japan)
World J Surg 35:815-821, 2008

Background.—Recently, somatic inactivating mutations in *HRPT2* have been reported in the majority of sporadic parathyroid carcinoma in primary hyperparathyroidism (HPT). Parafibromin is a tumor suppressor protein encoded by *HRPT2*, and loss of nuclear expression of parafibromin was found in approximately 70% of the carcinoma. In secondary HPT due to chronic kidney disease (CKD), parathyroid carcinoma is very rare and whether *HRPT2* plays a role in the carcinogenesis in these cases is not clear. We evaluated the expression of parafibromin in hemodialysis patients with distant metastatic parathyroid tumors.

Methods.—Between June 1973 and December 2006, 2,142 patients underwent parathyroidectomy (PTx) for secondary HPT in our department. We encountered five (0.23%) patients with distant metastatic parathyroid tumors. We evaluated the immunohistochemistry for parafibromin in eight primary parathyroid glands removed from the neck at the initial operation and/or at reoperation and seven distant metastatic tumors resected at reoperation.

Results.—In only one lung metastatic parathyroid tumor, negative staining for parafibromin was detected. In the other three lung, two regional node, and one chest wall metastatic parathyroid tumor, parafibromin was strongly stained in the nuclei of the parathyroid cells. Among eight primary glands, except for one with weakly positive staining, the expression of parafibromin was detected diffusely and strongly.

Conclusion.—We conclude that the inactivating mutations and/or allelic loss of the *HRPT2* gene may not play a major role in parathyroid carcinogenesis in secondary HPT due to CKD, but in these cases cancer development may be associated with a heterogeneous genetic disorder.

▶ Parathyroid carcinomas are among the rarest malignancies in the head and neck region and account for less than 1% of all primary hyperparathyroidism. The outcome with adequate surgical management is favorable. Those who succumb to disease usually do so secondary to intractable hypercalcemia rather than actual tumor burden. Recent molecular advances have consolidated the crucial role of the gene *HRPT2* in the carcinogenesis of both sporadic parathyroid carcinomas and carcinomas arising in the setting of familial hyperparathyroidism jaw tumor syndrome. The vast majority of parathyroid carcinomas arise in the setting of primary hyperparathyroidism. However, rare carcinomas arise in the setting of secondary or tertiary hyperparathyroidism. As such, the relevance of *HRPT2* in the carcinogenesis of these tumors is unclear. The authors here examine a fairly sizeable series of carcinomas arising in secondary hyperparathyroidism for immunohistochemical loss of parafibromin, the product of the *HRPT2* gene, to determine whether the molecular pathogenesis for these tumors is similar to that of carcinomas arising in primary hyperparathyroidism. Hyperplasia in secondary hyperparathyroidism may show atypical histologic features mimicking carcinoma. Thus, 1 major strength of this article is that all the tumors were unequivocally carcinoma as evidenced by distant metastases typically to lung. Loss of parafibromin by immunohistochemistry has been shown to be an acceptable surrogate for *HRPT2* gene mutations. The conclusions of this study are in keeping with the intuitive notion that carcinogenesis in primary and secondary hyperparathyroidism is different, in that *HRPT2* alterations do not contribute to the pathogenesis of carcinomas arising in secondary hyperparathyroidism.

For further reading on this subject I suggest articles by Cetani et al[1] and Schantz et al.[2]

R. Seethala, MD

References

1. Cetani F, Ambrogini E, Viacava P, et al. Should parafibromin staining replace HRTP2 gene analysis as an additional tool for histologic diagnosis of parathyroid carcinoma? *Eur J Endocrinol.* 2007;156:547-554.
2. Schantz A, Castleman B. Parathyroid carcinoma. a study of 70 cases. *Cancer.* 1973;31:600-605.

Hyalinizing trabecular tumors of the thyroid gland: quadruply described but not by the discoverer
Carney JA (Mayo Clinic, Rochester, MN)
Am J Surg Pathol:32:622-634, 2008

Hyalinizing trabecular tumors of the thyroid have been described on 4 occasions, by Carney and colleagues in 1987, by Ward and coworkers in 1982, by Pierre Masson in 1922, and by Rahel Zipkin in 1905. Zipkin credited her chief, Theodor Langhans (of Langhans giant cell fame), with identification of the cases she reported. Unaware of the 3 earlier descriptions, Carney and colleagues described 11 circumscribed or encapsulated thyroid tumors with elongated and polygonal cells arranged in trabeculae that contained a hyaline material resembling amyloid. The nuclei of the tumor cells had cytoplasmic invaginations and grooves similar to those of papillary carcinoma. Carney and colleagues labeled the neoplasms hyalinizing trabecular *adenomas* because of their microscopic appearance, absence of invasion, and benign natural history. Subsequently, the nuclear features of the tumor and the molecular genetic findings led to the introduction of equivocal designations for it, hyalinizing trabecular *tumor* and hyalinizing trabecular *neoplasm*, and later to its designation as a variant of papillary carcinoma. Experience has shown that most circumscribed or encapsulated follicular thyroid tumors with intratrabecular hyalin and nuclear features of papillary carcinoma behave as benign neoplasms. Hyalinizing trabecular carcinoma is a very rare tumor (Fig 8).

▶ Hyalinizing trabecular tumor (HTT) of the thyroid is a controversial entity of still undetermined biologic potential. Although primary investigative efforts to

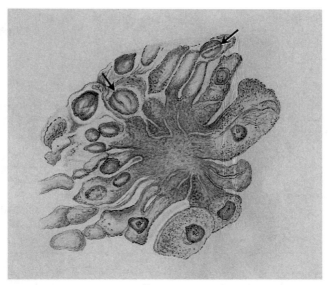

FIGURE 8.—Figure 3 from Zipkin's article.[57] Camera lucida drawing showed that van Gieson staining colored hyalin red. The legend read: "Beginning of sphere (of hyalin) formation, in which the narrowest parts of the basal ends of the cells flow together in the center of the circle." Comment: Elongated and polygonal cells had polygonal nuclei with peripherally condensed chromatin and prominent nucleoli showing perinucleolar clearing. Two nuclei exhibited roughly parallel bands of condensed chromatin separated by a clear zone (arrows), the type of structure illustrated by Casey et al.[12] Editor's note: Please refer to original journal article for full references. For interpretation of the references to color in this figure legend, the reader is referred to the web version of this article. (Reprinted from Carney JA, Hyalinizing trabecular tumors of the thyroid gland: quadruply described but not by the discoverer. *Am J Surg Pathol* 2008:32:622-634.)

clarify pathogenesis of this rare tumor are necessary, occasionally, historical investigative efforts may be as important. Here, one of the pathologists who lays claim to the description of this entity performs an exhaustive investigation into the origin of the description of this entity to lend perspective to the current investigative efforts. The author thus identifies that the description had already been in place almost a century before his description. Although current trends are to suggest that this tumor is benign, and "malignant" cases are different entities altogether, behaviorally malignant cases were initially described justifying the stance that this is a unique morphology with both benign and malignant variants based on evidence of capsular or vascular invasion. The author himself, based on his extensive experience, allows for both benign and malignant counterparts. His justification that one-third of his benign cases have over 10 years of follow-up, however, is not valid. Even bona fide papillary carcinomas that have been completely excised may have no evidence of disease at 10 years. Conversely, well-differentiated thyroid carcinomas of all types have been known to recur 20 to 40 years later. This is not to say that the author is incorrect, merely that his justification is misleading—well-differentiated thyroid carcinoma is difficult to study because of the requirement for extensive long-term follow-up—10 years is insufficient. Overall, historical investigations for rare entities such as this are as important as molecular or immunophenotypic investigations because the latter are meaningless if not grounded by the former (Fig 8).

For further reading on this subject, I suggest these important articles.[1,2]

R. Seethala, MD

References

1. Carney JA, Ryan J, Goellner JR. Hyalinizing trabecular adenoma of the thyroid gland. *Am J Surg Pathol*. 1987;11:583-591.
2. Cheung CC, Boerner SL, MacMillan CM, Ramyar L, Asa SL. Hyalinizing trabecular tumor of the thyroid: a variant of papillary carcinoma proved by molecular genetics. *Am J Surg Pathol*. 2000;24:1622-1626.

Calretinin Expression in the Differential Diagnosis of Human Ameloblastoma and Keratocystic Odontogenic Tumor
De Villiers P, Liu H, Suggs C, et al (Univ of Alabama, Birmingham, AL; Tianjin Union Medicine Centre, China; Univ of North Carolina at Chapel Hill; et al)
Am J Surg Pathol 32:256-260, 2008

Ameloblastoma is a benign, locally aggressive epithelial odontogenic tumor that has the potential to become malignant and produce metastasis to distant sites such as lungs and kidneys. The histologic presentation can be, in some instances, mistaken for keratocystic odontogenic tumor (KCOT) (formerly known as odontogenic keratocyst). The expression of calretinin [calbindin2 (CALB2)] was investigated on both ameloblastoma and KCOT. Nineteen cases of ameloblastoma and 17 cases of KCOT were stained with calretinin antiserum 18-0211 (Zymed, San Francisco, CA). All cases (100%) of ameloblastoma showed positive calretinin staining, restricted to the neoplastic epithelial component and none (0%) of the 17 KCOTs showed positive calretinin staining. Gene expression profiling of ameloblastomas showed *CALB2* expressed in the basal cell layer of

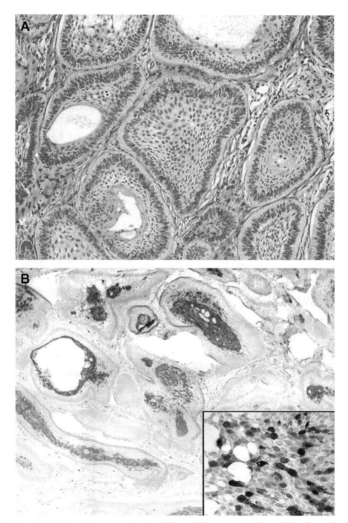

FIGURE 1.—A, B, Calretinin expression in solid ameloblastoma. A, Typical histology of solid ameloblastoma. Note the follicular pattern with acanthomatous differentiation. B, Calretinin expression in solid ameloblastoma. Prominent staining of the stellatelike reticulum showing emphasis on the areas of acanthomatous differentiation. The insert shows staining of nucleus and cytoplasm of individual cells. (Reprinted from De Villiers P, Liu H, Suggs C, et al. Calretinin expression in the differential diagnosis of human ameloblastoma and keratocystic odontogenic tumor. *Am J Surg Pathol.* 2008:32:256-260, with permission from Lippincott Williams & Wilkins.)

columnar cells resembling preameloblasts, in all 5 of the ameloblastomas evaluated. Taken together, the results of this study strongly support calretinin as a useful immunohistochemical marker for ameloblastoma and malignant ameloblastoma and it can also be used in the differential diagnosis of KCOT (Fig 1).

▶ Although the differentiation of cystic odontogenic lesions can usually be resolved with a combination of clinical, radiographic, and light microscopic features, occasionally, additional markers may be desirable. The differential diagnosis between unicystic ameloblastoma and keratocystic odontogenic tumors (KCOTs) may be important because of potential therapeutic differences. However, it is often challenging. Here the authors successfully confirm that calretinin is a useful marker in this distinction. The labeling of the stellate reticulum, particularly in the central more acanthomatous appearing areas (Fig 1), is characteristic of ameloblastoma. Thus, the luminal surface layer in a unicystic ameloblastoma is what will show the staining. None of the KCOTs were positive, though a photomicrograph of this finding would have been desirable in this article. The authors additionally confirm calretinin expression by array profiling of 5 tumors. It is interesting to note that these were formalin-fixed, paraffin-embedded specimens that were decalcified, yet yielded sufficient RNA to draw conclusions. The methodology of decalcification should have been mentioned because an acid decalcifying agent (which is standard in most gross laboratories) would likely not yield promising results. In our experience, calretinin can support an ameloblastic phenotype even in malignant tumors. These findings appear to be in keeping with other studies as well, in contrast to other markers such as amelogenin and enamelin, which may be seen in other tumor types. Other series of this type are still necessary for sufficient validation of this staining pattern by number.

R. Seethala, MD

CRTC1/MAML2 Fusion Transcript in Warthin's Tumor and Mucoepidermoid Carcinoma: Evidence for a Common Genetic Association

Bell D, Luna MA, Weber RS, et al (Univ of Texas MD Anderson Cancer Ctr, Houston, TX; et al)
Genes Chromosomes Cancer 47:309-314, 2008

Translocations and gene fusions have an important early role in tumorigenesis. The t(11;19) translocation and its *CRTC1/MAML2* fusion transcript have been identified in several examples of both Warthin's tumor and mucoepidermoid carcinoma and are believed to be associated with the development of a subset of these tumors. To determine whether Warthin's tumor and mucoepidermoid carcinoma are genetically related, we used reverse transcriptase-polymerase chain reaction and DNA sequencing to analyze microdissected components of three tumors consisting of Warthin's tumor and mucoepidermoid carcinoma. We also investigated a metastatic melanoma to Warthin's tumor and a Warthin's carcinoma of the parotid gland for comparison. The fusion transcript was identified in both Warthin's tumor and matching mucoepidermoid carcinoma components of all three tumors, in the Warthin's carcinoma, and in the Warthin's tumor component but not in the metastatic melanoma. The results provide evidence for a link between the t(11;19) fusion gene and the development of a subset of Warthin's tumors with concurrent mucoepidermoid carcinoma and possible malignant transformation to Warthin's carcinoma.

▶ The issue of whether a subset of Warthin tumors actually harbor the t(11;19) translocation resulting in the MECT1(CRTC1)/MAML2 is controversial. This translocation characterizes the more indolent lower-grade mucoepidermoid carcinomas, and thus the rare occurrence of this translocation in Warthin tumors suggested the possibility that Warthin tumors may be precursors to some mucoepidermoid carcinomas. Those who argue against this possibility counter that the translocation-positive Warthin tumors are actually misdiagnosed mucoepidermoid carcinomas with prominent lymphoid stroma, and that these tumors are unrelated. This study examines 3 "mucoepidermoid carcinomas ex Warthin tumor" to determine whether the Warthin component and the mucoepidermoid carcinoma component both harbored the translocation. The methodology for assessing the translocation status is technically sound and was performed on paraffin tissue with success. The authors have had extensive experience in this area as well.[1] The end result was that all 3 tumors tested showed the translocation, and additionally an entity they describe as "Warthin carcinoma" was also positive, whereas a Warthin tumor with an adjacent melanoma was negative. The conclusion was the Warthin tumor can serve as a precursor to mucoepidermoid carcinoma. The major flaw of this study is that the tumors were not morphologically well characterized. The photomicrographs of the mucoepidermoid carcinoma ex Warthin tumor appeared to me to merely show a mucoepidermoid carcinoma with oncocytic change and prominent lymphoid stroma. The "Warthin carcinoma" simply appeared to be a solid oncocytic mucoepidermoid carcinoma. This is an excellent example in which imprecise histopathologic characterization may potentially lead to false molecular assumptions. Criteria for defining mucoepidermoid carcinoma arising in Warthin tumor and Warthin carcinoma should have been better delineated, and more extensive photodocumentation of these histologic features would have been desirable. Nonetheless, this concept is intriguing and warrants further investigation.

For further reading on this subject, I suggest an article by Martins et al.[2]

R. Seethala, MD

References

1. Williamson JD, Simmons BH, el-Naggar A, et al. Mucoepidermoid carcinoma involving Warthin tumor. a report of five cases and review of the literature. *Am J Clin Pathol*. 2000;114:564-570.

2. Martins C, Cavaco B, Tonon G. A study of MECT1-MAML2 in mucoepidermoid carcinoma and Warthin's tumor of salivary glands. *J Mol Diagn.* 2004;6:205-210.

Differential Expression of Hormonal and Growth Factor Receptors in Salivary Duct Carcinomas: Biologic Significance and Potential Role in Therapeutic Stratification of Patients

Williams MD, Roberts D, Blumenschein GR Jr, et al (Univ of Texas M.D. Anderson Cancer Ctr, Houston, TX)

Am J Surg Pathol 31:1645-1652, 2007

Salivary duct carcinoma (SDC), a rare malignancy, manifests remarkable morphologic and biologic resemblance to high-grade mammary ductal carcinoma. We contend that, similar to mammary ductal carcinoma, hormones and growth factors may play a role in SDCs. Our aim was to determine the incidence and clinical significance of the expression of several hormone and growth factor receptors and evaluate their potential in therapeutic stratification of SDC patients in the largest cohort studied to date. Eighty-four archived tumor tissue blocks were analyzed immunohisto-chemically for expression of estrogen receptor-β (ERβ), androgen receptor (AR), and proline, glutamic acid, and leucine-rich protein-1 and growth factor receptors HER-2 and epidermal growth factor receptor. The results were correlated with available pathologic, demographic, and clinical data from 59 of 84 cases. Proline, glutamic acid, and leucine-rich protein-1, ERβ, and AR were expressed individually in 94% (71/76), 73% (57/80), and 67% (56/84) of SDCs, respectively, and coexpressed in 45% (34/75). AR was expressed significantly more often in SDCs of men than in SDCs of women [79% (35/57) vs. 33% (9/27), $P < 0.001$]. Epidermal growth factor receptor and HER-2 were overexpressed individually in 48% (40/83) and 25% (21/84), respectively, and co-overexpressed in 12% (10/83). Survival decreased significantly in patients with lymph node metastasis ($P = 0.002$) and positive surgical margins ($P = 0.006$). Lack of ERβ expression correlate with increased local and regional recurrence ($P = 0.05$ and $P = 0.002$, respectively). Together, these results indicate that (a) ERβ down-regulation is associated with adverse clinical features, (b) lymph node and surgical margin status are significant survival factors, and (c) the differential expression of these hormones and growth factor receptors may assist in triaging patients with SDC for novel therapies (Fig 1).

▶ Salivary duct carcinoma is a highly aggressive malignancy of the salivary gland that bears a morphologic resemblance to high-grade/apocrine ductal carcinoma of the breast. Most of these tumors present with advanced disease, and there is currently no satisfactory adjuvant treatment modality. The biology of this tumor is poorly understood, but available evidence suggests that, similar to mammary ductal carcinoma, HER family proteins and steroid hormones may contribute to salivary duct carcinoma tumorigenesis. Here, the authors investigate a variety of hormonal receptors as well as HER family proteins, EGFR, and

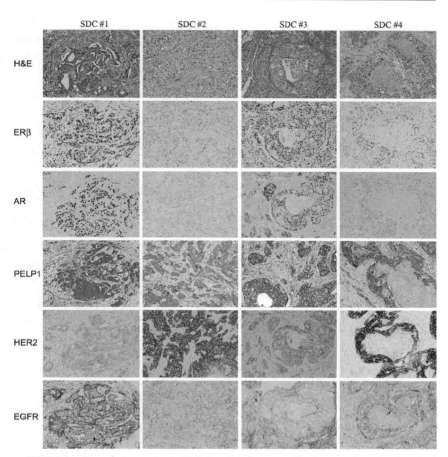

FIGURE 1.—Biomarker expression in SDCs (n = 4) and corresponding hematoxylin and eosin-stained sections. The parameters assessed were ERβ nuclear expression; AR nuclear expression; PELP1 cytoplasmic expression; HER-2 membranous expression; and EGFR membranous expression. (Reprinted from Williams MD, Roberts D, Blumenschein Jr GR, et al. Differential expression of hormonal and growth factor receptors in salivary duct carcinomas: biologic significance and potential role in therapeutic stratification of patients. *Am J Surg Pathol.* 2007;31:1645-1652, with permission from Lippincott Williams & Wilkins.)

HER-2/Neu. This is both a descriptive and correlative analysis on one of the largest series of salivary duct carcinomas ever reported. This alone is sufficient for this to be a must-read for pathologists and clinicians with an interest in salivary gland tumors. Because of the availability of targeted therapy to EGFR and HER-2/Neu, this immunohistochemical survey also supports the need for investigation of the application of these therapies toward this rare and aggressive malignancy. Additionally, the study validates the notion that salivary duct carcinoma is a hormonally driven malignancy, and that targeting these receptors may be even more important to the adequate treatment of these tumors. One question raised by this study is the accurate histologic and immunophenotypic classification of some of these tumors. Androgen receptor (AR) reactivity of only 67% is low for this tumor type, because in our experience this expression is nearly 100%. The authors suggest that estrogen receptor beta (ERβ)-negative and AR-negative tumors behave more aggressively, but the photomicrograph of one such tumor (Fig 1) has the appearance of an undifferentiated; that is, it lacks gland formation or apocrine morphology typical of salivary duct carcinoma. It would be interesting to see whether all the ERβ-and AR-negative "salivary duct carcinomas" showed morphologic differences from the remainder of the tumors. But overall, this study clearly illustrates the need to investigate the molecular mechanisms underlying the expression of these tumors and eventually perhaps even initiate a clinical trial with pharmacotherapeutic agents that target these markers.

For further reading on this subject I suggest articles by Vadlamudi et al[1] and Kapadia et al.[2]

R. Seethala, MD

References

1. Vadlamudi RK, Balasenthil S, Sahin AA, et al. Novel estrogen receptor coactivator PELP1/MNAR gene and ERβ expression in salivary duct adenocarcinoma: potential therapeutic targets. *Hum Pathol.* 2005;36:670-675.
2. Kapadia SB, Barnes L. Expression of androgen receptor, gross cystic disease fluid protein, and CD44 in salivary duct carcinoma. *Mod Pathol.* 1998;11:1033-1038.

Diagnostic utility of thyroid transcription factors Pax8 and TTF-2 (FoxE1) in thyroid epithelial neoplasms
Nonaka D, Tang Y, Chiriboga L, et al (Univ School of Medicine, New York, NY; et al)
Mod Pathol 21:192-200, 2008

Thyroid-specific transcription factors, Pax8, TTF-1, and TTF-2, are crucial for thyroid organogenesis and differentiation. Compared with TTF-1, the other two markers have scarcely been investigated in surgical pathology. The goal of this study is to evaluate the expressions of these markers in thyroid tumors of the full spectrum of differentiation, with special emphasis on anaplastic carcinomas. A total of 94 cases of thyroid neoplasms were studied: 17 papillary carcinomas, 18 follicular adenomas, 16 follicular carcinomas, 7 poorly differentiated carcinomas, 28 anaplastic carcinomas, and 8 medullary carcinomas. Immunostains for these three markers were performed. The antibodies to Pax8 and TTF-2 were also applied on 147 lung carcinomas as well as a variety of normal tissues and malignant tumors. All three markers were seen in papillary carcinomas, follicular adenomas and carcinomas, and poorly differentiated carcinomas in a diffuse manner, whereas their expressions in medullary carcinomas were variable. Pax8 was expressed in 79% of anaplastic carcinomas to a variable extent, whereas TTF-1 and TTF-2 were seen only in

18 and 7% of anaplastic carcinomas, respectively. TTF-2 was negative in all other neoplastic and non-neoplastic tissues including those of the lung. Pax8 was expressed in renal tubules, fallopian tubes, ovarian inclusion cysts, and lymphoid follicles as well as renal carcinoma, nephroblastoma, seminoma, and ovarian carcinoma, but not in normal tissue and carcinomas of the lung. Pax8 is a useful marker for the diagnosis of anaplastic carcinomas, particularly when the differential diagnosis includes pulmonary carcinoma. In differentiated thyroid neoplasms, no significant difference in expression was seen in all the three transcription factors (Fig 1).

▶ The transcription factor TTF-1 has been in clinical use for several years as a marker of thyroid differentiation. However, because it is expressed in lung

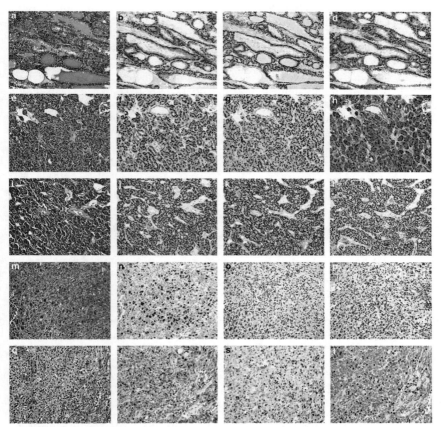

FIGURE 1.—Papillary carcinoma: (a) H&E stain, (b) Pax8, (c) TTF-1, (d) TTF-2. Follicular carcinoma: (e) H&E stain, (f) Pax8, (g) TTF-1, (h) TTF-2. Poorly differentiated carcinoma: (i) H&E stain, (j) Pax8, (k) TTF-1, (l) TTF-2. Anaplastic carcinoma: (m) H&E stain, (n) Pax8, (o) TTF-1, (p) TTF-2. Medullary carcinoma: (q) H&E stain, (r) Pax8, (s) TTF-1, (t) TTF-2. (Courtesy of Nonaka D, Tang Y, Chiriboga L, et al. Diagnostic utility of thyroid transcription factors Pax8 and TTF-2 (FoxE1) in thyroid epithelial neoplasms. *Mod Pathol.* 2008;21:192-200. Copyright © 2008, with permission from Macmillan Publishers.)

carcinomas, and even occasionally in other tumors, its use is occasionally limited in poorly differentiated tumors. More recently, commercially available antibodies to other transcription factors also expressed in thyroid, namely TTF-2 and PAX-8, have been developed. This study is a comprehensive survey of these markers in thyroid tumors using tissue microarray-based methodology. It is well known that TTF-1 is commonly lost in anaplastic thyroid carcinoma. What is surprising is that PAX-8 appears to be retained in most of these tumors. PAX-8 is negative in the lung tumors tested to date. The implications of the findings of this study are that 1) combined expression of TTF-1 and PAX-8 supports a thyroid origin even if thyroglobulin is negative, and that 2) PAX-8 immunoreactivity in a poorly differentiated malignancy may support the diagnosis of an anaplastic thyroid carcinoma over a lung primary. TTF-2 on the other hand does not appear as useful in this context because it is usually lost in anaplastic thyroid carcinoma. One caveat is that PAX-8 was not explored in detail in this series in sarcomatoid renal cell carcinoma. Because PAX-8 is also expressed in kidney, this marker may not be helpful when the differential diagnosis also includes metastatic renal cell carcinoma. The quality of staining (Fig 1) for PAX-8 appears acceptable for diagnostic use. This study provides supportive evidence for the use of PAX-8 in clinical practice to support a primary thyroid origin for poorly differentiated malignancies in the head and neck region and in lung nodules. In fact, at our laboratory, we had recently validated this antibody for clinical use, and our findings are in keeping with those of these authors.

For further reading on this subject I suggest important articles by Lacroix et al[1] and Miettinen et al.[2]

R. Seethala, MD

References

1. Lacroix L, Mian C, Barrier T, et al. PAX8 and peroxisome proliferator-activated receptor gamma 1 gene expression status in benign and malignant thyroid tissues. *Eur J Endocrinol.* 2004;151:367-374.
2. Miettinen M, Franssila KO. Variable expression of keratins and nearly uniform lack of thyroid transcription factor 1 in thyroid anaplastic carcinoma. *Hum Pathol.* 2000;31:1139-1145.

Sensitivity of direct immunofluorescence in oral diseases. Study of 125 cases

Sano SM, Quarracino MC, Aguas SC, et al (Universidad de Buenos Aires, Argentina; et al)
Med Oral Patol Cir Bucal 13:E287-E291, 2008

Direct immunofluorescence (DIF) is widely used for the diagnosis of bullous diseases and other autoimmune pathologies such as oral lichen planus. There is no evidence in the literature on how the following variants influence the detection rate of DIF: intraoral site chosen for the biopsy, perilesional locus or distant site from the clinical lesion, number of biopsies and instrument used.

Objectives.—to determine if the following variants influenced the sensitivity (detection rate): intraoral site chosen for the biopsy, perilesional or distant site from the clinical lesion, number of biopsies and instrument used (punch or scalpel).

Material and Methods.—A retrospective study was done at the Cátedra de Patología y Clínica Bucodental II at the Facultad de Odontología, Universidad de Buenos Aires; 136 clinical medical histories were revised for the period March 2000 – March 2005 corresponding to patients with clinical diagnosis of OLP and bullous diseases (vulgar pemphigus, bullous pemphigoid and cicatricial pemphigoid).

Results.—DIF detection rate was 65.8% in patients with OLP, 66.7% in cicatricial pemphigoid patients, in bullous pemphigoid 55.6%, in pemphigus vulgaris 100%, and in those cases in which certain diagnosis could not be obtained, the DIF positivity rate was 45.5% (Pearson $chi^2(4)= 21.5398$ Pr= 0.000). There was no statistically significant difference between the different sites of biopsy (Fisher exact test: 0.825). DIF detection rate in perilesional biopsies was 66.1% and in those distant from the site of clinical lesion was 64.7% (Pearson chi^2 (1)= 0.0073 Pr= 0.932). When the number of biopsies were incremented, DIF detection rate also incremented (Pearson $chi^2= 8.7247$ Pr= 0.003). The biopsies taken with punch had a higher detection rate than those taken with scalpel (39.1% versus 71.7%) (Pearson $chi^2= 49.0522$ Pr= 0.000).

Conclusion.—While not statistically significant, the tendency outlined in this study indicates there are intraoral regions in which the detection rate of the DIF technique is higher than others: mouth floor, hard palate, superior labial mucosa, ventral face of tongue. This finding could allow a choice of accessible locations and easy operator manipulation, even in distant places from the clinical lesion. Perilesional biopsies have a detection rate similar to those taken distant from the clinical lesion, and those taken with punch have a higher sensitivity rate than those taken with scalpel (both differences were statistically significant).

▶ Direct immunofluoresence (DIF) is a useful ancillary test in the diagnosis of a variety of vesicobullous diseases. The performance utility of this methodology has not been well studied in oral vesicobullous disease. Here, the authors report their experience with 125 cases. What is unique is that the authors attempt to demonstrate performance characteristics for each oral subsite and whether the biopsy was perilesional or distant. They found that gingival biopsies were less sensitive, although this difference was not statistically significant. Nonetheless, they also quote some practical considerations to support the recommendation not to use gingival biopsies for DIF. Interestingly, there was no difference between DIF use perilesionally or away from the lesion, suggesting that a biopsy does not always have to be near the lesion to be useful with this methodology. As expected, the detection rate improved with an increasing number of biopsies. Another finding was that punch biopsies were significantly more useful compared with scalpel biopsies. It would have been desirable for the authors to discuss this in more detail. In summary, these authors offer some practical guidelines on a rarely studied subject, although these findings need to be validated prospectively.

For further reading on this subject I suggest an article by Rinaggio et al.[1]

R. Seethala, MD

Reference

1. Rinaggio J, Crossland DM, Zeid MY. A determination of the range of oral conditions submitted for microscopic and direct immunofluorescence analysis. *J Periodontol.* 2007;78:1904-1910.

Sebaceous Epithelial-Myoepithelial Carcinoma of the Salivary Gland: Clinicopathologic and Immunohistochemical Analysis of 6 Cases of a New Histologic Variant

Shinozaki A, Nagao T, Endo H, et al (Univ of Tokyo; Tokyo Med Univ; International Med Ctr, Japan; et al)

Am J Surg Pathol 32:913-923, 2008

Epithelial-myoepithelial carcinoma (EMC) of the salivary glands is an uncommon, low-grade malignant tumor. A recent report demonstrates sebaceous differentiation in this tumor even though its significance has never been documented as a precise histologic variant. Six cases of EMC exhibiting sebaceous differentiation (sebaceous EMC) of the parotid gland were analyzed for their clinicopathologic features and immunohisto-chemical characteristics. In addition, primary salivary sebaceous carcinomas were also examined for comparison. In our series, the incidence of sebaceous EMC was 0.2% among 3012 cases of parotid gland tumors and 14.3% of all EMC cases. The 6 patients comprised 2 men and 4 women, age ranging from 77 to 93 years (mean, 83.7 y). Neither cervical lymph node nor distant organ metastases were found in any cases of sebaceous EMC and no patients died of disease, though local recurrences developed in 1 patient. Conversely, cervical lymph node metastasis was detected in 2 of 3 patients with sebaceous carcinoma, 1 of whom died of disease at 12 months. Histologically, all 6 tumors had an area of sebaceous differentiation admixed with features of bilayered ductal structures typical of EMC. A component of sebaceous differentiation was distributed diffusely in 4 tumors and focally in 2. Cytologic atypia of sebaceous EMCs was lesser than that of sebaceous carcinomas. Immunohistochemically, putative myoepithelial markers such as α-smooth muscle actin, calponin, p63, cytokeratin 14, S-100 protein, and vimentin were highly expressed in sebaceous EMC. However, the expression of the latter 4 markers was also observed in primary sebaceous carcinomas, whereas these tumors were all negative for α-smooth muscle actin and calponin. Positive immuno-reactivity for epithelial membrane antigen, adipophilin, and perilipin confirmed sebaceous differentiation in EMC. These results indicate that sebaceous EMC is a low-grade malignancy, similar to conventional EMC. Our data also suggest that immunohistochemical examination of specific myoepithelial markers is helpful in distinguishing sebaceous EMC from sebaceous carcinoma, which may occasionally be associated with an aggressive clinical course.

▶ Epithelial-myoepithelial carcinoma (EMC) is a rare but perhaps underdiagnosed low-grade salivary gland malignancy. Recently, several morphologic variants of this tumor have been described but not well characterized. The authors characterize 6 new cases of EMC with sebaceous elements and contrast them with pure sebaceous salivary gland tumors. The prevalence of this variant is similar to what we had reported previously. Regarding behavior, the authors conclude that sebaceous EMC behaves in a similarly indolent fashion to conventional EMC. This appears valid, but in previous series, time to recurrence in conventional EMC is about 11 years, whereas the longest follow-up in this series was 51 months, thus this issue is not fully resolved. Additionally, in previous series, sebaceous elements in EMC were more closely associated with the oncocytic variant rather than the conventional variant; this was not addressed here. One clinically relevant conclusion is that these should not be confused with sebaceous carcinoma, which appears to have a more aggressive biologic behavior based on the few cases reported. Of interest, the markers adipophilin and perilipin are shown to be useful markers of sebaceous differentiation. Although this was not discussed in detail, sebaceous differentiation in salivary gland does not appear to be androgenically-driven in contrast to sebaceous lesions of the skin—all cases were negative for androgen receptor. In summary, this is a detailed update on a newly described histologic variant of an already rare tumor that will be useful to pathologists who encounter a large volume of salivary gland tumors.

For further reading on this subject I suggests articles by Seethala et al[1] and Gnepp et al.[2]

R. Seethala, MD

References

1. Seethala RR, Barnes EL, Hunt JL. Epithelial-myoepithelial carcinoma: a review of the clinicopathologic spectrum and immunophenotypic characteristics in 61 tumors of the salivary glands and upper aerodigestive tract. *Am J Surg Pathol.* 2007;31:44-57.
2. Gnepp DR, Brannon R. Sebaceous neoplasms of salivary gland origin. report of 21 cases. *Cancer.* 1984;53:2155-2170.

13 Neuropathology

The Familial Parkinsonism Gene *LRRK2* Regulates Neurite Process Morphology
MacLeod D, Dowman J, Hammond R, et al (Columbia Univ, New York)
Neuron 52:587-593, 2006

Mutations in *LRRK2* underlie an autosomal-dominant, inherited form of Parkinson's disease (PD) that mimics the clinical features of the common "sporadic" form of PD. The *LRRK2* protein includes putative GTPase, protein kinase, WD40 repeat, and leucine-rich repeat (LRR) domains of unknown function. Here we show that PD-associated *LRRK2* mutations display disinhibited kinase activity and induce a progressive reduction in neurite length and branching both in primary neuronal cultures and in the intact rodent CNS. In contrast, *LRRK2* deficiency leads to increased neurite length and branching. Neurons that express PD-associated *LRRK2* mutations additionally harbor prominent phospho-tau-positive inclusions with lysosomal characteristics and ultimately undergo apoptosis.\

▶ Cloning of leucine-rich repeat kinase 2 (*LRRK2*) led to the identification of several *LRRK2* mutations in the PARK8 locus of autosomal dominant Parkinsonism. Recent studies of mutations in the kinase domain (G2019S[1]) and Roc domain (R1441C[2]) demonstrate that the resulting LRRK2 protein has enhanced kinase activity accounting for its toxicity in several in vitro cell-culture models. MacLeod and colleagues present evidence supporting the role of *LRRK2* in regulating neurite morphology and demonstrate that PD-associated mutations in LRRK2 result in neuritic toxicity with inclusions.

The authors expressed wild-type and PD-associated mutant *LRRK2* cDNAs in several in vitro and in vivo systems. Overexpression of the wild-type *LRRK2* in primary rat cortical cultures was innocuous; however, expression of mutated LRRK2 resulted in a progressive decline in neurite length and complexity preceding morphologic or functional indicators of cell death. Deletion analysis indicated that the kinase domain of LRRK2 is sufficient to cause neurite blunting in cell culture. Further analysis of neurites from cells transfected with PD-associated *LRRK2* mutants revealed abnormal neurite morphology with inclusions. Confocal microscopic analysis demonstrated colocalization of LRRK2 and immunoreactivities to tau-protein and lysosomal markers. A-synuclein was not detected in the varicosities. Consistent findings were shown in the substantia nigra of adult rats transduced with *LRRK2* mutants via AAV-2 vectors and in developing cortical neurons of rat embryos following in utero lentiviral transduction.

The authors suggest a pathologic schema in which the enhanced kinase activity of PD-associated *LRRK2* mutants results in phosphorylation of tau, inhibiting its ability to stabilize microtubules in neuritic processes and resulting in tau-positive lysosomal inclusions. This proposal is exciting with regard to potential roles for LRRK2 in a spectrum of Parkinsonian movement disorders and neurodegenerative diseases characterized by tauopathy.

Interestingly, the authors also demonstrate in several systems that knockdown of endogenous *LRRK2* gene expression via RNA interference results in enhanced neuritic outgrowth and branching complexity. These observations are consistent with possible roles of LRRK2 as negative regulator of neurite outgrowth and branching in physiologic and pathologic contexts. Important roles of LRRK2 in neurite remodeling and plasticity, in addition to its pathologic role in Parkinsonian movement disorders, make this gene product an exciting focus of neuropathology and neuroscience research.

C. Wiley, MD, PhD

References

1. Smith WW, Pei Z, Jiang H, Dawson VL, Dawson TM, Ross CA. Kinase activity of mutant *LRRK2* mediated neuronal toxicity. *Nat Neurosci.* 2006;9:1231-1233.
2. West AB, Moore DJ, Choi C, et al. Parkinson's disease-associated mutations in *LRRK2* link enhanced GTP-bonding and kinase activities to neuronal toxicity. *Hum Mol Genet.* 2007;16:223-232.

A Review of Changes Introduced by the *WHO Classification of Tumours of the Central Nervous System*, 4th Edition

Brat DJ, Parisi JE, Kleinschmidt-DeMasters BK, et al (Emory Univ, Atlanta, GA; Mayo Clinic, Rochester, MN; Univ of Colorado at Denver and Health Sciences Center; et al)
Arch Pathol Lab Med 132:993-1007, 2008

Context.—The World Health Organization (WHO) recently published its 4th edition of the classification of tumors of the central nervous system, incorporating a substantial number of important changes to the previous version (WHO 2000). The new WHO classification introduces 7 changes in the grading of central nervous system neoplasms, ranging in significance from minor to major, in categories of anaplastic oligoastrocytomas, meningiomas, choroid plexus tumors, pineal parenchymal tumors, ganglioglioma, cerebellar liponeurocytoma, and hemangiopericytomas. The 4th edition also introduces 10 newly codified entities, variants, and patterns, as well as 1 new genetic syndrome. A number of established brain tumors are reorganized, including medulloblastomas and primitive neuroectodermal tumors, in an attempt to more closely align classification with current understanding of central nervous system neoplasia.

Objective.—To summarize and discuss the most significant updates in the 4th edition for the practicing surgical pathologist, including (1) changes in grading among established entities; (2) newly codified tumor entities, variants, patterns, and syndromes; and (3) changes in the classification of existing brain tumors.

Data Sources.—The primary source for this review is the *WHO Classification of Tumours of the Central Nervous System*, 4th edition. Other important sources include the 3rd edition of this book and the primary literature that supported changes in the 4th edition.

Conclusions.—The new edition of the WHO blue book reflects advancements in the understanding of brain tumors in terms of classification, grading, and new entities. The changes introduced are substantial and will have an impact on the practice of general surgical pathologists and neuropathologists.

▶ The fourth edition of the World Health Organization (WHO) classification of tumors of the central nervous system (CNS) was published in 2007, updating and supplanting the third edition published in 2000.[1] This publication, like its predecessors, provides a consensus classification scheme and criteria for the standardized, optimal diagnosis and grading of neoplasms affecting the central nervous system. Although controversies remain,[2] the fourth edition, like its predecessors, provides concisely compiled clinicopathologic, histologic, immunohistochemical, and genetic data about each neoplastic "entity" (unique, distinct morphology, location, age of occurrence, and/or biologic behavior, eg, ependymoma, WHO grade II) and its (a) "variants" (histologic subtypes of an entity, reliably identified, but with different biologic properties or clinical behavior that justifies their distinction, eg, cellular, papillary, and clear cell variants of ependymoma, all WHO grade II) and (b) histologic patterns of differentiation (distinct histologic features or differentiation without a distinct difference clinically or pathologically to justify classification as either a variant or a distinct entity, eg, the newly recognized "small cell glioblastoma" histologic pattern of differentiation within the entity "glioblastoma," WHO grade IV).

The fourth edition introduced a substantial number of changes. Some of these changes are prominent, such as the introduction of 7 new entities, variants, and patterns of differentiation including angiocentric glioma, pituicytoma, papillary glioneuronal tumor, pilomyxoid astrocytoma, and others. However, other critically important changes are subtle, and a close comparison of the third and fourth editions would be necessary to identify them. Such changes include the controversial designation of anaplastic oligoastrocytomas with any degree of necrosis, previously classified in most instances as WHO grade III, as glioblastoma with oligodendroglial component, WHO grade IV; the introduction of brain invasion by a meningioma as an independent criterion sufficient for designation of the tumor as WHO grade II; the introduction of criteria for the diagnosis of atypical choroid plexus papilloma, WHO grade II; and changes in the diagnosis of pineal parenchymal tumors with pineocytoma now classified as WHO grade I, pineal parenchymal tumor of intermediate differentiation classified as WHO grade II or III, and pineoblastoma classified as WHO grade IV.

This publication by Brat et al thoroughly and concisely summarizes, and in some instances illustrates, the changes. Particularly helpful, the modifications from the third edition are summarized in a tabular form. It supplements several other publications which highlight the various new entities and changes in the fourth edition[3-5] and associated controversies.[2] In summary, this publication helps update the diagnostic pathologist and oncologist as she/he makes the transition to practical application of the fourth edition's classifications of tumors of the CNS.

P. Boyer, MD, PhD

References

1. Louis DN, Ohgaki H, Wiestler OD, Cavenee WK. *WHO Classification of Tumours of the Central Nervous System.* Albany: WHO Publications Center; 2007.
2. Scheithauer BW, Fuller GN, VandenBerg SR. The 2007 WHO classification of tumors of the nervous system: controversies in surgical neuropathology. *Brain Pathol.* 2008;18:307-316.
3. Louis DN, Ohgaki H, Wiestler OD, et al. The 2007 WHO classification of tumours of the central nervous system. *Acta Neuropathol (Berl).* 2007;114: 97-109.
4. Brat DJ, Scheithauer BW, Fuller GN, Tihan T. Newly codified glial neoplasms of the 2007 WHO Classification of Tumours of the Central Nervous System: angiocentric glioma, pilomyxoid astrocytoma and pituicytoma. *Brain Pathol.* 2007;17: 319-324.
5. Rosenblum MK. The 2007 WHO Classification of Nervous System Tumors: newly recognized members of the mixed glioneuronal group. *Brain Pathol.* 2007;17: 308-313.

Gray Zones in Brain Tumor Classification: Evolving Concepts
Trembath D, Miller CR, Perry A (Laboratory Medicine; Univ of North Carolina, Chapel Hill; Washington Univ School of Medicine, St Louis)
Adv Anat Pathol 15:287-297, 2008

The World Health Organization recently updated its classification of central nervous system tumors, adding 8 entities, as well as defining new variants and morphologic patterns of existing entities. Despite the continued refinement of brain tumor histologic classification and grading, there remain some diagnostic "gray zones" that challenge general surgical pathologists and neuropathologists alike. These include the presence of oligodendroglial features in (mixed) oligoastrocytomas and glioblastomas (GBMs), GBM variants (such as small cell GBM), meningioma classification and grading, medulloblastoma variants, ependymoma grading, the presence of "neuronal features" in otherwise morphologically classic gliomas, and low-grade gliomas with high Ki-67 labeling indices. In the current review, we discuss these issues and offer some practical guidelines for dealing with problematic cases.

▶ The diagnosis and grading of the multiple variations of primary glial, neuronal, and glioneuronal central nervous system tumors are challenging and require distinction among the various types of tumors. Distinction is critical for both appropriate classification and then treatment of an individual patient's neoplasm and for optimizing the research of CNS tumors.

The World Health Organization (WHO)-sponsored Working Group of neuro-oncology experts apply a uniform, consensus classification and grading system to CNS neoplasms, based on peer-reviewed studies, for use in clinical and research settings throughout the world.[1] The CNS tumor "Blue Book" provides concisely compiled clinicopathologic, histologic, immunohistochemical, and genetic data about CNS neoplasms. Critically, the WHO CNS tumor Working Group has, over the years, helped to establish criteria for the diagnosis and grading of these tumor entities and their variants and histologic patterns of differentiation. As an example, the provision of specific diagnostic criteria for the grading of meningiomas has immensely facilitated the consistent sign-out of such neoplasms. New in the 2007 edition, identification of "brain invasion" by meningioma on histologic examination is sufficient in and of itself to confer a "WHO grade II" on a tumor, regardless of other features identified in the neoplasm, clearing up an issue that had been contentious for years.

Nevertheless, despite the excellent guidance of the WHO text, multiple "gray zones" exist in the diagnosis and grading of tumors. This article provides an excellent overview and illustration of remaining controversies and offers suggestions about how to approach tumors within this zone. Critical topics include (1) identification of an oligodendroglial component within a glial neoplasm sufficient to make the diagnosis of oligoastrocytoma or glioblastoma with oligodendroglial features; (2) identification of variants of glioblastoma distinction including the small-cell variant and distinction from oligodendroglioma (and small-cell astrocytoma); (3) distinction of variants of medulloblastoma; (4) grading of ependymomas; (5) classification of neuronal features in otherwise classic gliomas; and (6) dealing with high MIB-1/Ki-67 labeling indices in low-grade neoplasms. This article provides a succinct review of these topics and offers practical guidance when they are encountered.

P. Boyer, MD, PhD

Reference

1. Louis DN, Ohgaki H, Wiestler OD, Cavenee WK. *WHO Classification of Tumours of the Central Nervous System.* Albany: WHO Publications Center; 2007.

14 Cytopathology

Interobserver Variability in Human Papillomavirus Test Results in Cervicovaginal Cytologic Specimens Interpreted as Atypical Squamous Cells

Geisinger KR, Vrbin C, Grzybicki DM, et al (Wake Forest Univ School of Medicine, Winston-Salem, NC; Univ of Pittursburgh School of Medicine, PA)
Am J Clin Pathol 128:1010-1014, 2007

We studied interobserver variability in the proportions of human papillomavirus (HPV)-positive results for atypical squamous cells of undetermined significance (ASCUS) and atypical squamous cells, cannot exclude high-grade squamous intraepithelial lesion (ASC-H) diagnoses among 5 pathologists from the same laboratory during a 2-year period. These proportions were compared with individual pathologist's ASCUS/squamous intraepithelial lesion (SIL) ratios.

Of 1,299 ASCUS diagnoses, 32.3% had HPV testing; 49.4% were HPV+. Positive findings by individual pathologists ranged from 38% to 67% ($P = .057$). There was a difference in the proportions of high-risk HPV results for individual pathologists ($P < .001$). For the pathologist who diagnosed 38% (23/61) of samples as HPV+, the ASCUS/SIL was 0.58; the pathologist who diagnosed 67% (28/42) as HPV+ had a ratio of 1.02. Of the ASC-H diagnoses, 32.9% were tested for HPV; 63% (46/73) were positive. Although the HPV+ proportion by pathologist ranged from 54% to 83%, no significant differences were identified.

Within the same laboratory, interobserver variability exists in the proportions of HPV positivity for ASCUS and ASC-H interpretations.

▶ As the diagnosis of atypical squamous cells – undetermined significance (ASC-US) is the most frequently used Bethesda System epithelial cell abnormality diagnosis, it is important that labs standardize on how this diagnosis is used. A major benefit of human papillomavirus (HPV) testing is that individual pathologists (and cytotechnologists) may be evaluated in terms of the frequency of high-risk HPV positivity rates. Geisinger et al showed a statistically significant difference among cytopathologists in HPV positivity rates for ASC-US diagnoses. Ideally, the next step would be to determine how pathologists behave when these data are presented to them and to see if the HPV positivity rate of an ASC-US diagnosis changes. This feedback could allow labs to standardize on national HPV positive rates and prevent the occurrence of over- or under-diagnosis. In some labs, a low ASC-US HPV positivity rate could indicate that there is an over-diagnosis of ASC-US.

S. S. Raab, MD

Accuracy of Fine-Needle Aspiration Cytology of Axillary Lymph Nodes in Breast Cancer Patients: A Study of 115 Cases With Cytologic-Histologic Correlation
Alkuwari E, Auger M (McGill Univ Health Ctr, Montreal, Quebec, Canada)
Cancer 114:89-93, 2008

Background.—Fine-needle aspiration (FNA) cytology of axillary lymph nodes is a simple, minimally invasive technique that can be used to improve preoperative determination of the status of the axillary lymph nodes in patients with breast cancer, thereby serving as a tool with which to triage patients for sentinel versus full lymph node dissection procedures. The aim of the current study was to determine the sensitivity and specificity of FNA cytology to detect metastatic breast carcinoma in axillary lymph nodes.

Methods.—A total of 115 FNAs of axillary lymph nodes of breast cancer patients with histologic follow-up (subsequent sentinel or full lymph node dissection) were included in the current study. The specificity and sensitivity, as well as the positive and negative predictive values, were calculated.

Results.—The positive and negative predictive values of FNA cytology of axillary lymph nodes for metastatic breast carcinoma were 1.00 and 0.60, respectively. The overall sensitivity of axillary lymph node FNA in all the cases studied was 65% and the specificity was 100%. The sensitivity of FNA was lower in the sentinel lymph node group than in the full lymph node dissection group (16% vs 88%, respectively), which was believed to be attributable to the small size of the metastatic foci in the sentinel lymph node group (median, 0.25 cm). All false-negative FNAs, with the exception of 1 case, were believed to be the result of sampling error. There was no 'true' false-positive FNA case in the current study.

Conclusions.—FNA of axillary lymph nodes is a sensitive and very specific method with which to detect metastasis in breast cancer patients. Because of its excellent positive predictive value, full axillary lymph node dissection can be planned safely instead of a sentinel lymph node dissection when a preoperative positive FNA result is rendered.

▶ Alkuwari and Auger report the sensitivity and the specificity of fine needle aspiration (FNA) cytology of axillary lymph nodes for metastatic carcinoma. As expected, most false negatives are secondary to problems in sampling, generally related to small size of metastases, the low number of lymph nodes positive for metastases, or the failure to observe the lymph nodes during axillary ultrasound examination. The question is how can we improve the sampling process and eliminate, or at least effectively decrease, these types of errors— possible solutions include obtaining additional passes if the first passes are negative (assuming that an immediate interpretation is performed, which in itself may help to reduce false-negative diagnoses compared with when it is not performed), using immunohistochemical staining, preparing cell blocks, or perhaps using technologies such as monolayer preparations. The difficulty in addressing this issue is that false negative diagnoses are relatively few in number, and a large number of single institutional cases (or cases from several institutions) would be needed to study this issue. We also need to study the clinical effect of missing micrometastatic disease by FNA.

For further reading on this subject I suggest an article by Raab et al.[1]

S. S. Raab, MD

Reference

1. Raab SS, Vrbin CM, Grzybicki DM, et al. Errors in thyroid gland fine needle aspiration. *Am J Clin Pathol.* 2006;125:873-882.

The role of breast FNAC in diagnosis and clinical management: a survey of current practice

Kocjan G, Bourgain C, Fassina A, et al (Univ College London, London, UK; Dept of Pathology and Ctr for Reproductive Medicine, Brussels, Belgium; Univ of Padova, Italy; et al)
Cytopathology 19:271-278, 2008

Most participating countries have now adopted a triple assessment approach, i.e. clinical,imaging and pathology, to breast diagnosis, with FNAC as the first-line pathological investigation in both screening and symptomatic populations, with the exception of microcalcifications. Pathologists specialized in cytopathology are best qualified to collect and interpret FNAC samples, but this is not always possible or practical. Radiologists involved in breast imaging should ensure that they have the necessary skills to carry out FNAC under all forms of image guidance. Best results are achieved by a combination of both techniques, as shown in the image-guided FNAC in the presence of the cytopathologist. The majority of European countries use similar reporting systems for breast FNAC (C1–C5), in keeping with European Guidelines for Quality Assurance in Breast Cancer Screening and Diagnosis, although some still prefer descriptive reporting only. When triple assessment is concordant, final treatment may proceed on the basis of FNAC, without a tissue biopsy. ER and PR assessment can be done safely on FNAC material. However, not all institutions may have expertise in doing this. HER-2 protein expression on direct cytological preparations is insufficiently reliable for clinical use, although its use for FISH is possible, if expertise is available. The majority of participants practise a degree of one-stop diagnosis with a cytopathologist present in the out-patient clinic. Formal recognition of the importance of the time spent outside the laboratory, both for cytopathologist and cytotechnologist, is necessary in order to ensure appropriate resourcing. The use of core biopsy (CB) has increased, although not always for evidence-based reasons. CB and FNAC are not mutually exclusive. FNAC should be used in diagnosis of benign, symptomatic lesions and CB in microcalcifications, suspicious FNAC findings and malignancies where radiology cannot guarantee stromal invasion.

▶ Kocjan and colleagues report the differences in the practice of fine needle aspiration biopsy (FNAB) for breast lesions in various settings in Europe and the United States. Clearly, some areas of breast FNAB are more standardized than others. In almost all countries, the use of the triple assessment is critical in determining appropriate follow-up. The triple assessment involves the use of clinical examination findings, radiologic findings, and the FNAB results. If all 3 findings are concordant (eg, the radiologic, clinical, and FNAB findings are malignant), then final treatment may rest without obtaining additional tissue. If not concordant, then clinical decision-making must rest on all 3 components. The use of the triple test depends on close communication of the clinician, radiologist, and pathologist. This communication helps to improve all aspects of care including triage of the patient and better understanding of the more difficult cases. Additional benefits of this close cooperation are improved reporting and preclinical assessments.

For further reading on this subject I suggest an article by Perry et al.[1]

S. S. Raab, MD

Reference

1. Perry N, Broeders M, de Wolf C, et al. European guidelines for quality assurance in breast cancer screening and diagnosis. Fourth edition—summary document. *Ann Oncol.* 2008;19:614-622.

The Use of Fine Needle Aspiration Cytology for the Distinction of Pancreatic Mucinous Neoplasia

Stelow EB, Shami VM, Abbott TE, et al (Univ of Virginia, Charlottesville, VA; et al)
Am J Clin Pathol 129:67-74, 2008

Cytology frequently has some role in preoperatively distinguishing pancreatic mucus-producing neoplasia (intraductal papillary mucinous neoplasms [IPMNs] and mucinous cystic neoplasms [MCNs]) from other pancreatic cysts. We evaluated all cytologic specimens at our institutions from resected pancreatic cystic lesions for lesional extracellular and cellular material. Lesional extracellular material was identified in 32 of 38 of the cytologic samples from cystic pancreatic mucus-producing neoplasms (28 of 31 IPMNs and 4 of 7 MCNs). Lesional cellular material was seen in 22 of 38 cases (17 of 31 IPMNs and 5 of 7 MCNs). Lesional material was more commonly identified in higher grade and invasive lesions. Lesional extracellular material was seen in 3 of 14 samples of other pancreatic cysts, and lesional cellular material was seen in 6 of 14 cases.

▶ The diagnosis of pancreatic cystic lesions is a difficult one, especially when very little material is obtained. The ability to diagnose these lesions depends not only on cytopathologist expertise but also clinician expertise in radiologic interpretation and aspiration technique. Stelow et al report that nonspecific negative findings do not preclude the presence of mucinous neoplasia (such as an intraductal pancreatic mucinous neoplasm [IPMN]) or even a malignant mucinous tumor. True positive and true negative predictive values of these cystic lesions are generally unknown, as most cystic lesions are never resected. Selection bias of using a histologic gold standard results in artificially high sensitivities. Stelow et al demonstrate that by using extracellular and cellular material they were able to identify most neoplastic pancreatic cysts that were resected. However, it is difficult to determine if lesions are not resected because they were diagnosed as benign when they were, or could have been, neoplastic. It would appear that long-term follow-up would be useful in these lesions.

S. S. Raab, MD

Assessing New Technologies for Cervical Cancer Screening: Beyond Sensitivity

Massad LS (Washington Univ School of Medicine, St Louis)
J Low Genit Tract Dis 12:311-315, 2008

New technologies have been proposed to replace cervical cytology as the medium for cervical cancer screening, especially testing for human papillomavirus (HPV). Many of these alternatives have been endorsed because their single-test sensitivity is superior to that of cytology. The sensitivity of a single Pap test may be as low as 50%, but lifetime testing has significantly greater sensitivity, and other parameters are also important in defining the optimal screening test. Test accuracy depends not only on sensitivity but also on specificity and disease prevalence; both of these are problematic when considering HPV as a screen. A screening test also must be acceptable to both clinicians and patients. HPV testing is regarded as test for a sexually transmitted disease by many women. Clinicians often fail to appreciate the transient nature of HPV infection, prompting overly aggressive treatment that risks future preterm birth, and there is no consensus about strategies for follow-up of abnormal HPV screening results when obtained without concomitant cytology. An emphasis on sensitivity also may be inappropriate when most cervical cancers occur in unscreened women, for whom the sensitivity of testing is irrelevant. HPV testing and other technologies have substantial promise as tests that may replace cytology in cervical cancer screening, but obstacles are significant, and premature adoption of these methods may result in patient harm.

▶ Currently, the best method to screen for cervical cancer is being debated. With the introduction of new technologies such as human papillomavirus (HPV) testing and the HPV vaccine, the traditional paradigm of screening (Pap test followed by colposcopy for specific abnormal diagnosis) is being questioned. The article by Massad raises many important points in the transformation for the cervical cancer screening industry in both the United States and throughout the world. One aspect of the traditional system is that a great deal of quality assurance and sociological issues have been in place for a while, and altering the paradigm has profound issues in the medical system. For example, Massad correctly points out that there is no general agreement on an appropriate triage test for a positive HPV result. In addition, Massad writes that excellent screening systems minimize complexity, although some have suggested that different screening paradigms should be in place for different subgroups of women (eg, younger women with a high prevalence of HPV and older women with a low prevalence). The obstacles to altering the traditional system are high and additional consensus and study are needed about technology implementation and acceptance.

S. S. Raab, MD

Changes in Specimen Preparation Method May Impact Urine Cytologic Evaluation
Voss JS, Kipp BR, Krueger AK, et al (Mayo Clinic and Foundation, Rochester, MN)
Am J Clin Pathol 130:428-433, 2008

This study was performed to identify differences in the frequency of specific cytologic diagnoses obtained between specimens prepared by the filtration and ThinPrep (Cytyc, Marlborough, MA) techniques and to assess how these cytologic diagnoses correlated with pathologic findings. Data were collected from 2,347 voided urine specimens analyzed 8 months before and after ThinPrep implementation. Urine cytologic and bladder biopsy specimens were obtained as part of clinical follow-up, and positive diagnoses were considered evidence of malignancy. After ThinPrep implementation, the proportion of specimens diagnosed as negative significantly decreased (85.5% vs 78.6%; $P < .001$), clusters (5.8% vs 5.6%; $P = .597$) and positive (2.8% vs 3.3%; $P = .143$) diagnoses remained similar, and atypical (3.1% vs 8.4%; $P < .001$) and "suspicious" diagnoses (2.7% vs 4.1%; $P < .001$) increased. After 1 year of follow-up, there was no significant difference in the percentage of patients diagnosed with bladder carcinoma between the 2 methods for all cytologic categories.

▶ Voss et al wrote a nice article on how diagnostic category use changes with the introduction of new technology. In this case, the use of indeterminate diagnostic categories increased with the use of a monolayer technology in urine cytology. There has been little study of the use of indeterminate diagnostic categories, although many cytologists tend to use these categories to classify lesions of which they are unsure. From these data, it is unclear if the monolayer technology is better at detecting cells that are more worrisome or if the cytologists were less certain about particular cells because they were using a new technology. It is critical to know how clinicians behave with the use of indeterminate categories and if they either obtain additional specimens or if they refer patients for a cystoscopic examination. If either of these behaviors are true, the use of indeterminate categories led to additional testing without an increase in the diagnosis of cancer.

For further reading on this subject I suggest an article by Wright and Halford.[1]

S. S. Raab, MD

Reference

1. Wright RG, Halford JA. Evaluation of thin-layer methods in urine cytology. *Cytopathology*. 2001;12:306-313.

Bladder Cancer Detection Using FISH (UroVysion Assay)
Halling KC, Kipp BR (Mayo Clinic and Foundation, Rochester, MN)
Adv Anat Pathol 15:279-286, 2008

UroVysion is a fluorescence in situ hybridization assay that was developed for the detection of bladder cancer in urine specimens. It consists of fluorescently labeled DNA probes to the pericentromeric regions of chromosomes 3 (red), 7 (green), and 17 (aqua) and to the 9p21 band (gold) location of the *P16* tumor suppressor gene. The UroVysion assay works by detecting urinary cells that have chromosomal abnormalities consistent with a diagnosis of bladder cancer. Studies have shown that UroVysion is more sensitive than urine cytology for the detection of all stages and grades of bladder cancer. UroVysion is Food and Drug Administration-approved for the detection of recurrent bladder cancer in voided urine specimens from patients with a history of bladder cancer and for the detection of bladder cancer in voided urine specimens from patients with gross or microscopic hematuria, but no previous history of bladder cancer. Recent studies also suggest that UroVysion may be useful for assessing superficial bladder cancer patients' response to bacillus Calmette-Guerin therapy and in detecting upper tract urothelial carcinoma.

▶ In cases of bladder cancer, life-long surveillance is required to detect subsequent tumor recurrence. Current surveillance protocols consist of cystoscopic evaluation and urine cytology every 3 to 4 months for the first 2 years and at longer intervals in the following years. As discussed earlier, voided urine cytology has excellent sensitivity for high-grade bladder cancers and lower sensitivity for low-grade cancers. Cystoscopic examination has a sensitivity as low as 70%, is expensive, and causes considerable patient discomfort. For these reasons, noninvasive and accurate biomarkers are needed for the surveillance of patients who have a history of bladder cancer and also for primary screening. The use of biomarkers is generally assessed by comparing the sensitivity and specificity with urine cytology. For example, the UroVysion test relies on chromosomal alterations associated with bladder cancer by the use of fluorescent probes to centromeres on chromosomes 3, 7, 17, and 9p21. The protocol for test performance is both labor-intensive and operator-dependent, requiring expertise of the person who counts and examines the slides. In a meta-analysis of diagnostic accuracy, Hadjdinjak reported that excluding Ta tumors, the sensitivity for UroVysion and cytology was 86% and 61%, respectively.[1] Differences in test performance disappeared when superficial cases were excluded from the analysis. Hajdinjak concluded that cytology results were highly specific, although a negative cytology result did not meaningfully change the post-test probability of urothelial cancer. UroVysion results did not provide conclusive evidence of the presence or absence of cancer, but both positive and negative results altered the post-test probability of malignancy.

S. S. Raab, MD

Reference

1. Hajdinjak T. UroVysion FISH test for detecting urothelial cancers: meta-analysis of diagnsotic accuracy and comparison with urinary tract cytology testing [published online ahead of print]. *Urol Oncol.* 2008 Jan 14; 2008 Jan 14.

15 Hematolymphoid

CD33 Detection by Immunohistochemistry in Paraffin-Embedded Tissues: A New Antibody Shows Excellent Specificity and Sensitivity for Cells of Myelomonocytic Lineage.
Hoyer JD, Grogg KL, Hanson CA, et al (Mayo Clinic, Rochester, MN)
Am J Clin Pathol 129:316-323, 2008

A new monoclonal antibody to CD33 that reacts in paraffin-embedded tissue samples was evaluated. The expected reactivity in granulocytic and monocytic cells was found in a tissue microarray composed of multiple tissue sites. There was no unexpected reactivity found in a wide variety of hematolymphoid and nonhematolymphoid disorders. In cases of acute leukemia, the CD33 antibody showed equivalent results by immunohistochemical analysis compared with flow cytometric analysis. The CD33 antibody was also found to be a useful marker in the workup of myeloid sarcomas. This anti-CD33 antibody will be a useful marker in the workup of acute leukemias and myeloid sarcomas on paraffin-embedded tissue samples.

▶ Assessment of myeloid lineage in formalin-fixed paraffin-embedded (FFPE) tissue may sometimes present problems. Most available antibodies including myeloperoxidase, CD68 KP1, CD68 PG-M1, CD43, lysozyme, and CD117 are either positive mostly in more mature cells or lineage nonspecific. CD33 antigen along with CD13 has been a mainstay marker for myeloid lineage assessment in flow cytometric (FC) analysis. In this article, Hoyer and colleagues evaluate a newly available anti-CD33 antibody for use in FFPE. The antibody may be used for both formalin- and B5-fixed tissue. The evaluation of antibody in tissue microarrays of normal tissues as well as a spectrum of hematolymphoid and non-hematolymphoid cancers revealed no unexpected reactivity. Anti-CD33 antibody was highly specific for myeloid and monocytic precursors of all maturational stages including blasts. There was a high degree of correlation between CD33 immunohistochemistry and FC in immunophenotypic analysis of leukemia including all major myeloid leukemia types and lymphoblastic leukemia with aberrant CD33 expression. CD33 antibody also showed high sensitivity for myeloid sarcoma. With increasing use of anti-CD33 targeted therapy (gemtuzumab ozogamicin), which is conditioned on CD33 expression by neoplastic cells, this marker may offer a valuable alternative to FC.

M. Djokic, MD

Monoclonal B-Cell Lymphocytosis and Chronic Lymphocytic Leukemia

Rawstron AC, Bennett FL, O'Connor SJM, et al (Leeds Teaching Hosps, UK)
N Engl J Med 359:575-583, 2008

Background.—A diagnosis of chronic lymphocytic leukemia (CLL) requires a count of over 5000 circulating CLL-phenotype cells per cubic millimeter. Asymptomatic persons with fewer CLL-phenotype cells have monoclonal B-cell lymphocytosis (MBL). The goal of this study was to investigate the relation between MBL and CLL.

Methods.—We investigated 1520 subjects who were 62 to 80 years of age with a normal blood count and 2228 subjects with lymphocytosis (>4000 lymphocytes per cubic millimeter) for the presence of MBL, using flow cytometry. Monoclonal B cells were further characterized by means of cytogenetic and molecular analyses. A representative cohort of 185 subjects with CLL-phenotype MBL and lymphocytosis were monitored for a median of 6.7 years (range, 0.2 to 11.8).

Results.—Monoclonal CLL-phenotype B cells were detected in 5.1% of subjects (78 of 1520) with a normal blood count and 13.9% (309 of 2228) with lymphocytosis. CLL-phenotype MBL had a frequency of 13q14 deletion and trisomy 12 similar to that of CLL and showed a skewed repertoire of the immunoglobulin heavy variable group (*IGHV*) genes. Among 185 subjects presenting with lymphocytosis, progressive lymphocytosis occurred in 51 (28%), progressive CLL developed in 28 (15%), and chemotherapy was required in 13 (7%). The absolute B-cell count was the only independent prognostic factor associated with progressive lymphocytosis. During follow-up over a median of 6.7 years, 34% of subjects (62 of 185) died, but only 4 of these deaths were due to CLL. Age above 68 years and hemoglobin level below 12.5 g per deciliter were the only independent prognostic factors for death.

Conclusions.—The CLL-phenotype cells found in the general population and in subjects with lymphocytosis have features in common with CLL cells. CLL requiring treatment develops in subjects with CLL-phenotype MBL and with lymphocytosis at the rate of 1.1% per year.

▶ Monoclonal B-cell lymphocytosis (MBL) is defined as the presence of less than 5000 monoclonal B-lymphocytes per microliter in the absence of history or symptoms of chronic lymphocytic leukemia (CLL) or any other lymphoproliferative disorder or autoimmune disease.[1] Rawstron et al studied 2 large cohorts of patients by flow cytometric immunophenotypic analysis of peripheral blood—1520 patients with normal blood counts and 2228 patients with lymphocytosis. They found monoclonal B-cells with CLL-like phenotype (CD19+, CD5+, CD23+, dim CD20+, kappa- or lambda-restricted surface light chain expression) in 5.1% and 13.9% of subjects, respectively. Further investigation revealed that frequencies of del13q14 and trisomy 12 in the MBL populations were similar to those in CLL. Eighty-eight percent of investigated cases with CLL-like MBL had more than 2% immunoglobulin heavy variable (IGHV) mutation similar to indolent CLL with mutated IGHV. Progressive lymphocytosis was observed in 28% of subjects with CLL-like MBL (defined as > 4000 monoclonal B-lymphocytes per microliter), 15% developed classic CLL, mostly lymphadenopathy, and 7% required chemotherapy during a median follow-up of 6.7 years. These results suggest that MBL is a premalignant condition with an estimated risk of progression to CLL requiring chemotherapy of 1.1% per year, analogous to the rate of progression to myeloma in patients with monoclonal gammopathy of undetermined significance.

M. Djokic, MD

Reference

1. Marti GE, Abbasi F, Raveche E, et al. Overview of monoclonal B-cell lymphocytosis. *Br J Haematol.* 2007;139:701-708.

A Subset of CD5– Diffuse Large B-Cell Lymphomas Expresses Nuclear Cyclin D1 With Aberrations at the *CCND1* Locus

Ehinger M, Linderoth J, Christensson B, et al (Lund Univ Hosp, Sweden; Karolinska Univ Hosp Huddinge, Stockholm)
Am J Clin Pathol 129:630-638, 2008

In 231 diffuse large B-cell lymphomas, the expression of cyclin D1 and CD5 was evaluated. All cases were CD5–. Ten (4.3%) were positive for cyclin D1 and were subjected to fluorescence in situ hybridization at the *CCND1* locus. One case showed the t(11;14). In another case, the telomeric probe signal for cyclin D1 was lost in most tumor cells, and in a small proportion of the cells, there were fluorescence signals indicative of the t(11;14). Two other cases displayed additional cyclin D1 signals in the absence of the t(11;14). All cases but 1 were positive for bcl-6 or MUM1, disfavoring the possibility of misdiagnosed blastoid variants of CD5– mantle cell lymphomas. Thus, contrary to the current view, there seems to exist a certain number of cyclin D1+ and CD5– diffuse large B-cell lymphomas, some of which have structural aberrations at the *CCND1* locus, including the t(11;14).

▶ Rearrangement of cyclin D1 (*CCND1*) gene is a critical biological event in the lymphomagenesis of mantle cell lymphoma. Overexpression of CCND1 protein is also present in a subset of cases of plasma cell myeloma and hairy cell leukemia, although the majority of positive cases, at least in the latter category, may not have *CCND1* gene rearrangement. Diffuse large B-cell lymphoma (DLBCL) is considered to be *CCND1*-negative lymphoma, although at least 1 smaller study demonstrated scattered weakly *CCND1*-positive neoplastic cells.[1] Ehinger and coworkers examine *CCND1* expression in a large series of CD5– diffuse large B-cell lymphoma (DLBCL) using multiple antibody clones for immunohistochemical staining. They found 10 *CCND1*+ cases (4.3%), with 3 cases showing diffuse staining and the remaining 7 cases with focal staining. Fluorescence in situ hybridization (FISH) analysis showed 1 case with immunoglobulin heavy chain (IGH)/*CCND1* rearrangement (strong, diffuse staining for CCND1). Another case had evidence of fusion signal only in a subset of neoplastic cells (10%), whereas 2 other cases had multiple copies of *CCND1* signal suggestive of *CCND1* amplification. The remaining 3 cases with available tissue had normal FISH pattern with multiple probes, suggesting possible post-translational mechanism of *CCND1* overexpression. These results indicate that dysregulation of *CCND1* expression may be seen in a small subset of DLBCL, possibly as a nonprimary event in pathogenesis. The authors remind us that no hematolymphoid malignancy can be defined by a single genetic abnormality, and that integration of clinical, morphologic, immunophenotypic, and genetic findings is necessary for complete pathologic diagnosis.

M. Djokic, MD

Reference

1. Sánchez-Beato M, Camacho FI, Martínez-Montero JC, et al. Anomalous high p27/KIP1 expression in a subset of aggressive B-cell lymphomas is associated with cyclin D3 overexpression. p27/KIP1-cyclin D3 colocalization in tumor cells. *Blood.* 1999;94:765-772.

Genome-wide analysis of genetic alterations in acute lymphoblastic leukaemia

Mullighan CG, Goorha S, Radtke I, et al (St Jude Children's Res Hosp, Memphis, TN)

Nature 446:758-764, 2007

Chromosomal aberrations are a hallmark of acute lymphoblastic leukaemia (ALL) but alone fail to induce leukaemia. To identify cooperating oncogenic lesions, we performed a genome-wide analysis of leukaemic cells from 242 paediatric ALL patients using high-resolution, single-nucleotide polymorphism arrays and genomic DNA sequencing. Our analyses revealed deletion, amplification, point mutation and structural rearrangement in genes encoding principal regulators of B lymphocyte development and differentiation in 40% of B-progenitor ALL cases. The *PAX5* gene was the most frequent target of somatic mutation, being altered in 31.7% of cases. The identified *PAX5* mutations resulted in reduced levels of PAX5 protein or the generation of hypomorphic alleles. Deletions were also detected in *TCF3* (also known as *E2A*), *EBF1*, *LEF1*, *IKZF1* (*IKAROS*) and *IKZF3* (*AIOLOS*). These findings suggest that direct disruption of pathways controlling B-cell development and differentiation contributes to B-progenitor ALL pathogenesis. Moreover, these data demonstrate the power of high-resolution, genome-wide approaches to identify new molecular lesions in cancer.

▶ High-density DNA microarrays provide an invaluable tool for precise mapping of genomic amplifications and deletions allowing a systematic search for recurring genetic abnormalities and identification of genes that are mutated in cancer. Mullighan et al use high-density DNA microarrays to study recurrent genetic alterations in childhood acute lymphoblastic leukemia. They discover deletions of short arm of chromosome 9 involving *PAX5* gene in 57 of 192 (30%) patients with precursor B-cell acute lymphoblastic leukemia (ALL). *PAX5* gene is an important transcription factor regulating B-cell differentiation. There are 4 distinct patterns of deletions: a) focal deletions involving only *PAX5* gene; b) broader deletions involving *PAX5* and a variable number of flanking genes; c) large 9p deletions involving 3' end of *PAX5*; and d) deletion of entire 9p or monosomy 9. Sequencing of *PAX5* reveals point mutations in an additional 14 cases involving primarily DNA-binding or transcriptional regulatory domains of the protein. Interestingly, in most cases with *PAX5* deletions or functionally inactivating mutations the remaining copy of the gene was not affected, suggesting "haploinsufficiency" as the most likely mechanism of *PAX5* dysregulation. Deletions were also discovered in other genes involved in B-cell development, indicating that pathways controlling B-cell differentiation are important for pathogenesis of precursor B-cell ALL.

M. Djokic, MD

Intravascular Large T-cell or NK-cell Lymphoma: A Rare Variant of Intravascular Large Cell Lymphoma With Frequent Cytotoxic Phenotype and Association With Epstein-Barr Virus Infection
Cerroni L, Massone C, Kutzner H, et al (Med Univ of Graz, Austria; Dermatopathologische Gemeinschaftspraxis, Friedrichshafen, Germany; et al)
Am J Surg Pathol 32:891-898, 2008

Most cases of intravascular large cell lymphoma have a B-cell phenotype, but rare T-cell and natural killer (NK)-cell variants have been reported. We describe the clinicopathologic features of 4 patients (M:F = 3:1; age range: 63 to 87; median age: 65) with intravascular large NK/T-cell lymphoma. The skin was the site of presentation in all patients (leg: 1 case; trunk: 1 case; trunk and extremities: 2 cases). Two patients had lesions confined to the skin; in 1 case concomitant involvement of the brain was detected and in 1 case no further studies were carried out. Immunohistology showed positivity for cytotoxic markers in 3/4 cases. One case had an NK phenotype similar to NK/T-cell lymphoma, nasal-type, whereas the other cases could not be precisely classified into specific categories (peripheral T-cell lymphoma, NOS). One of these cases was negative for cytotoxic markers and was positive only for CD2 and CD3 epsilon. Association with Epstein-Barr virus (EBV) was demonstrated in 2 cases by in situ hybridization, whereas 1 case was negative. All our patients had aggressive disease and died between 2 weeks and 7 months from presentation. Analysis of our cases and of those published in the literature shows that intravascular large NK/T-cell lymphoma is a rare, aggressive lymphoma with variable phenotypic features, frequent expression of cytotoxic proteins, true NK-cell phenotype and association with Epstein-Barr virus infection, and common presentation in the skin. Homogeneous studies on larger number of patients and reevaluation of cases published with incomplete phenotypic data would be necessary to gather more information on this extremely rare type of lymphoma.

▶ This article is the first published series of intravascular large NK/T-cell lymphoma, an extremely rare type of non-Hodgkin lymphoma. The authors have collected a series of 4 cases, which presented as skin lesions and in 2 cases involved other organs. The lesions consisted of medium- or large-sized pleomorphic cells contained within lumina of the vessels. Immunophenotypic characterization demonstrated NK/T-cell phenotype with expression of CD2 and CD3ε chain (all 4 cases), expression of cytotoxic markers (3 of 4 cases), and association with Epstein-Barr virus (EBV) infection (2 of 4). Two cases had monoclonal rearrangement of T-cell receptor g chain, whereas the other 2 cases had T-cell receptor in germline configuration. All 4 subjects had an aggressive course and died within 7 months. A review of the literature revealed an additional 33 cases published mostly as case reports. Cutaneous involvement was observed in 54% of cases and in 41% of cases the disease was confined to the skin. In most cases the disease had a very aggressive course with slightly worse prognosis in multiple organ involvement. These characteristics are analogous to the picture in intravascular large B-cell lymphoma. Larger studies are necessary to further characterize this entity. Considering the rarity of the disease, probably the best chance of collecting a sufficient number of cases would be through an international workshop.

M. Djokic, MD

Instability of Immunophenotype in Plasma Cell Myeloma

Cao W, Goolsby CL, Nelson BP, et al (Northwestern Univ, Chicago, IL)
Am J Clin Pathol 129:926-933, 2008

Little information has been reported describing antigen stability in plasma cell myeloma. In this study, the expression frequency and stability of 2 potential therapeutic targets, CD20 and CD52, along with the frequently aberrantly expressed CD56 antigen, were evaluated by flow cytometric analyses in 56 patients with plasma cell myeloma. Of the 56 patients, 23 (41%) showed immunophenotype change, including CD56 in 6 cases, CD20 in 7 cases, and CD52 in 17 cases. Combined CD56/CD52 change was seen in 3 cases and combined CD20/CD52 in 4 cases. No correlation was found between immunophenotype change and age, sex, stage, plasma cell morphologic features, extent of marrow involvement, time between analyses, type of therapy, or response to therapy. Immunophenotype shift was more common in patients with IgA than in patients with IgG paraprotein. Recognition of lack of stability in immunophenotype may be important, especially in antigen-directed treatment decisions and when specific phenotypes are used to detect residual disease.

▶ Plasma cell myeloma is a clonal proliferation of plasma cells. Flow cytometry is frequently used for immunophenotypic characterization of plasma cells in cases of suspected plasma cell neoplasia. Neoplastic plasma cells usually have an aberrant phenotype at diagnosis characterized by expression of CD56 and loss of CD19 in addition to expression of CD138, bright CD38, and monotypic cytoplasmic immunoglobulin. There is variable expression of CD20 and CD45. Combinations of these markers have been used both for diagnosis and in minimal residual monitoring of myeloma patients. This study by Cao and coworkers focuses on a different aspect of plasma cell immunophenotype, namely on the stability of potential therapeutic targets including CD20 and CD52 and stability of aberrant CD56 expression. Overall, they see immunophenotypic shifts in 75% of cases with IgA myeloma and in 28% of cases with IgG myeloma. Shifts in CD20 antigen expression were observed in 13% of cases, and CD52 expression was modulated in 30% of cases. Expression of CD56 was altered in 11% of cases. None of the patients in their study were treated with rituximab or alemtuzumab, so these antigenic shifts are not because of the effects of therapeutic antibody. Antigen instability may have important consequences in the choice of targeted therapy with monoclonal antibody and in residual disease monitoring.

M. Djokic, MD

Subcutaneous panniculitis-like T-cell lymphoma: definition, classification, and prognostic factors: an EORTC Cutaneous Lymphoma Group Study of 83 cases
Willemze R, Jansen PM, Cerroni L, et al (Leiden Univ Med Ctr, Leiden, The Netherlands; Univ of Graz, Austria; et al)
Blood 111:838-845, 2008

In the WHO classification, subcutaneous panniculitis-like T-cell lymphoma (SPTL) is defined as a distinct type of T-cell lymphoma with an aggressive clinical behavior. Recent studies suggest that distinction should be made between SPTL with an α/β T-cell phenotype (SPTL-AB) and SPTL with a γδ T-cell phenotype (SPTL-GD), but studies are limited. To better define their clinicopathologic features, immunophenotype, treatment, and survival, 63 SPTL-ABs and 20 SPTL-GDs were studied at a workshop of the EORTC Cutaneous Lymphoma Group. SPTL-ABs were generally confined to the subcutis, had a CD4⁻, CD8⁺, CD56⁻, βF1⁺ phenotype, were uncommonly associated with a hemophagocytic syndrome (HPS; 17%), and had a favorable prognosis (5-year overall survival [OS]: 82%). SPTL-AB patients without HPS had a significantly better survival than patients with HPS (5-year OS: 91% vs 46%; $P < .001$). SPTL-GDs often showed (epi)dermal involvement and/or ulceration, a CD4⁻, CD8⁻, CD56⁺/⁻, betaF1⁻ T-cell phenotype, and poor prognosis (5-year OS:

11%), irrespective of the presence of HPS or type of treatment. These results indicate that SPTL-AB and SPTL-GD are distinct entities, and justify that the term SPTL should further be used only for SPTL-AB. SPTL-ABs without associated HPS have an excellent prognosis, and multiagent chemotherapy as first choice of treatment should be questioned.

▶ The World Health Organization (WHO) defines subcutaneous panniculitis-like T-cell lymphoma (SPTL) as a cytotoxic T-cell lymphoma that preferentially infiltrates subcutaneous tissue. Some patients also present with hemophagocytic syndrome (HPS) accompanied with fever, hepatosplenomegaly, and pancyto-penia. Recent studies have indicated that presence of HPS or an uncommon γ/δ-phenotype may be associated with more aggressive disease and worse prog-nosis. The European Organization for Research and Treatment of Cancer (EORTC) Cutaneous Lymphoma Group collected 83 cases of SPTL and studied their clinicopathologic features, immunophenotype, treatment, and survival. Their findings clearly indicate that SPTL with α/β and γ/δ phenotype are 2 sepa-rate entities with distinct histologic features (subcutaneous vs subcutaneous and dermal epidermal involvement), immunophenotypes (bF1 +, TCRd1 −, CD4−, CD8 +, CD56− versus (bF1 −, TCRd1 +, CD4−, CD8−, CD56 mostly +), clin-ical features (rare ulceration, association with autoimmune disorders, HPS uncommon vs. ulceration common, HPS common), and overall survival (5-yr 82% vs 11%). Presence of HPS is a significant indicator of poorer prognosis in SPTL with α/β phenotype, but not in SPTL with γ/δ phenotype. SPTL with α/β phenotype without HPS has an excellent prognosis and may not need multi-agent chemotherapy. The authors also suggest that SPTL diagnosis should be limited to cases that have α/β phenotype, whereas γ/δ cases should be renamed cutaneous γ/δ T-cell lymphoma (CGD-TCL).

M. Djokic, MD

***BCL6* gene amplification/3q27 gain is associated with unique clinicopathological characteristics among follicular lymphoma without *BCL2* gene translocation**
Karube K, Ying G, Tagawa H, et al (Kurume Univ, Japan; Fourth Military Med Univ, Xi'an, Shannxi, People's Republic of China; Aichi Cancer Ctr Inst, Nagoya, Japan; et al)
Mod Pathol 21:973-978, 2008

Although approximately 10–20% cases of follicular lymphoma lack *BCL2* gene rearrangement, there are few reports having described the alternative genetic aberrations and their association about clinicopatho-logical features. In this study, analysis by Fluorescence *in situ* hybridiza-tion of *BCL6* gene aberrations in 100 follicular lymphoma cases without *IGH/BCL2* rearrangement resulted in the identification of four subgroups. Group I: *BCL6* gene rearrangement ($n = 41$); Group II: *BCL6* gene amplification/3q27 gain ($n = 30$); Group III: the absence of both ($n = 23$); and Group IV: the presence of both ($n = 6$). Group II showed higher grade morphology (Grade 3a/b: 93%), higher bcl2 and MUM1 expression (73 and 57%, respectively), and more frequent combination with BCL2 gene amplification/18q21 gain (90%) than the other groups. BCL6 gene aberration, especially amplification/3q27 gain, indicates the presence of certain morphological and phenotypical findings in follicular lymphoma cases without *IGH/BCL2* rearrangement.

▶ *BCL2* gene rearrangement, usually present in the form of translocation t(14;18), is a genetic hallmark of follicular lymphoma and is thought to play a critical role in lymphomagenesis. Follicular lymphomas that lack *BCL2* rearrangement have high-grade morphologic features with reduced expression of CD10 and bcl2. Most of these cases were thought to have rearrangement of *BCL6* gene on chromosome 3q27. Karube and coworkers have studied 100 cases of follicular lymphoma without *IGH/BCL2* rearrangement looking for *BCL6* rearrangement or copy number change by fluorescence in-situ hybridization. *BCL6* gene rearrangement was found in 41% of cases. Most cases with BCL6 rearrangement had low-grade morphologic features. These cases were morphologically and phenotypically similar to cases that had no *BCL6* aberration. In 30% of cases, there was 3q27 gain/*BCL6* amplification. These cases showed higher grade morphology and stronger expression of bcl2 and MUM1. Strong bcl2 expression in this group was thought to be due to frequent 18q21 gain/*BCL2* amplification. These results indicate that the *BCL6* gene rearrangement may not play an important role in follicular lymphoma, as was previously thought.

M. Djokic, MD

Immunohistochemical Expression of Langerin in Langerhans Cell Histiocytosis and Non-Langerhans Cell Histiocytic Disorders
Lau SK, Chu PG, Weiss LM (City of Hope Natl Med Ctr, Duarte, CA)
Am J Surg Pathol 32:615-619, 2008

Langerin is a type II transmembrane C-type lectin associated with the formation of Birbeck granules in Langerhans cells. Langerin is a highly selective marker for Langerhans cells and the lesional cells of Langerhans cell histiocytosis. Although Langerin protein expression in Langerhans cell histiocytosis has been previously documented, the specificity of Langerin expression as determined by immunohistochemistry in the context of other histiocytic disorders has not been well established. In the present study, Langerin immunoreactivity was examined in a series of histiocytic disorders of monocyte/macrophage and dendritic cell derivation to assess the specificity and utility of Langerin as a diagnostic marker for Langerhans cell histiocytosis. Immunohistochemical expression of CD1a was also evaluated for comparison. Seventeen cases of Langerhans cell histiocytosis and 64 cases of non-Langerhans cell histiocytic disorders were examined. Langerin and CD1a were uniformly expressed in all cases of Langerhans cell histiocytosis, with the exception of one case that was positive for Langerin and negative for CD1a. Among the non-Langerhans cell histiocytic disorders evaluated, focal Langerin immunoreactivity was observed only in 2 of 10 cases of histiocytic sarcoma. All non-Langerhans cell histiocytic disorders showed no expression of CD1a. Langerin expression seems to be a highly sensitive and relatively specific marker of Langerhans cell histiocytosis. Immunohistochemical evaluation of Langerin expression may have utility in substantiating a diagnosis of Langerhans cell histiocytosis and separating this disorder from other non-Langerhans cell histiocytic proliferations.

▶ Diagnosis of histiocytic and dendritic tumors usually poses a challenge. These are very uncommon tumors that may present with variable morphologic features. Pathologists rely heavily on immunohistochemical staining to make a specific diagnosis. Langerin is a protein associated with Birbeck granules in Langerhans cells. Langerin antibody (anti-CD207) is highly sensitive for Langerhans cells and useful for diagnosis of Langerhans cell histiocytosis (LCH). Lau and colleagues have characterized the immunohistochemical expression of Langerin in a wide variety of histiocytic and dendritic disorders to determine its specificity and diagnostic use. Langerin immunoreactivity was tested in 17 previously diagnosed cases of LCH, 46 cases of malignant and nonmalignant histiocytic disorders, and 18 cases of dendritic cell neoplasia, and compared its expression profile with CD1a. Langerin staining was present in all cases of LCH including a single case, which was CD1a negative, but showed the presence of Birbeck granules by electron microscopy. The immunohistochemical staining was absent in most cases of non-Langerhans cell histiocytic disorders with the exception of 2 of 10 cases of histiocytic sarcoma where focal staining (less than 5% of neoplastic cells) was observed. These 2 cases of histiocytic disorders were CD1a negative. Lau et al conclude that Langerin is a highly sensitive marker for LCH and may serve as adjunct to CD1a staining. It may be of particular value for those cases lacking CD1a reactivity where it can serve as an alternative to electron microscopy. Langerin specificity for histiocytic disorders other than LCH appears to be somewhat lower than CD1a.

M. Djokic, MD

Marrow fibrosis predicts early fatal marrow failure in patients with myelodysplastic syndromes
Buesche G, Teoman H, Wilczak W, et al (Medizinische Hochschule Hannover, Germany; Universitätsklinikum Hamburg-Eppendorf, Germany; et al)
Leukemia 22:313-322, 2008

Marrow fibrosis (MF) has rarely been studied in myelodysplastic syndromes (MDS). There are no data on occurrence and significance of MF in the context of the World Health Organization (WHO) classification of disease. In total, 349 bone marrow biopsies from 200 patients with primary MDS were examined for MF and its prognostic relevance. MF correlated with multilineage dysplasia, more severe thrombopenia, higher probability of a clonal karyotype abnormality, and higher percentages of blasts in the peripheral blood ($P < 0.002$). Its frequency varied markedly between different MDS types ranging from 0 (RARS) to 16% (RCMD, RAEB, $P < 0.007$). Two patients with MF showed a Janus kinase-2 mutation (V617F). Patients with MF suffered from marrow failure significantly earlier with shortening of the survival time down to 0.5 (RAEB-1/-2), and 1–2 (RCMD, RA) years in median ($P < 0.00005$). The prognostic relevance of MF was independent of the International Prognostic Scoring System and the classification of disease. Conclusion: The risk of MF Differs markedly between various subtypes of MDS. MF indicates an aggressive course with a significantly faster progression to fatal marrow failure and should therefore be considered in diagnosis, prognosis and treatment of disease.

▶ The WHO classification considers multiple criteria for stratification of myelo-dysplastic syndromes (MDS) including the presence of multilineage dysplasia, blast count, and recurrent cytogenetic abnormalities. It devotes scant attention to prevalence and extent of myelofibrosis (MF) and its effect on disease course and survival. In a retrospective study, Buesche and coworkers evaluate the occurrence and significance of MF and relate the results to the WHO classification and the International Prognostic Scoring System (IPSS). To improve the reproducibility of grading of fibrosis they use a novel scoring system evaluating the extent of fibrosis in the marrow—"normal fiber content" if > 95% of marrow does not show any fiber increase; "MF" when ≥15% of bone marrow shows increased reticulin fibers, and "extensive diffuse MF" when ≥50% of area is affected by fibrosis. "Foci with an increased fiber deposition" (FFI) represented 5% to 14% of marrow area with increased fibrosis. MF correlates with multilineage dysplasia, severe thrombocytopenia, clonal karyotype, and higher blast counts. Presence of MF at initial diagnostic marrow for MDS had independent prognostic significance for overall survival, risk for AML transformation, and MDS-related death in multivariate analysis. This study indicates that we should be regularly evaluating MF in bone marrow biopsies of MDS patients.

M. Djokic, MD

Detection of phospho-STAT5 in mast cells: a reliable phenotypic marker of systemic mast cell disease that reflects constitutive tyrosine kinase activation

Zuluaga Toro T, Hsieh FH, Bodo J, et al (Cleveland Clinic, OH; et al)
Br J Haematol 139:31-40, 2007

Systemic mastocytosis (SM) is characterized by the abnormal proliferation and accumulation of mast cells (MCs). Constitutive activation of kit, a receptor tyrosine kinase (TK), has been associated with all types of SM. Signal transducers and activators of transcription (STATs), such as STAT5, mediate downstream kit signalling. We hypothesized that nuclear phospho-STAT5 (pSTAT5) in MCs might reflect TK activation and would be a marker of abnormal MCs in SM. Expression of tryptase, CD25, CD2 and pSTAT5 was evaluated by immunohistochemistry (IHC) on archival cases of SM and cutaneous mastocytosis (CM). pSTAT5 was detected in 23/23 of SM and 1/9 of CM MC nuclei. 23/23 SM had CD25 + MCs. Control tissue MCs were negative for pSTAT5. Nuclear pSTAT5 in MCs from SM reflects abnormal TK activation. We propose nuclear pSTAT5 positivity in MCs as an additional minor phenotypic criterion for diagnosis of SM in future World Health Organization classification schemes.

▶ Systemic mastocytosis (SM) is an abnormal mast cell (MC) proliferation involving 1 or more extracutaneous organs, which usually presents in adults older than 30 years. Bone marrow is usually involved. Clinicopathologic criteria for diagnosis of SM include presence of multifocal dense infiltrates of MCs, abnormal MC morphology, KIT mutation at codon 816, aberrant MC expression of CD2 and/or CD25, and total serum tryptase > 20 ng/ml. The pathogenesis of SM is characterized by constitutive c-kit tyrosine kinase signaling, which leads to the activation of downstream transducers. Phospho-STAT5 (pSTAT5), a known transducer of tyrosine kinase signaling, was previously noted to be a target of constitutively activated tyrosine kinase JAK2 V617F in chronic myeloproliferative disorders.[1] Zuluaga Toro and colleagues studied the expression of pSTAT5 in archival cases of SM and cutaneous mastocytosis (CM). They found that abnormal nuclear pSTAT5 was expressed in all cases of SM, whereas only a single case of CM and all non-neoplastic MCs lacked pSTAT5. Immunohistochemical staining for nuclear pSTAT5 was superior to CD2 immunohistochemical staining of neoplastic MCs. Moreover, dual immunohistochemical staining with mast cell tryptase is possible because of nuclear localization of pSTAT5. The authors argue that nuclear expression of pSTAT5 should be used as another criterion for diagnosis of SM.

M. Djokic, MD

Reference

1. Aboudola S, Murugesan G, Szpurka H, et al. Bone marrow phospho-STAT5 expression in non-CML chronic myeloproliferative disorders correlates with JAK2 V617F mutation and provides evidence of in vivo JAK2 activation. *Am J Surg Pathol.* 2007;31:233-239.

ALK⁻ anaplastic large-cell lymphoma is clinically and immunophenotypically different from both ALK⁺ ALCL and peripheral T-cell lymphoma, not otherwise specified: report from the International Peripheral T-Cell Lymphoma Project
Savage KJ, for the International Peripheral T-Cell Lymphoma Project (British Columbia Cancer Agency, Vancouver, Canada; et al)
Blood 111:5496-5504, 2008

The International Peripheral T-Cell Lymphoma Project is a collaborative effort designed to gain better understanding of peripheral T-cell and natural killer (NK)/T-cell lymphomas (PTCLs). A total of 22 institutions in North America, Europe, and Asia submitted clinical and pathologic information on PTCLs diagnosed and treated at their respective centers. Of the 1314 eligible patients, 181 had anaplastic large-cell lymphoma (ALCL; 13.8%) on consensus review: One hundred fifty-nine had systemic ALCL (12.1%) and 22 had primary cutaneous ALCL (1.7%). Patients with anaplastic lymphoma kinase–positive (ALK$^+$) ALCL had a superior outcome compared with those with ALK$^-$ ALCL (5-year failure-free survival [FFS], 60% vs 36%; $P=.015$; 5-year overall survival [OS], 70% vs 49%; $P=.016$). However, contrary to prior reports, the 5-year FFS (36% vs 20%; $P=.012$) and OS (49% vs 32%; $P=.032$) were superior for ALK$^-$ ALCL compared with PTCL, not otherwise specified (PTCL-NOS). Patients with primary cutaneous ALCL had a very favorable 5-year OS (90%), but with a propensity to relapse (5-year FFS, 55%). In summary, ALK$^-$ ALCL should continue to be separated from both ALK$^+$ ALCL and PTCL-NOS. Although the prognosis of ALK$^-$ ALCL appears to be better than that for PTCL-NOS, it is still unsatisfactory and better therapies are needed. Primary cutaneous ALCL is associated with an indolent course.

▶ Anaplastic large-cell lymphoma (ALCL) was first described as a proliferation of CD30-positive large anaplastic cells with cohesive growth pattern and tendency for invasion of lymph node sinuses. Subsequent studies demonstrated overexpression of anaplastic lymphoma kinase (ALK) protein in 50% to 85% of cases with systemic disease (cutaneous ALCL is by definition limited to skin and ALK−). The ALK+ cases have deregulated expression of ALK gene because of chromosomal rearrangement usually involving t(2;5)(p23;q35). ALK+ ALCL usually presents at younger age and has more favorable prognosis than ALK− cases. There have been suggestions that ALCL as entity should be limited to ALK-positive cases. International Peripheral T-Cell Lymphoma Project has examined a large number of patients with peripheral T-cell lymphoma (PTCL) from North America, Europe, and Asia to try to define characteristic features of ALCL subtypes and compare them with PTCL, not otherwise specified (NOS). They found that supposedly more favorable prognosis of ALK+ cases may be largely due to patients' younger age because ALK+ cases in subjects who are 40 years or older had similar outcome as ALK− cases. Extranodal involvement of bone marrow, bone, subcutaneous tissue, and spleen was more common in ALK+ cases, whereas ALK− cases had more frequent involvement of skin, liver, and gastrointestinal tract. ALK− ALCL differed from PTCL-NOS both in terms of pathologic features and clinical presentation. In distinction from PTCL-NOS, ALK− ALCL had worse performance status and more frequent B-symptoms, although bone marrow or spleen involvement and thrombocytopenia were less common. Somewhat surprisingly, ALK− ALCL had better failure-free survival and overall survival than PTCL-NOS, supporting the notion that it should be diagnosed as a distinct entity.

M. Djokic, MD

The impact of Epstein-Barr virus status on clinical outcome in diffuse large B-cell lymphoma.

Park S, Lee J, Ko YH, et al (Sungkyunkwan Univ School of Medicine, Seoul, Korea)
Blood 110:972-978, 2007

To define prognostic impact of Epstein-Barr virus (EBV) infection in diffuse large B-cell lymphoma (DLBCL), we investigated EBV status in patients with DLBCL. In all, 380 slides from paraffin-embedded tissue were available for analysis by EBVencoded RNA-1 (EBER) in situ hybridization, and 34 cases (9.0%) were identified as EBER-positive. EBER positivity was significantly associated with age greater than 60 years ($P = .005$), more advanced stage ($P < .001$), more than one extranodal involvement ($P = .009$), higher International Prognostic Index (IPI) risk group ($P = .015$), presence of B symptom ($P = .004$), and poorer outcome to initial treatment ($P = .006$). The EBER$^+$ patients with DLBCL demonstrated substantially poorer overall survival (EBER$^+$ vs EBER$^-$ 35.8 months [95% confidence interval (CI), 0-114.1 months] vs not reached, $P = .026$) and progression-free survival (EBER$^+$ vs EBER$^-$ 12.8 months [95% CI, 0-31.8 months] vs 35.8 months [95% CI, 0-114.1 months], respectively ($P = .018$). In nongerminal center B-cell–like subtype, EBER in situ hybridization positivity retained its statistical significance at the multivariate level ($P = .045$). Nongerminal center B-cell–like patients with DLBCL with EBER positivity showed substantially poorer overall survival with 2.9-fold (95% CI, 1.1-8.1) risk for death. Taken together, DLBCL patients with EBER in situ hybridization$^+$ pursued more rapidly deteriorating clinical course with poorer treatment response, survival, and progression-free survival.

▶ Epstein–Barr virus (EBV) is associated with multiple types of malignant lymphoma including Hodgkin lymphoma, Burkitt lymphoma, diffuse large B-cell lymphoma (DLBCL), senile EBV+ B-cell lymphoma, and NK/T-cell lymphoma, nasal type. However, the incidence of EBV infection and its impact on outcome in DLBCL has not been investigated in large series of patients. This study by Park and colleagues is the largest single institution series to look at the significance of EBV positivity on treatment outcome and survival in patients with DLBCL. Using EBV-encoded RNA-1 (EBER-1) in situ hybridization, they have evaluated archival material (paraffin blocks of formalin-fixed tissue) of 380 cases of DLBCL. Nine percent of cases were EBER +, similar to findings in other studies. These patients tended to be older than 60 years, at higher stage, in higher International Prognostic Index risk group, and with presence of extranodal disease. The EBER + patients had poorer response to initial therapy, lower overall survival, and lower progression-free survival. In nongerminal center B-cell-like DLBCL group, EBER positivity was an independent indicator of poor prognosis in a multivariate analysis. These findings suggest that this group of patients may need more effective therapy, possibly including anti-EBV therapy. The pathologists may soon be asked to assess EBV status in all elderly patients with DLBCL.

M. Djokic, MD

Bone Marrow Biopsies in Patients 85 Years or Older
Manion EM, Rosenthal NS (Univ of Iowa Carver College of Medicine, IA)
Am J Clin Pathol 130:832-835, 2008

Increasing numbers of bone marrow aspirates and core biopsies are done in very elderly people; there is little published literature regarding the usefulness of bone marrow biopsies in these patients. We undertook a retrospective review of 119 bone marrow aspirates and biopsies from patients 85 years or older. These procedures were performed for a variety of abnormalities, including unexplained cytopenias; evaluation of a known myelodysplastic syndrome; suspicion or follow-up of plasma cell myeloma, thrombocytosis, or leukocytosis; and suspicion or staging of lymphoma. When staging or follow-up biopsies were excluded, 34 (43%) of 79 yielded specific diagnoses. Follow-up was available for 45 patients, and of these 45, 20 patients received therapy: 17 were treated with an abbreviated or modified regimen, and 12 were treated for leukemia/lymphoma. Therapy failed in all patients. As a result of these biopsies, relatively few patients received more than supportive treatment, suggesting that higher thresholds for biopsy for cytopenias may be indicated.

▶ Many of us who look at bone marrow biopsies have noticed a slight but steady increase of procedures done in elderly patients with vague symptoms and unexplained cytopenias. Manion and Rosenthal have asked the question that has vexed many of us at one time or another: How likely is it that the findings in the bone marrow biopsy will lead to a specific diagnosis and alter the therapy course for these patients? They come up with some interesting findings—the elderly patients who underwent biopsy for leukocytosis or thrombocytosis were likely to be given a specific diagnosis in 80% or more instances. In contrast, the patients who were biopsied because of unexplained cytopenias (1 or more) or suspicion of multiple myeloma were likely to receive a specific diagnosis in 30% and 38% of cases, respectively. However, 85% of patients who were treated as categorized by the given diagnosis had to receive abbreviated or modified therapy because of poor performance status or drug intolerance. It seems that bone marrow examination was not likely to alter the management or outcome in most elderly patients with cytopenias. This may suggest that a higher threshold for bone marrow biopsy may be indicated for elderly patients.

M. Djokic, MD

PD-1, a Follicular T-cell Marker Useful for Recognizing Nodular Lymphocyte-Predominant Hodgkin Lymphoma.

Nam-Cha SH, Roncador G, Sanchez-Verde L, et al (Spanish Natl Cancer Ctr, Madrid, Spain; et al)
Am J Surg Pathol 32:1252-1257, 2008

The nodularity and presence of T-cell rosettes surrounding the neoplastic cells has been described as a defining feature of nodular lymphocyte-predominant Hodgkin lymphoma (NLPHL). We have explored the potential diagnostic value of a new marker (NAT105) that recognizes the antigen PD-1 in a series of 152 cases diagnosed as nodular sclerosis Hodgkin lymphoma, mixed cellularity Hodgkin lymphoma, lymphocyterich classic Hodgkin lymphoma, NLPHL, and T-cell/histiocyterich B-cell lymphoma (T/HRBCL). All the cases were immunostained with a panel of antibodies against CD10, bcl-6, CXCL13, CD57, and PD-1 (NAT-105). The series includes a set of cases diagnosed as NLPHL with diffuse areas, and a group of borderline cases with features between those of NLPHL and T/HRBCL. Results show that PD-1 (NAT-105) is an excellent immunomarker not only of follicular T-cell rosettes in NLPHL, but also of a subset of lymphocyte-rich classic Hodgkin lymphomas. However, it is not a unique and defining feature of NLPHL. The presence of PD-1–positive (NAT-105) T-cell rosettes seems to be an additional useful feature in the differential diagnosis of NLPHL and T/HRBCL, which is normally a controversial and difficult task. The standard T/HRBCL cases lack follicular T-cell rosettes, whereas most of the borderline cases between the 2 entities have follicular T-cell rosettes, thus suggesting a closer relation with NLPHL.

▶ Nodular lymphocyte-predominant Hodgkin lymphoma (NLPHL) is a distinct clinical entity that usually presents in younger, predominantly male patients and has good prognosis. Therefore, pathologic distinction from classical Hodgkin lymphoma (CHL) and T-cell/histiocyte-rich B-cell lymphoma (T/HRBCL), an aggressive type of non-Hodgkin lymphoma, has significant clinical and therapeutic implications. NLPHL is thought to arise from transformed germinal center B-cell, and is morphologically characterized by the presence of large nodules comprised mostly of small, nonmalignant B-cells, extensive dendritic cell meshworks, and rosettes of follicular T-cells, positive for CD57 and bcl6. PD-1 antigen is member of CD28 receptor family with limited distribution in lymphoid tissue, mostly restricted to follicular T-cells in tonsil. Nam-Cha and colleagues have evaluated expression of PD-1 in 152 cases of nodular sclerosis and mixed cellularity CHL, NLPHL, and T/HRBCL. This antigen seems to be the most sensitive marker of follicular T-cells and was consistently reliable in outlining follicular T-cell rosettes in NLPHL. These rosettes were not found in any cases of T/HRBCL, which is thought to have lost the features of germinal center microenvironment. This marker may be useful in outlining follicular T-cell subset in other types of lymphoma where these cells may play a significant role such as lymphocyte-rich CHL and angioimmunoblastic T-cell lymphoma.

M. Djokic, MD

Lymphomas Involving the Breast: A Study of 106 Cases Comparing Localized and Disseminated Neoplasms

Talwalkar SS, Miranda RN, Valbuena JR, et al (Univ of Texas M.D. Anderson Cancer Ctr, Houston)
Am J Surg Pathol 32:1299-1309, 2008

Lymphomas involving the breast account for approximately 2% of extranodal and < 1% of all non-Hodgkin lymphomas. Our aim in this study was to classify breast lymphomas using the World Health Organization classification and then compare this classification with clinical, histologic, and radiologic findings as well as survival. The study group included 106 patients with breast lymphoma (105 women and 1 man). The neoplasms were divided into 2 groups based on extent of disease at initial diagnosis: localized disease (n = 50) and disseminated disease (n = 56). The follow-up period ranged from 4 to 252 months (median, 49 mo). Almost all (97%) patients presented with a palpable breast mass or masses. In the localized group, diffuse large B-cell lymphoma (DLBCL) was most frequent (n = 32, 64%). In the disseminated group, follicular lymphoma was most frequent and exclusive to this group (*P* = 0.0004). Mucosa-associated lymphoid tissue lymphomas occurred in both groups without a significant difference in frequency. A variety of other types of B-cell and T-cell non-Hodgkin lymphomas and classical Hodgkin lymphoma involved the breast at much lower frequency; most of these neoplasms involved the breast as part of disseminated disease. The clinical presentation correlated with radiologic findings: localized lymphomas presented as solitary masses, whereas disseminated lymphomas commonly presented as multifocal masses. There was a significant difference in the disease-free survival between patients with localized and disseminated DLBCL (*P* = 0.003). In the disseminated group, patients with DLBCL had a worse disease-free survival compared with patients with mucosa-associated lymphoid tissue lymphoma or follicular lymphoma (*P* = 0.01).

▶ Non-Hodgkin lymphomas (NHLs) are the most common nonepithelial tumors of breast. Talwalkar and colleagues have compiled a large series of breast lymphomas from a single institution (University of Texas M.D. Anderson Cancer Center) and classified them according to the current WHO classification system. Morphologic and immunohistochemical characteristics of breast lymphomas across the entire histologic spectrum are very similar to their nodal and extranodal counterparts found at other sites. Fifty-three percent of cases in their series were disseminated lymphomas, which presumably have arisen elsewhere and secondarily involve the breast. The most common histologic subtypes include diffuse large B-cell lymphoma (DLBCL), mucosa-associated lymphoid tissue (MALT) lymphoma, follicular lymphoma, and precursor-B lymphoblastic leukemia/lymphoma. Interestingly, all cases of follicular lymphoma and mantle cell lymphoma in this series were disseminated at the time of diagnosis and it was not clear if any had arisen in the breast. In the localized group, DLBCL was, somewhat unexpectedly, a more common histologic subtype than mucosa-associated lymphoid tissue (MALT) lymphoma. This is contrary to what most hematopathologists and general pathologists anecdotally notice in their practice. One wonders if there is a selection bias considering that the institution where the study originated is one of the largest treatment reference centers in the country.

M. Djokic, MD

Clinical significance of minimal residual disease in childhood acute lymphoblastic leukemia and its relationship to other prognostic factors: a Children's Oncology Group study
Borowitz MJ, Devidas M, Hunger SP, et al (Johns Hopkins Med Inst, Baltimore; Univ of Florida, Gainesville; Univ of Colorado Denver and The Children's Hosp, Aurora)
Blood 111:5477-5485, 2008

Minimal residual disease (MRD) is an important predictor of relapse in acute lymphoblastic leukemia (ALL), but its relationship to other prognostic variables has not been fully assessed. The Children's Oncology Group studied the prognostic impact of MRD measured by flow cytometry in the peripheral blood at day 8, and in end-induction (day 29) and end-consolidation marrows in 2143 children with precursor B-cell ALL (B-ALL). The presence of MRD in day-8 blood and day-29 marrow MRD was associated with shorter event-free survival (EFS) in all risk groups; even patients with 0.01% to 0.1% day-29 MRD had poor outcome compared with patients negative for MRD patients (59% ± 5% vs 88% ± 1% 5-year EFS). Presence of good prognostic markers TEL-AML1 or trisomies of chromosomes 4 and 10 still provided additional prognostic information, but not in National Cancer Institute high-risk (NCI HR) patients who were MRD⁺. The few patients with detectable MRD at end of consolidation fared especially poorly, with only a 43% plus or minus 7% 5-year EFS. Day-29 marrow MRD was the most important prognostic variable in multi-variate analysis. The 12% of patients with all favorable risk factors, including NCI risk group, genetics, and absence of days 8 and 29 MRD, had a 97% plus or minus 1% 5-year EFS with nonintensive therapy. These studies are registered at www.clinicaltrials.gov as NCT00005585, NCT00005596, and NCT00005603.

▶ Minimal residual disease (MRD), as assessed by PCR-based molecular methods or flow cytometric immunophenotypic analysis, is the best prognostic indicator of relapse in pediatric and adult acute lymphoblastic leukemia. However, the relationship between MRD and other prognostic indicators such as age, white blood cell count, and cytogenetic profile of blasts is not clear. Another open question is the best time period after the start of therapy to assess MRD. This study by Borowitz et al on behalf of Children's Oncology Group on 2143 children with precursor B-cell acute lymphoblastic leukemia (ALL) demonstrates that day-29 MRD in the bone marrow sample is the most important prognostic indicator in multivariate analysis. Additional prognostic information was provided by day-8 peripheral blood MRD, which, if negative and in combination with day-29 negative MRD and favorable cytogenetic profile, defines a subset of patients who have extremely low propensity to relapse and may benefit from least toxic chemotherapy. Conversely, patients who have detectable MRD at the end of consolidation have the worst event-free survival (EFS). Importantly, only 24-marker combinations (CD20-FITC/CD10-PE/CD45-PerCP/CD19-APC and CD9-FITC/CD34-PE/CD45PerCP/CD19-APC) were sufficient to identify leukemic cells in most cases and results were routinely available within 24 hours of sample arrival to the laboratory.

M. Djokic, MD

16 Pediatrics

Common variable immunodeficiency disorders: division into distinct clinical phenotypes
Chapel H, Lucas M, Lee M, et al (Univ of Oxford, UK; Univ of California at Los Angeles; Sahlgrenska Univ Hosp, Gothenberg, Sweden; et al)
Blood 15;112:277-286, 2008

The European Common Variable Immunodeficiency Disorders registry was started in 1996 to define distinct clinical phenotypes and determine overlap within individual patients. A total of 7 centers contributed patient data, resulting in the largest cohort yet reported. Patients (334), validated for the diagnosis, were followed for an average of 25.6 years (9461 patient-years). Data were used to define 5 distinct clinical phenotypes: no complications, autoimmunity, polyclonal lymphocytic infiltration, enteropathy, and lymphoid malignancy. A total of 83% of patients had only one of these phenotypes. Analysis of mortality showed a considerable reduction in the last 15 years and that different phenotypes were associated with different survival times. Types of complications and clinical phenotypes varied significantly between countries, indicating the need for large, international registries. Ages at onset of symptoms and diagnosis were shown to have a Gaussian distribution, but were not useful predictors of phenotype. The only clinical predictor was polyclonal lymphocytic infiltration, which was associated with a 5-fold increased risk of lymphoid malignancy. There was widespread variation in the levels of serum immunoglobulin isotypes as well as in the percentages and absolute numbers of B cells, confirming the heterogeneity of these conditions. Higher serum IgM and lower circulating CD8 proportions were found to be predictive markers for polyclonal lymphocytic infiltration and autoimmunity, respectively.

▶ This article is the result of a 10-year study by The European Common Variable Immunodeficiency Disorders Registry/The European Society of Immunodeficiencies that was put together to define clinical phenotypes of common variable immunodeficiency disorders (CVID). As indicated by its name, CVID is a common disorder of children with fairly variable clinical presentations; hence, it presents an everyday diagnostic challenge for pediatric caregivers. This comprehensive study involved 334 children with CVID who were followed for an average of 25.6 years. They were able to group patients into 5 distinct clinical phenotypes including autoimmunity, polyclonal lymphocytic infiltration with or without epithelioid granulomas, enteropathy, lymphoid malignancy, and

CVID with no clinical manifestation. The results of this article send an important reminder to practicing pediatric pathologists—any atypical lymphoid proliferation, epithelioid granulomas ("sarcoid"), early onset of lymphoma, or early onset of enteropathy (such as early Crohn's disease) should raise a suspicion for CVID. In such cases, the recommendation of a comprehensive workup of CVID is indispensable.

C. Galambos, MD, PhD

Heterozygous nonsense SCN5A mutation W822X explains a simultaneous sudden infant death syndrome
Turillazzi E, La Rocca G, Anzalone R, et al (Univ of Foggia, Italy; Univ of Palermo, Italy)
Virchows Arch 453:209-216, 2008

The sudden, unexpected, and unexplained death of both members of a set of healthy twins (simultaneous sudden infant death syndrome (SSIDS)) is defined as a case in which both infants meet the definition of sudden infant death syndrome individually. A search of the world medical literature resulted in only 42 reported cases of SSIDS. We report the case of a pair of identical, male, monozygotic twins, 138 days old, who suddenly died, meeting the full criteria of SSIDS and where a genetic screen was performed, resulting in a heterozygous nonsense SCN5A mutation (W822X) in both twins. Immunohistochemistry was performed on cardiac tissue samples utilizing polyclonal antibodies anti-Na$^+$ CP type V α (C-20) and a terminal deoxynucleotidyl transferase deoxyuridine triphosphate nick end labeling assay. The cellular localization of the Na$^+$ CP type V α (C-20) demonstrated by confocal microscopy on staining pattern of myocytes was concentrated in the intercalated disks of ventricular myocytes. These findings suggest that defective ion channels represent viable candidates for the pathogenesis of SIDS and, obviously, of SSIDS, supporting a link between sudden infant death syndrome and cardiac channelopathies.

▶ This case report is a nice example of modern molecular medicine applied to a previously unexplained phenomenon. The rapid evolution of molecular biology in cardiac pathology has led to the incorporation of ion channelopathies to the primary cardiomyopathy disease category. The defective proteins of ion channels have been shown to cause conduction alterations of the heart that can lead to arrhythmias of various degrees. Patients with channelopathies could have signs of benign disease, but could also suffer more aggressive ventricular dysfunction, and there are cases of sudden cardiac death as well. Turillazzi et al, using a combination of molecular and immunohistochemical techniques, demonstrated that a heterozygous nonsense SCN5A mutation was present in previously healthy twin infants who died unexpectedly. The circumstances of deaths, along with clinical and pathologic findings, met the criteria for simultaneous sudden infant death syndrome. Heterozygote expression in twin hearts showed a nearly 50% reduction in Na^+ channel protein type Valpha in ventricular myocytes detected by confocal laser scanning microscope when compared with that of control case. The impaired expression of the Na-channel protein in the heart muscle of both infants, therefore, offered an explanation for the sudden deaths and supports a link between some instances of "sudden infant death syndrome" and cardiac channelopathies.

C. Galambos, MD, PhD

Genetic causes of vascular malformations
Brouillard P, Vikkula M (Université catholique de Louvain, Brussels, Belgium)
Hum Mol Genet 16:R140-R149, 2007

Vascular malformations are localized defects of vascular development. They usually affect a limited number of vessels in a restricted area of the body. Although most malformations are sporadic, inheritance is observed, enabling genetic analysis. Usually, sporadic forms present with a single lesion whereas multiple lesions are observed in familial cases. The last decade has seen unraveling of several causative genes and beginning of elucidation of the pathophysiological pathways involved in the inherited forms. In parallel, definition of the clinical phenotypes has improved and disorders such as Parkes-Weber syndrome (PKWS), first thought to be sporadic, is now known to be part of a more common inheritable phenotype. In addition, the concept of double-hit mechanism that we proposed earlier to explain the incomplete penetrance, variable expressivity and multifocality of lesions in inherited venous anomalies is now becoming confirmed, as some somatic mutations have been identified in venous, glomuvenous and cerebral cavernous malformations. It is thus tempting to suggest that familial forms of vascular malformations follow paradominant inheritance and that sporadic forms, the etiopathogenic causes of which are still unelucidated, are caused by somatic mutations in the same genes.

▶ Vascular malformations are commonly encountered lesions in pediatric pathology practice. The vast majority of them are sporadic with good prognosis. Recent increase in our understanding of the mechanisms of angiogenesis and lymphangiogenesis, however, has shed some light on certain factors and molecules that are involved in the pathomechanism of vascular malformations. The discovery of new causative factors and genes has led to a better understanding of disease mechanisms, and an expansion of inherited/syndromic vascular malformation group by inclusions of new disease entities. The outcome of inherited and/or syndromic vascular malformations can be quite variable; some are without worrisome prognosis, but others could evoke fatal systemic hemorrhage. Therefore, awareness of these entities is essential in today's practice.

This review article by Brouillard and Vikkula provides an update on the genetic cause of vascular malformation with clinical details including outcome in regard of sporadic and inhered vascular malformations.

C. Galambos, MD, PhD

Clinical, radiological and pathological features of ABCA3 mutations in children

Doan ML, Guillerman RP, Dishop MK, et al (Texas Children's Hospital, Houston, Texas, USA; et al)
Thorax 63:366-373, 2008

Background.—Mutations in the ABCA3 gene can result in fatal surfactant deficiency in term newborn infants and chronic interstitial lung disease in older children. Previous studies on ABCA3 mutations have focused primarily on the genetic abnormalities and reported limited clinical information about the resultant disease. A study was undertaken to analyse systematically the clinical presentation, pulmonary function, diagnostic imaging, pathological features and outcomes of children with ABCA3 mutations.

Methods.—The records of nine children with ABCA3 mutations evaluated at Texas Children's Hospital between 1992 and 2005 were reviewed and their current clinical status updated. Previous diagnostic imaging studies and lung biopsy specimens were re-examined. The results of DNA analyses were confirmed.

Results.—Age at symptom onset ranged from birth to 4 years. Cough, crackles, failure to thrive and clubbing were frequent findings. Mean lung function was low but tended to remain static. CT scans commonly revealed ground-glass opacification, septal thickening, parenchymal cysts and pectus excavatum. Histopathological patterns included pulmonary alveolar proteinosis, desquamative interstitial pneumonitis and non-specific interstitial pneumonitis, and varied with age. Dense abnormalities of lamellar bodies, characteristic of ABCA3 mutations, were seen by electron microscopy in all adequate specimens. Outcomes varied with the age at which the severity of lung disease warranted open lung biopsy, and some patients have had prolonged survival without lung transplantation.

Conclusions.—The presentation and course of interstitial lung disease due to ABCA3 mutations are variable, and open lung biopsy and genetic testing are warranted early in the evaluation of children with a consistent clinical picture.

▶ Childhood interstitial lung disease is a heterogenous group of pediatric diseases that present diagnostic and management challenges for pediatric pulmonologists, radiologists, and pathologists. Recently, interstitial lung disease of infants and older children has become the focus of a pediatric pulmonology study and a standardized terminology classification system has been developed to aid in diagnosis and prognostication.[1] One disease category, inborn errors in surfactant metabolism, is still expanding. In addition to the well-known surfactant protein A, B, and C mutations, there is now a report of an effect caused by a mutation to the third member of the superfamily of ATP-binding cassette transporters, ABCA3 mutation. Doan and coworkers present a systematic review of the clinical features, lung function, imaging changes, and histopathology of children with ABCA3 mutations. An important point of the article is that although the disease has its characteristic clinical, imaging, and pathologic features, the age of presentation, disease progression, and survival are quite variable. Thus, the diagnostic workup of older children with interstitial lung disease should also include this entity. The wide variation in gene mutations among the patients is likely responsible for the variability of the disease characteristics; further research will hopefully predict those with severe outcome. The article emphasizes the need for electron microscopic (EM) studies because of the presence of characteristic small dense lamellar bodies. The authors suggest that this finding may be a sensitive and rapidly diagnostic feature of ABCA3 mutation. The critical role of EM in the diagnostic workup of interstitial lung disorders such as ABCA3 mutation further points out that use of established protocols for correct handling of lung biopsies is essential in pediatric pathology laboratories.[2]

C. Galambos, MD, PhD

References

1. Deutsch GH, Young LR, Deterding RR, et al. Diffuse lung disease in young children: application of a novel classification scheme. *Am J Respir Crit Care med.* 2007;176:1120-1128.
2. Langston C, Patterson K, Dishop MK, et al. A protocol for the handling of tissue obtained by operative lung biopsy: recommendations of the chILD pathology co-operative group. *Pediatr Dev Pathol.* 2006;9:173-180.

RNA-Containing Cytoplasmic Inclusion Bodies in Ciliated Bronchial Epithelium Months to Years after Acute Kawasaki Disease

Rowley AH, Baker SC, Shulman ST, et al (Northwestern Univ Feinberg School of Medicine, USA; Loyola Univ Stritch School of Medicine, Maywood, IL; et al)
PLoS ONE 3:e1582, 2008

Background.—Kawasaki Disease (KD) is the most common cause of acquired heart disease in children in developed nations. The KD etiologic agent is unknown but likely to be a ubiquitous microbe that usually causes asymptomatic childhood infection, resulting in KD only in genetically susceptible individuals. KD synthetic antibodies made from prevalent IgA gene sequences in KD arterial tissue detect intracytoplasmic inclusion bodies (ICI) resembling viral ICI in acute KD but not control infant ciliated bronchial epithelium. The prevalence of ICI in late-stage KD fatalities and in older individuals with non-KD illness should be low, unless persistent infection is common.

Methods and Principal Findings.—Lung tissue from late-stage KD fatalities and non-infant controls was examined by light microscopy for the presence of ICI. Nucleic acid stains and transmission electron microscopy (TEM) were performed on tissues that were strongly positive for ICI. ICI were present in ciliated bronchial epithelium in 6/7 (86%) late-stage KD fatalities and 7/27 (26%) controls ages 9–84 years (p = 0.01). Nucleic acid stains revealed RNA but not DNA within the ICI. ICI were also identified in lung macrophages in some KD cases. TEM of bronchial epithelium and macrophages from KD cases revealed finely granular homogeneous ICI.

Significance.—These findings are consistent with a previously unidentified, ubiquitous RNA virus that forms ICI and can result in persistent infection in bronchial epithelium and macrophages as the etiologic agent of KD.

▶ Kawasaki disease is the most frequent cause of acquired cardiac disorders of children in developed countries. Although the cause of the disease remains mysterious, clinical and epidemiologic studies strongly support an infectious etiology. The results of an ongoing research effort led by Dr Rowley's group have identified an antigen-driven IgA response directed against cytoplasmic inclusion bodies present in ciliated bronchial epithelial cells of patients with acute Kawasaki disease. The group's most recent finding is that the previously identified cytoplasmic inclusion bodies contain RNA (not DNA), and are present even in the late stage of lethal Kawasaki disease in the vast majority patients but not in control individuals. Transmission electron microscopic studies demonstrated the presence of inclusion bodies (granular spheroid bodies) not only in ciliary bronchial epithelial cells but also in alveolar macrophages and in macrophages of peribronchial lymph nodes. The findings strongly support the notion that a ubiquitous RNA virus drives the pathology of Kawasaki disease, most likely only in genetically susceptible individuals.

C. Galambos, MD, PhD

17 Techniques/Molecular

Standard Mutation Nomenclature in Molecular Diagnostics: Practical and Educational Challenges

Ogino S, for the Association for Molecular Pathology Training and Education Committee (Brigham and Women's Hosp, Boston; et al)

J Mol Diagn 9:1-6, 2007

To translate basic research findings into clinical practice, it is essential that information about mutations and variations in the human genome are communicated easily and unequivocally. Unfortunately, there has been much confusion regarding the description of genetic sequence variants. This is largely because research articles that first report novel sequence variants do not often use standard nomenclature, and the final genomic sequence is compiled over many separate entries. In this article, we discuss issues crucial to clear communication, using examples of genes that are commonly assayed in clinical laboratories. Although molecular diagnostics is a dynamic field, this should not inhibit the need for and movement toward consensus nomenclature for accurate reporting among laboratories. Our aim is to alert laboratory scientists and other health care professionals to the important issues and provide a foundation for further discussions that will ultimately lead to solutions.

▶ With more sequence variations identified as the cause of congenital and acquired disorders, more molecular diagnostics laboratories are performing sequencing assays. As more patients get tested it is more likely that laboratories will encounter novel variants. As pointed out by the authors of this article, even well-established colloquial terms of mutations might be incorrect and thus there is a need for all laboratories and physicians to speak the same language as it refers to DNA sequence variations.

This article reviews the recommendations for standardized sequence variation nomenclature and, with examples based on a common sequence-based test for cystic fibrosis, it reviews the more common nomenclature issues that arise in a clinical laboratory. The authors do a short and concise review of the guidelines established by the Human Genome Variation Society and also discuss the need for applying this nomenclature in the clinical environment. This article is required reading for all laboratories performing genetic tests and/or reporting sequence variations.

F. A. Monzon, MD

Rapid SNP diagnostics using asymmetric isothermal amplification and a new mismatch-suppression technology

Mitani Y, Lezhava A, Kawai Y, et al (RIKEN Yokohama Inst, Kanagawa, Japan; K.K. Dnaform, Kanagawa, Japan; RIKEN Wako Inst, Saitama, Japan; et al)
Nat Methods 4:257-262, 2007

We developed a rapid single nucleotide polymorphism (SNP) detection system named smart amplification process version 2 (SMAP 2). Because DNA amplification only occurred with a perfect primer match, amplification alone was sufficient to identify the target allele. To achieve the requisite fidelity to support this claim, we used two new and complementary approaches to suppress exponential background DNA amplification that resulted from mispriming events. SMAP 2 is isothermal and achieved SNP detection from whole huma n blood in 30 min when performed with a new DNA polymerase that was cloned and isolated from *Alicyclobacillus acidocaldarius* (*Aac* pol). Furthermore, to assist the scientific community in configuring SMAP 2 assays, we developed software specific for SMAP 2 primer design. With these new tools, a high-precision and rapid DNA amplification technology becomes available to aid in pharmacogenomic research and molecular-diagnostics applications.

▶ Speed and performance are concepts usually associated with automobiles and not with clinical tests. However, it seems that the need for faster and better performing diagnostic assays keeps driving innovation in molecular methods. In this article, the authors describe an isothermal amplification assay for single nucleotide polymorphism in (SNP) diagnostics that can be performed on whole blood, under 20 min, and with suppression of random mismatch priming to reduce (or eliminate) false positives. The authors use a combination of self-priming primer design, strand displacement, and mismatch detection and blockage by a DNA polymerase (TaqMutS) to achieve an assay, termed SMAP2, capable of distinguishing SNP alleles in whole blood and in a reliable fashion and with fast turnaround time.

Although this is not the only method out there that achieves similar results such as the LAMP assay,[1] this article is a good example of developments on alternatives to PCR for diagnostic assay development. One of the stated goals of this type of assay is the possibility of enabling point-of-care (POC) molecular testing. Isothermal assays that can be done on whole blood specimens are ideal for POC tests and thus it is very likely that some of these techniques will be incorporated into diagnostic assays in the future. Suddenly, bedside assays for Factor V Leiden within minutes of a patient suffering a thromboembolic event seem entirely possible.

F. A. Monzon, MD

Reference

1. Iwasaki M, Yonokawa T. Validation of the loop-mediated isothermal amplification method for single nucleotide polymorphism genotyping with whole blood. *Genome Lett.* 2003;2:119-126.

Diagnosis of the Small Round Blue Cell Tumors Using Multiplex Polymerase Chain Reaction

Chen Q-R, Vansant G, Oades K, et al (Natl Cancer Inst, Gaithersburg, MD; Natl Cancer Inst-Frederick, MD; Althea Technologies, San Diego, CA)
J Mol Diagn 9:80-88, 2007

The small round blue cell tumors of childhood, which include neuroblastoma, rhabdomyosarcoma, non-Hodgkin's lymphoma, and the Ewing's family of tumors, are so called because of their similar appearance on routine histology. Using cDNA microarray gene expression profiles and artificial neural networks (ANNs), we previously identified 93 genes capable of diagnosing these cancers. Using a subset of these, together with some additional genes (total 39), we developed a multiplex polymerase chain reaction (PCR) assay to diagnose these cancer types. Blinded testing of 96 new samples (26 Ewing's family of tumors, 29 rhabdomyosarcomas, 24 neuroblastomas, and 17 lymphomas) using ANNs in a complete leave-one-out analysis demonstrated that all except one sample were accurately diagnosed as their respective category. Moreover, using an ANN-based gene minimization strategy in a separate analysis, we found that the top 31 genes could correctly diagnose all 96 tumors. Our results suggest that this molecular test based on a multiplex PCR reaction may assist the physician in the rapid confirmation of the diagnosis of these cancers.

▶ The diagnosis of pediatric small round blue cell tumors (SRBCT) requires extensive workup to confirm a morphologic diagnostic impression. The most common ancillary method is immunohistochemistry for protein markers of the tumors in this group (Ewing's sarcoma, rhabdomyosarcoma, neuroblastoma, non-Hodgkin's lymphoma, and others). This article describes a 31-target multiplexed RT-PCR method for the diagnostic workup of pediatric SRBCT.

The authors use an artificial neuron network (ANN) approach to classify samples into the diagnostic categories. The transcripts measured by the assay were obtained from previous gene expression studies performed by the authors. The authors claim that because the list of 31 genes was obtained from an independent study, this study is in itself a validation of the approach. However, because the authors derive the ANN for RT-PCR data from the same samples tested and because this same methodology (RT-PCR and ANN) has not been applied to other samples not used in the development of the algorithm, this assay should not be considered validated. There is a risk for over-fitting by including the same samples used for algorithm development as the validation set. Although this algorithm performs well in this study, it is not known if this approach would be successful in a separate site or with different samples. In addition, although not clearly stated, it appears that the test was developed with the use of frozen tissue samples. The feasibility and performance of this assay in paraffin-embedded tissue samples needs to be established.

There is no question that there is a need for assays that help surgical pathologist distinguish between the categories of small round blue cell tumors in the pediatric population. Other authors have actually approached the problem by developing real-time PCR assays that target the fusion gene products from the chromosomal translocations characteristic of some of these entities.[1] Although this approach might not be able to categorize samples into as many diagnostic categories as the multiplexed PCR, it can detect the major neoplasms in the pediatric SRBCT group and can readily be applied to paraffin-embedded samples.

F. A. Monzon, MD

Reference

1. Lewis TB, Coffin CM, Bernard PS. Differentiating Ewing's sarcoma from other round blue cell tumors using a RT-PCR translocation panel on formalin-fixed paraffin-embedded tissues. *Mod Pathol.* 2007;20:397-404.

Replacing PCR with COLD-PCR enriches variant DNA sequences and redefines the sensitivity of genetic testing

Li J, Wang L, Mamon H, et al (Harvard Med School, Boston, MA; et al)
Nat Med 14:579-584, 2008

PCR is widely employed as the initial DNA amplification step for genetic testing. However, a key limitation of PCR-based methods is the inability to selectively amplify low levels of mutations in a wild-type background. As a result, downstream assays are limited in their ability to identify subtle genetic changes that can have a profound impact in clinical decision-making and outcome. Here we describe co-amplification at lower denaturation temperature PCR (COLD-PCR), a novel form of PCR that amplifies minority alleles selectively from mixtures of wild-type and mutation-containing sequences irrespective of the mutation type or position on the sequence. We replaced regular PCR with COLD-PCR before sequencing or genotyping assays to improve mutation detection sensitivity by up to 100-fold and identified new mutations in the genes encoding p53, KRAS and epidermal growth factor in heterogeneous cancer samples that had been missed by the currently used methods. For clinically relevant microdeletions, COLD-PCR enabled exclusive amplification and isolation of the mutants. COLD-PCR will transform the capabilities of PCR-based genetic testing, including applications in cancer, infectious diseases and prenatal identification of fetal alleles in maternal blood.

▶ Detection of germline mutations in the context of genetic diseases is relatively straightforward given the fact that half of the alleles will be mutated (heterozygous). However, in situations where acquired mutations are being tested (eg, cancer or microbiology), the sensitivity of current sequencing technologies is often limited and low percentages of mutant alleles are usually missed.

In this article, Li and collaborators describe a modification of the polymerase chain reaction (PCR) method that selectively favors the amplification of mutant alleles. As shown in Fig 1 in the original article, the modification takes advantage of the change in melting temperature (T_m) created when mixtures of mutant and wild-type alleles pair together. With this modification the PCR reaction is enriched in mutant alleles. The authors convincingly show that this method increases the sensitivity of various mutation detection techniques such as restriction fragment length polymorphism (RFLP), Sanger dideoxy-sequencing, pyrosequencing, and matrix-assisted laser desorption/ionization time-of-flight (MALDI-TOF) in which a PCR reaction is needed previous to mutation detection. Although other approaches to this problem have been proposed, the method shown in this article has the advantage that is easily applied to currently established assays in any molecular diagnostics laboratory.

The detection of low-prevalence mutations is quickly becoming a significant issue for situations in which therapeutic decisions must be made based on the presence of a mutation. Examples of this are the detection of *KRAS* mutations in colon cancer (as discussed in another commentary) or detection of antibiotic resistance. However, in many instances, the clinical significance of a mutation present in a small percentage of tumor cells or microorganisms is not fully understood. Therefore, the use of more sensitive assays for mutation detection has to be carefully evaluated in its clinical context.

F. A. Monzon, MD

Inter-Laboratory Comparison of Chronic Myeloid Leukemia Minimal Residual Disease Monitoring: Summary and Recommendations
Zhang T, and the Association for Molecular Pathology Hematopathology Subdivision (Univ Health Network, Toronto, Ontario, Canada)
J Mol Diagn 9:421-430, 2007

In patients with chronic myeloid leukemia, the use of real-time quantitative reverse transcription-polymerase chain reaction (qRT-PCR) for measuring *BCR-ABL1* transcripts has become standard methodology for the diagnosis and monitoring of minimal residual disease. In 2004 and 2005, 38 different laboratories from North America participated in three separate sample exchanges using real-time qRT-PCR to measure RNA transcript levels in unknown diluents of a *BCR-ABL1*-positive cell line, K562. In this study we compared results of quantitative testing for *BCR-ABL1* from laboratories using different platforms, internal controls, reagents, and calculation methods. Our data showed that there can be considerable variability of results from laboratory to laboratory, with log reduction calculations varying from 1.6 to 3 log between laboratories at the same dilution. We found that none of the variables tested had a significant impact on the results reported, except for the use of *ABL1* as the internal control ($P < 0.001$). Laboratories that used *ABL1* consistently underreported their log reduction values. Regardless of the specific methodology and platform used for real-time qRT-PCR testing, it is important for laboratories to participate in proficiency testing to ensure consistent and acceptable test accuracy and sensitivity. Our study emphasizes the need for optimization of real-time qRT-PCR before offering clinical testing and the need for widely available universal standards that can be used for test calibration.

▶ The use of quantitative polymerase chain reaction (PCR) to monitor therapeutic response and minimal residual disease in patients with chronic myeloid leukemia (CML) is now a standard of care. However, in the United States, there has not been an attempt to standardize assays that measure levels of BCR-ABL1 transcripts. This is a problem that is underscored by the results of this article by Zhang and collaborators from the Hematopathology Subdivision of the Association for Molecular Pathology.

In this article, the authors describe significant variability in results from different laboratories in the United States and Canada. It is important to note that the protocols used by all laboratories are different in multiple aspects, including instrumentation, controls for standard curve, and choice of internal control. Although the design of the study precludes a detailed analysis on the specific factors that are responsible for the interlaboratory variability observed, the results showed that laboratories using ABL1 as an internal control consistently under-reported results. Interestingly, ABL1 was the internal control chosen by the European BIOMED group in their efforts to standardize molecular tests for hematologic malignancies.[1] However, many other authors have shown that other internal controls (GUS, BCR) show better performance.[2,3]

Given the importance of accurate determination of BCR-ABL1 transcript levels for patient management, it is imperative that efforts to standardize these assays are undertaken. In this context, articles like this one are valuable to highlight the extent of the problem, and should be followed by efforts in the diagnostics community to develop of standards and commercially available controls.

F. A. Monzon, MD

References

1. Beillard E, Pallisgaard N, van der Velden VH, et al. Evaluation of candidate control genes for diagnosis and residual disease detection in leukemic patients using 'real-time' quantitative reverse-transcriptase polymerase chain reaction (RQ-PCR):a Europe against cancer program. *Leukemia*. 2003;17:2474-2486.
2. Wang YL, Lee JW, Cesarman E, Jin DK, Csernus B. Molecular monitoring of chronic myelogenous leukemia: identification of the most suitable internal control gene for real-time quantification of BCR-ABL transcripts. *J Mol Diagn*. 2006;8: 231-239.
3. Lee JW, Chen Q, Knowles DM, Cesarman E, Wang YL. beta-Glucuronidase is an optimal normalization control gene for molecular monitoring of chronic myelogenous leukemia. *J Mol Diagn*. 2006;8:385-389.

Successful Application of a Direct Detection Slide-Based Sequential Phenotype/Genotype Assay Using Archived Bone Marrow Smears and Paraffin Embedded Tissue Sections

Bedell V, Forman SJ, Gaal K, et al (City of Hope Natl Med Ctr, Duarte, California)
J Mol Diagn 9:589-597, 2007

Identification of genetic abnormalities in pathological samples is critical for accurate diagnosis, risk stratification, detection of minimal residual disease, and assessment of response to therapy. Interphase fluorescence *in situ* hybridization analysis is the standard cytogenetic assay used by many laboratories to detect specific clonal karyotypic aberrations in formalin-fixed, paraffin-embedded tissue. However, direct correlation with immunophenotype or morphology in individual cells is rarely performed because the procedural steps are labor intensive and usually require extensive troubleshooting. In this study, we present a sequential fluorescence *in situ* hybridization-based technique that uses the identical archived bone marrow smears or paraffin-embedded tissue sections previously evaluated by a pathologist for morphological or immunohistochemical characteristics. This approach is relatively straightforward, using uncomplicated pretreatment and hybridization conditions and basic equipment attached to an automated image analyzer with image capture software to record the location of targeted cells for genotypic/phenotype correlation. Furthermore, the method has proved reliable and reproducible on test samples regardless of specimen age, tissue type, or referring institution.

▶ Molecular assays such as fluorescence in situ hybridization (FISH) are useful for detection of chromosomal rearrangements for diagnosis or prognosis in hematologic malignancies. Unfortunately, in many instances, all material collected is used for diagnosis and no remaining specimen is left for these assays.

In this article, Bedell and coworkers describe a method to perform FISH analysis on the same bone marrow smear or paraffin section used for morphologic diagnosis. Although the authors show that it is possible to achieve these results, the technologies used (imaging instrumentation) and laborious protocols make it unlikely that this technique could be performed in most laboratories. It is thus a development that could be available in the reference laboratory setting as a resource for cases in which correlation of morphology and genotype at the cell level is necessary.

A nice feature of this article is the detailed description of the clinical scenarios in which this technique can be applied and the significance of how these results can impact patient management.

F. A. Monzon, MD

Locked Nucleic Acids Can Enhance the Analytical Performance of Quantitative Methylation-Specific Polymerase Chain Reaction

Gustafson KS (John's Hopkins Univ, Baltimore, MD)
J Mol Diagn 10:33-42, 2008

Aberrant DNA methylation of tumor suppressor genes is a frequent epigenetic event that occurs early in tumor progression. Real-time quantitative methylation-specific polymerase chain reaction (QMSP) assays can provide accurate detection and quantitation of methylated alleles that may be potentially useful in diagnosis and risk assessment for cancer. Development of QMSP requires optimization to maximize analytical specificity and sensitivity for the detection of methylated alleles. However, in some cases challenges encountered in primer and probe design can make optimization difficult and limit assay performance. Locked nucleic acids (LNAs) demonstrate increased affinity and specificity for their cognate DNA sequences. In this proof-of-principle study, LNA residues were incorporated into primer and probe design to determine whether LNA-modified oligonucleotides could enhance the analytical performance of QMSP for *IGSF4* promoter methylation in human cancer cell lines using either SYBR Green or fluorogenic probe detection methods. Use of LNA primers in QMSP with SYBR Green improved analytical specificity for methylated alleles and eliminated the formation of nonspecific products because of mispriming from unmethylated alleles. QMSP using LNA probe and primers showed an increased amplification efficiency and maximum fluorescent signal. QMSP with LNA oligonucleotides and either detection method could reliably detect five genome equivalents of methylated DNA in 1000- to 10,000-fold excess unmethylated DNA. Thus, LNA oligonucleotides can be used in QMSP optimization to enhance analytical performance.

▶ Promoter methylation is a gene silencing mechanism common to many human tumors. Detection of promoter methylation for specific genes has been shown to have diagnostic or prognostic use. An example of this is the use of methylation in promoters of genes associated with prostate cancer in a urine-based assay for prostate cancer as discussed in another commentary.

The detection of methylated DNA sites is based on a chemical reaction that changes unmethylated cytosines to uracils (bisulfite conversion) and then detects the sequence difference between methylated and unmethylated sites. When the site assayed has a high frequency of methylation sites, the technique is quite reliable. However, when the frequency of methylated sites is low, it affects performance of the assay and design of primers.

In this article, the author uses locked nucleic acids (LNAs) to improve the performance of quantitative methylation assays. LNAs are structurally modified nucleotides that have higher affinity to their complementary bases (A/G and C/T) and thus improve the sensitivity and specificity of primer/probe binding. The results indicate that LNAs significantly improve the performance of methylation-specific polymerase chain reaction (MSP) in 2 quantitative real-time

PCR assay formats using SYBR Green detection or using hydrolysis probes. The assay performed a comprehensive assessment of how the use of LNAs affects different parameters of quantitative methylation assays.

It is expected that methylation assays will be used clinically in the near future and, thus, efforts to improve these assays are important.

F. A. Monzon, MD

Wild-Type *KRAS* Is Required for Panitumumab Efficacy in Patients With Metastatic Colorectal Cancer

Amado RG, Wolf M, Peeters M, et al (Thousand Oaks, CA; Ghent Univ Hosp, Belgium; Univ Hosp Gasthuisberg, Leuven, Belgium; et al)
J Clin Oncol 26:1626-1634, 2008

Purpose.—Panitumumab, a fully human antibody against the epidermal growth factor receptor (EGFR), has activity in a subset of patients with metastatic colorectal cancer (mCRC). Although activating mutations in KRAS, a small G-protein downstream of EGFR, correlate with poor response to anti-EGFR antibodies in mCRC, their role as a selection marker has not been established in randomized trials.

Patients And Methods.—KRAS mutations were detected using polymerase chain reaction on DNA from tumor sections collected in a phase III mCRC trial comparing panitumumab monotherapy to best supportive care (BSC). We tested whether the effect of panitumumab on progression-free survival (PFS) differed by KRAS status.

Results.—KRAS status was ascertained in 427 (92%) of 463 patients (208 panitumumab, 219 BSC). KRAS mutations were found in 43% of patients. The treatment effect on PFS in the wild-type (WT) KRAS group (hazard ratio [HR], 0.45; 95% CI: 0.34 to 0.59) was significantly greater ($P < .0001$) than in the mutant group (HR, 0.99; 95% CI, 0.73 to 1.36). Median PFS in the WT KRAS group was 12.3 weeks for panitumumab and 7.3 weeks for BSC. Response rates to panitumumab were 17% and 0%, for the WT and mutant groups, respectively. WT KRAS patients had longer overall survival (HR, 0.67; 95% CI, 0.55 to 0.82; treatment arms combined). Consistent with longer exposure, more grade III treatment-related toxicities occurred in the WT KRAS group. No significant differences in toxicity were observed between the WT KRAS group and the overall population.

Conclusion.—Panitumumab monotherapy efficacy in mCRC is confined to patients with WT KRAS tumors. KRAS status should be considered in selecting patients with mCRC as candidates for panitumumab monotherapy.

▶ The use of companion tests to determine eligibility for specific targeted therapies is quickly becoming commonplace in the management of patients with cancer. The first example of this type of test was the detection of Her2-Neu (ERBB2) in breast cancer patients to determine eligibility for the humanized antibody Herceptin. In this article, the authors confirm that in patients with metastatic colon cancer, there is an association between mutations in the KRAS gene and resistance to therapy based on anti-epidermal growth factor receptor (EGFR) antibodies. This is so far, the largest retrospective study that has tried to confirm this association. The results indicate that panitumumab, and anti-EGFR antibody, has a modest response rate and confers increased overall survival in patients with metastatic colon cancer when compared with best supportive care. Importantly, only patients with wild-type KRAS showed response. Although this is a retrospective study, performed on tissue samples from the clinical trial, the strength of the association was sufficient for the European equivalent of the Food and Drug Administration (FDA) to approve this drug for patients with EGFR expressing metastatic colorectal carcinoma with nonmutated (wild-type) KRAS. Interestingly, in the United States, the FDA has considered that there was insufficient data to warrant labeling of panitumumab for use in patients with wild-type KRAS. However, judging by the recent number of requests to perform KRAS mutation analysis in our laboratory, it appears that the oncology community is not going to wait for the FDA's approval to incorporate this test into their algorithms for metastatic colorectal patient management. Importantly, this association has also been shown in 2 independent studies where cetuximab, another anti-EGFR antibody, was used,[1,2] strongly suggesting that the lack of response in tumors with mutated KRAS is a feature that might be found in all agents that target EGFR. Although some groups have manifested concerns about standardization of assays for these mutations, the great majority of published methods seem to have adequate sensitivity and specificity to be used in a clinical setting. In Europe, a specific kit has been designed and approved to be used in the selection of patients for panitumumab therapy. It is likely that, as more targeted therapies are developed, we will see more companion tests being performed in our laboratories.

F. A. M. Bordonaba, MD

References

1. Lievre A, Bachet J-B, Boige V. KRAS mutations as an independent prognostic factor in patients with advanced colorectal cancer treated with cetuximab. *JCO.* 2008;26:374-379.
2. Lievre A, Bachet JB, Le Corre D, et al. KRAS mutation status is predictive of response to cetuximab therapy in colorectal cancer. *Cancer Res.* 2006;66: 3992-3995.

Clinical Testing Experience and Relationship to EGFR Gene Copy Number and Immunohistochemical Expression

Li AR, Chitale D, Riely GJ, et al (Memorial Sloan-Kettering Cancer Ctr, NY)
J Mol Diagn 10:242-248, 2008

Lung adenocarcinomas responsive to epidermal growth factor receptor (EGFR) tyrosine kinase inhibitors possess *EGFR* mutations and often increased *EGFR* copy number. We prospectively studied 334 clinical cases using polymerase chain reaction-based assays to detect deletions within exon 19 and the L858R mutation in exon 21, which together account for approximately 90% of *EGFR* mutations. Seventy-eight (23%) of these tumors had an *EGFR* mutation, with 55 (71%) exon 19 deletions and 23 (29%) exon 21 L858R mutations. We were able to compare mutant and normal *EGFR* alleles and found a preferential amplification of the mutant allele. The association of mutations with *EGFR* amplification (determined by chromogenic *in situ* hybridization) and EGFR expression (determined by immunohistochemistry) was further examined in a subset of 60 tumors. *EGFR* amplification (≥ 5 *EGFR* signals per nucleus) was seen in 15 of 29 (52%) *EGFR*-mutated tumors but in only five of 31 (6%) non-mutated tumors ($P = 0.006$). EGFR overexpression was strongly associated with amplification but was statistically independent of *EGFR* mutation. Most patients with *EGFR* mutations (17 of 29, 59%) never smoked compared with 13% (four of 31) of patients lacking such mutations ($P = 0.0003$). The association of amplification with smoking status was marginal and was non-existent with EGFR expression. Thus, these results indicate that *EGFR* amplification, preferentially of the mutant allele, often accompanies *EGFR* mutation, whereas EGFR immunohistochemical staining associates with amplification but cannot predict *EGFR* mutation status.

▶ Another companion test that predicts responsiveness to a targeted drug is the determination of mutations in the epidermal growth factor receptor (EGFR) gene. As opposed to mutations in KRAS which predict resistance to therapy, mutations in the EGFR gene are predictive for response to treatment with the tyrosine kinase inhibitors (TKIs), gefitifinib and erlotinib, in patients with lung adenocarcinoma. In this article Li and coauthors summarize their experience in performing testing for EGFR mutations in a 12-month period with PCR-based tests. Although most laboratories performing this testing use sequencing to detect these mutations, the authors describe 2 PCR assays that together detect over 90% of mutations in this gene. The authors also compare their results to detection of EGFR amplification by in situ hybridization and by immunohistochemistry. The assay presented seems to be a reproducible method that increases the sensitivity over sequencing. It is expected that more sensitive mutation detection would identify cases in which only a minor fraction of tumor cells actually carry a mutation. It is unknown if people whose tumors carry only a minor fraction of cells with EGFR mutations respond to TKIs in the same way as patients identified with other less sensitive methodologies (those used in the clinical trials). A follow-up study in which outcomes for these patients are evaluated would be desirable. The authors also discuss the clinical significance of EGFR mutation detection for therapeutic selection and for decisions to maintain or withdraw TKI-based therapy in the event of progression. These are all important issues that all pathologists should be familiar with to provide adequate support to the clinical oncology community.

F. A. Monzon, MD

Translational Genomics to Develop a *Salmonella enterica* Serovar Paratyphi A Multiplex Polymerase Chain Reaction Assay
Ou H-Y, Ju CTS, Thong K-L, et al (Shanghai Jiaotong Univ, China; Univ of Malaya, Kuala Lumpur, Malaysia; et al)
J Mol Diagn 9:624-630, 2007

The use of pathogen genome sequence data for the control and management of infections remains an ongoing challenge. We describe a broadly applicable, web-enabled approach that can be used to develop bacteria-specific polymerase chain reaction (PCR) assays. *Salmonella enterica* Paratyphi A has emerged as a major cause of enteric fever in Asia. Culture-based diagnosis is slow and frequently negative in patients with suspected typhoid and paratyphoid fever, potentially compromising patient management and public health. We used the MobilomeFINDER web-server to perform *in silico* subtractive hybridization, thus identifying 43 protein-coding sequences (CDSs) that were present in two Paratyphi A strains but not in other sequenced *Salmonella* genomes. After exclusion of 29 CDSs found to be variably present in Paratyphi A strains by microarray hybridization and grouping of remaining CDSs by genomic location, four dispersed targets (*stkF, spa2473, spa2539, hsdM*) were used to develop a highly discriminatory multiplex PCR assay. All 52 Paratyphi A strains within the diverse panel investigated produced one of two pathognomonic four-band signatures. Given rapid and ongoing expansion of DNA and comparative genomics databases, our universally accessible web-server-supported do-it-yourself approach offers the potential to contribute significantly to the rapid development of species-, serovar-, or pathotype-specific PCR assays targeting pre-existing and emerging bacterial pathogens.

▶ This is an interesting article that highlights how new genomic information can impact the development of molecular assays. In this article, the authors mined genomic databases to identify differences between different strains of *Salmonella* Paratyphi and designed a PCR-based assay based on the information obtained. Although the topic is not necessarily relevant to our United States readers (*Salmonella* Paratyphi A is not as prevalent in the United States as in Asia), the importance of this article is the demonstration that genomic information can be harnessed to solve a diagnostic problem of public health importance.

In recent years, there has been an explosion in the amount of genomic information available. However, the translation of this information into clinically useful assays has been slow. This article shows how a well thought out multidisciplinary effort can lead to the successful development of clinical assays. This is particularly important in certain areas of microbiology, such as the diagnosis of organisms that are difficult to culture or for which phenotypic identification is cumbersome and/or practically impossible.

F. A. Monzon, MD

Whole genome SNP arrays as a potential diagnostic tool for the detection of characteristic chromosomal aberrations in renal epithelial tumors

Monzon FA, Hagenkord JM, Lyons-Weiler MA, et al (Univ of Pittsburgh, PA; et al)
Mod Pathol 21:599-608, 2008

Renal tumors with complex or unusual morphology require extensive workup for accurate classification. Chromosomal aberrations that define subtypes of renal epithelial neoplasms have been reported. We explored if whole-genome chromosome copy number and loss-of-heterozygosity analysis with single nucleotide polymorphism (SNP) arrays can be used to identify these aberrations and classify renal epithelial tumors. We analyzed 20 paraffin-embedded tissues representing clear cell, papillary renal and chromophobe renal cell carcinoma, as well as oncocytoma with Affymetrix GeneChip 10K 2.0 Mapping arrays. SNP array results were in concordance with known genetic aberrations for each renal tumor subtype. Additional chromosomal aberrations were detected in all renal cell tumor types. The unique patterns allowed 19 out of 20 tumors to be readily categorized by their chromosomal copy number aberrations. One papillary renal cell carcinoma type 2 did not show the characteristic 7/17 trisomies. Clustering using the median copy number of each chromosomal arm correlated with histological class when using a restricted set of chromosomes. In addition, three morphologically challenging tumors were analyzed to explore the potential clinical utility of this method. In these cases, the SNP array-based copy number evaluation yielded information with potential clinical value. These results show that SNP arrays can detect characteristic chromosomal aberrations in paraffin-embedded renal tumors, and thus offer a high-resolution, genome-wide method that can be used as an ancillary study for classification and potentially for prognostic stratification of these tumors.

▶ Specific genetic abnormalities have been found in different subtypes of renal cell tumors and have been well characterized in the literature. However, this knowledge has not been routinely used in the diagnostic evaluation of these tumors. More than a decade ago, Steiner and Sidransky[1] proposed the use of loss of heterozygosity (LOH) analysis with microsatellites to detect specific chromosomal deletions in renal tumors. However, these assays were not incorporated into clinical practice. Correct pathological classification of renal cell tumors is critical for prognosis, management, therapy, and (in the age of targeted therapy) for eligibility to clinical trials. In this article, the authors assess the use of single nucleotide polymorphism (SNP) arrays in the detection of chromosomal abnormalities in formalin-fixed paraffin-embedded (FFPE) tissues from renal epithelial tumors. Although the number of cases analyzed in this study is small (total 20 with 5 tumors on each tumor subtype), the authors show that each tumor subtype can be accurately identified based on its profile of chromosomal imbalances obtained with SNP microarrays. Furthermore, the authors show examples of how this technique can be used to identify the tumor subtypes for cases that are not readily classifiable by standard histopathologic evaluation. A larger study expanding the application to classic cases, other subtypes, and tumors with uncertain classification by morphology is desirable to confirm the results of this study. Given the relevance of accurately classifying patients for prognostic implications and therapeutic decisions, there is a need for diagnostic tools that reliably detect and quantify genetic lesions that are diagnostic for each subgroup of renal epithelial neoplasms. Several techniques have been used for genome-wide scanning of chromosomal aberrations in renal tumors, including comparative genomic hybridization (CGH), array CGH, and SNP arrays. One of the limitations of array CGH is that it cannot detect regions of "copy neutral LOH" or uniparental disomy (UPD), which has been reported to constitute 50% to 80% of the LOH in human cancers. SNP arrays also provide genotypes, which can be used to determine regions of LOH and thus presents an advantage over array CGH. It is important to note that an inherent limitation of all array-based technologies is the inability to detect balanced chromosomal translocations. The SNP array is a robust platform that can be used with fresh or paraffin-embedded tissue, has relatively low costs and is amenable to automation. In fact, SNP arrays are already being used for detection of inherited chromosomal aberrations in cases of mental retardation and other genetic diseases in multiple laboratories. Although chromosomal analysis of human tumors presents different challenges from constitutional genetics, such as tumor heterogeneity and polyploidy, the potential clinical applications for SNP microarrays in molecular oncology are suggested in this article and by other authors.[2,3]

F. A. Monzon, MD

References

1. Steiner G, Sidransky D. Molecular differential diagnosis of renal carcinoma: from microscopes to microsatellites. *Am J Pathol.* 1996;149:1791-1795.
2. Gondek LP, Dunbar AJ, Szpurka H, McDevitt MA, Maciejewski JP. SNP array karyotyping allows for the detection of uniparental disomy and cryptic chromosomal abnormalities in MDS/MPD-U and MPD. *PLoS ONE.* 2007;2:e1225. PMID: 18030353.

3. Lehmann S, Ogawa S, Raynaud SD, et al. Molecular allelokaryotyping of early-stage, untreated chronic lymphocytic leukemia. *Cancer.* 2008;112:1296-1305. PMID: 18246537.

Sentinel node staging for breast cancer: intraoperative molecular pathology overcomes conventional histologic sampling errors
Blumencranz P, Whitworth PW, Deck K, et al (Morton Plant Mease Health Care, Clearwater, FL; Nashville Breast Cancer, Nashville, TN; South Orange County Surgical Med Group, Laguna Hills, CA; et al)
Am J Surg 194:426-432, 2007

Background.—When sentinel node dissection reveals breast cancer metastasis, completion axillary lymph node dissection is ideally performed during the same operation. Intraoperative histologic techniques have low and variable sensitivity. A new intraoperative molecular assay (Gene-Search BLN Assay; Veridex, LLC, Warren, NJ) was evaluated to determine its efficiency in identifying significant sentinel lymph node metastases (>.2 mm).

Methods.—Positive or negative BLN Assay results generated from fresh 2-mm node slabs were compared with results from conventional histologic evaluation of adjacent fixed tissue slabs.

Results.—In a prospective study of 416 patients at 11 clinical sites, the assay detected 98% of metastases >2 mm and 88% of metastasis greater >.2 mm, results superior to frozen section. Micrometastases were less frequently detected (57%) and assay positive results in nodes found negative by histology were rare (4%).

Conclusions.—The BLN Assay is properly calibrated for use as a stand alone intraoperative molecular test.

▶ The evaluation of sentinel lymph nodes (SLNs) for detection of metastatic breast cancer during intraoperative evaluation has practical limitations on the amount of tissue that is actually examined. It is estimated that only 1% of lymph node tissue is evaluated and, thus, it is possible that a significant number of false negative diagnoses are routinely being done. This results in the need to perform a completion axillary lymph node dissection (ALND) in a second surgery. In this article, Blumencranz and coauthors evaluated a molecular test that attempts to address this shortcoming by molecularly evaluating 50% of lymph node tissue. The GeneSearch BLN Assay is an RT-PCR test that detects the presence of mRNA transcripts for mammaglobin and cytokeratin 19 in lymph node tissue. The test is intended to be run in parallel to frozen section or touch prep evaluation of sentinel lymph nodes. The primary objective of the test is to reduce the number of false negatives and thus avoid a second surgery for these patients. The study has significant strengths such as being multi-institutional, using a test and validation cohorts, having central review of histology, and having well-defined endpoints. The results show that the test is able to detect 98% of metastasis > 2 mm and 88% of metastasis > .2 mm. Importantly, 4% of cases showed a positive test result in the absence of histologically confirmed metastasis. Should all pathologists implement this test in their frozen section laboratories? The results indicate that it is possible that the implementation of this test would decrease second surgeries in 2% to 3% of cases (cases negative by frozen section that were positive on permanent histology), and that its use might be best for difficult to diagnose tumor types such as lobular carcinoma. However, in 4% of patients the test yielded a positive result in the absence of histologically confirmed metastatic disease. The appropriateness of doing an ANLD in this patient group has not been evaluated. Thus, the implementation of this test could modestly reduce the number of second surgeries, whereas potentially increasing the number of unnecessary ALNDs, which is a surgical procedure with significant comorbidity. As pathologists, another important issue to consider is the technical, personnel, and space requirements to implement this molecular test in the frozen section area of a surgical pathology laboratory. The setup requires a significant amount of space and a dedicated molecular technologist to perform the test whenever it's required (2 technologists are recommended by those already performing the test). It is unlikely that many laboratories will be able to assign these types of resources to a single laboratory test without significant improvement in patient outcomes. Another consideration is the added time to perform the assay, which might extend surgical time, especially in cases with large lymph nodes in which multiple runs need to be done to test 50% of lymph node tissue. It is important to note that molecular staging (detection of occult metastasis by molecular methods) is an area of active current research in assay development. A commercial assay for the detection of colon cancer metastasis in lymph nodes (Previstage GCC, DiagnoCure, LLC) has completed a prospective trial and should be in the market soon. It is likely that similar molecular assays will be developed for other malignancies. Note: At the time of submission of this commentary, a new article with more detail on the performance of theGene-Search BLN assay was published.[1] Readers are referred to this article for more details.

F. A. Monzon, MD

Reference

1. Julian TB, Blumencranz P, Deck K, et al. Novel intraoperative molecular test for sentinel lymph node metastases in patients with early-stage breast cancer. *J Clin Oncol.* 2008;26:3338-3345.

A First-Generation Multiplex Biomarker Analysis of Urine for the Early Detection of Prostate Cancer

Laxman B, Morris DS, Yu J, et al (Univ of Michigan Med School, Ann Arbor, MI)

Cancer Res 68:645-649, 2008

Although prostate-specific antigen (PSA) serum level is currently the standard of care for prostate cancer screening in the United States, it lacks ideal specificity and additional biomarkers are needed to supplement or potentially replace serum PSA testing. Emerging evidence suggests that monitoring the noncoding RNA transcript *PCA3* in urine may be useful in detecting prostate cancer in patients with elevated PSA levels. Here, we show that a multiplex panel of urine transcripts outperforms *PCA3* transcript alone for the detection of prostate cancer. We measured the expression of seven putative prostate cancer biomarkers, including *PCA3*, in sedimented urine using quantitative PCR on a cohort of 234 patients presenting for biopsy or radical prostatectomy. By univariate analysis, we found that increased *GOLPH2*, *SPINK1*, and *PCA3* transcript expression and *TMPRSS2:ERG* fusion status were significant predictors of prostate cancer. Multivariate regression analysis showed that a multiplexed model, including these biomarkers, outperformed serum PSA or *PCA3* alone in detecting prostate cancer. The area under the receiver-operating characteristic curve was 0.758 for the multiplexed model versus 0.662 for *PCA3* alone ($P = 0.003$). The sensitivity and specificity for the multiplexed model were 65.9% and 76.0%, respectively, and the positive and negative predictive values were 79.8% and 60.8%, respectively. Taken together, these results provide the framework for the development of highly optimized, multiplex urine biomarker tests for more accurate detection of prostate cancer.

▶ Prostate-specific antigen (PSA) testing changed the landscape of prostate cancer diagnosis by increasing the number of tumors detected in an early fashion. However, the PSA test has low specificity (~20%) and thus the rate of false positives is quite high. Many research groups have focused their efforts in finding biomarkers that can substitute for PSA, or be used in conjunction with it, to increase the specificity of prostate cancer detection methods. Recently, an assay for detection of *PCA3*, a specific biomarker for prostate cancer, has been evaluated in a multicenter study for use as a reflex test in patients with elevated PSA.[1] In the present article, Laxman et al evaluated multiple biomarkers, including *PCA3*, in an effort to develop a multiplex test with better specificity compared with PSA or *PCA3* alone. The authors selected 7 markers overexpressed in prostate cancer, and developed a 4-marker test that showed specificity of 76% and a positive predictive value of 79.8%. Importantly, the negative predictive value is 60.8%, which was reduced to 58.1% when a leave-one-out validation strategy (to reduce overfitting) was used. This indicates that close to 40% of patients with a negative test result still harbor prostate cancer. This parameter will need to be improved in future assays if the intent is to reduce the number of biopsies performed on patients with elevated PSA. As mentioned above, this is an area of intense research and a group of researchers from Veridex, LLC recently reported the performance of a similar multiplex assay based on the methylation status of 3 markers. The performance of this assay is comparable with the one reported by Laxman but appears to have better specificity. Clearly, this is an area that should be followed closely by pathologists since it is very likely that new multiplex assays to be used in conjunction with PSA testing will be in use in the near future.

F. A. Monzon, MD

Reference

1. Vener T, Derecho C, Baden J, et al. Development of a multiplexed urine assay for prostate cancer diagnosis. *Clin Chem.* 2008;54:874-882.

PART II

LABORATORY MEDICINE

Introduction

Laboratory medicine continues to flourish and expand, under the aegis of its many scientific disciplines. This year we have continued to monitor not only the standard lab medicine journals, but also the broad array of other basic and clinical scientific publications with direct relevance to this field; not only specialty and subspecialty medical journals, but also major publications in the physical, chemical, and biological sciences. Literally thousands of laboratory medicine-related articles, published across this broad spectrum, are scanned to provide you with those most relevant to current and future clinical laboratory practice, along with commentary on their relevance and context for today's laboratorians. We hope you continue to find this coverage useful in your practice.

Michael G. Bissell, MD, PhD, MPH

18 Laboratory Management and Outcomes

Establishing a Simple and Sustainable Quality Assurance Program and Clinical Chemistry Services in Eritrea

Scott MG, Morin S, Hock KG, et al (Washington Univ School of Medicine, St Louis, MO; Natl Health Lab, Asmara, Eritrea; et al)

Clin Chem 53:1945-1953, 2007

Background.—As chronic diseases become more prevalent in developing nations, establishment of sustainable clinical chemistry services will become increasingly important. The complexity of automated instruments, coupled with a lack of resources and skilled workers, will present a challenge for these countries.

Methods.—A system emphasizing simplified instrumentation, single source reagents, technical education and support, and simple QC algorithms was established in the small African nation of Eritrea. The same reagents were used on different analyzers, as well as the same lot numbers of QC material. To allow traceability of Eritrea results to an accredited US laboratory, the reagents and QC materials were identical to those used in a large university hospital in the US, and patient samples were frequently exchanged between locations.

Results.—QC values for 23 clinical chemistry tests in the Eritrean National Health Laboratory compared well to values obtained in the US, showing some statistically different values but no clinically significant differences. QC values were also stable over time in Eritrea. Patient sample values from Eritrea correlated well to values from the US, with *r* values ranging from 0.71 to 0.99. For 9 chemistry tests, small regional laboratories in Eritrea produced QC and patient values that usually compared well to those from the Eritrea National Health Laboratory, but markedly discrepant values were occasionally observed that prompted investigation.

Conclusion.—A simple but sustainable national laboratory system has been established in the developing nation of Eritrea.

▶ Imagine setting up clinical laboratory services for the first time in a third-world nation that has never had them before. Only when one makes the mental effort to visualize this process in complete detail does the complexity of the infrastructure we take for granted here begin to become apparent. What tests are most needed, and which of these can actually be performed "on the ground" in the third-world environment? What instrumentation is actually (a) available, and (b) supportable, technically, in this environment? How are reagents going to be supplied, and how will their steady supply be assured? How are operators of the equipment going to be trained? Who will provide equipment maintenance and repairs? How will specimens be transported? This article is an excellent laboratory management case history of how this feat was accomplished in the African nation of Eritrea by a volunteer group, Pathologists Overseas, Inc, in collaboration with a major United States academic medical center.

M. G. Bissell, MD, PhD, MPH

Is flow cytometry accurate enough to screen platelet autoantibodies?
Hézard N, Simon G, Macé C, et al (Laboratoire d'Hématologie, CHU Robert Debré, Reims, France; Institut Natl de Transfusion Sanguine, Paris, France)
Transfusion 48:513-518, 2008

Background.—The diagnosis of immune thrombocytopenic purpura (ITP) is a diagnosis of exclusion, as stated by international guidelines. Nevertheless, the assessment of platelet (PLT) antibodies has been reported as helpful for the diagnosis and the follow-up of ITP patients. PLT antibodies are detected by highly specialized assays, such as monoclonal antibody-specific immobilization of PLT antigen (MAIPA) test. Flow cytometry for PLT-associated immunoglobulin G (PAIgG) detection has been described more recently. This study was meant to evaluate the utility of flow cytometry to screen accurately patients needing further MAIPA testing.

Study Design and Methods.—PAIgG, PAIgM, and PAIgA were determined in 107 consecutive patients and in 147 healthy controls in parallel. MAIPA testing was performed in all patients. The accuracy of flow cytometry was assessed with a receiver operating characteristics (ROC) curve analysis versus MAIPA.

Results.—MAIPA assay found PLT-specific IgG in 27 patients (25%). The ROC curve analysis showed that no false-negative result in flow cytometry was obtained for a mean fluorescence intensity (MFI) cutoff of 0.2. With this cutoff, PAIgG were positive in 61 patients (57%). In this series, MAIPA was unnecessary in 42 percent of patients (corresponding to true-negative results). When MAIPA was positive, PAIgM values ranged from 0.1 to 1.0, and PAIgA from 0.1 to 2.

Conclusion.—Flow cytometry for PAIgG assessment may be used to accurately decide whether or not MAIPA must be subsequently performed. In this series, MAIPA was unnecessary in 42 percent of patients. Moreover,

PAIgM results suggested that its determination combined with PAIgG may be of interest in ITP investigation.

▶ Prostate cancer is the most commonly diagnosed cancer in males in the United Kingdom, and screening for this condition is the subject of national discussion regarding the advisability and cost effectiveness of setting up a universal national screening program. To date, the British National Health Service does not believe that there is sufficient evidence that the risk benefit ratio is favorable enough overall to justify such an undertaking. In the context of such considerations, it is important to develop an accounting of the induced costs of screening. This article discusses this aspect of a multicenter pharmaceutical industry trial of cancer chemoprevention in which eligible men were randomized between placebo and active drug. The authors studied the process of subject recruitment to this study, which involved PSA screening followed up by referrals for patients with abnormalities (those PSA 3-10 ng/mL to TRUS-guided prostate biopsy; and those with PSA > 10 ng/mL to further workup and management).

M. G. Bissell, MD, PhD, MPH

Studying Critical Values: Adverse Event Identification Following a Critical Laboratory Values Study at the Ohio State University Medical Center
Jenkins JJ II, Crawford JM, Bissell MG (Doctors Hosp (Ohio Health); The Ohio State Univ, Columbus)
Am J Clin Pathol 128:604-609, 2007

No study to date has used laboratory critical values to evaluate variations in patient adverse events. We retrospectively analyzed a database of critical values to determine their distribution by hospital unit over time. The data were drawn from the Ohio State University Medical Center Information Warehouse (Columbus) for a 58-month period. Critical values were plotted over time on statistical control charts and analyzed for unusual peaks in monthly occurrence rates. Chart review of individual patient results yielded several predictor variables for the unusual peaks. Of these, occurrence of patient adverse events was the most relevant independent predictor variable for a month with an unusual number of critical values vs a normal month. This result epidemiologically confirms the basic premise of critical value reporting and suggests that the control-chart method of this type could be a new statistical tool to compare clinical activity of different hospital locations at different times (Fig1).

▶ All of us in laboratory medicine know something about critical values. We know, for example, how critical values are supposed to represent ranges of values for certain analytes that are generally believed to be associated with increased risk of immediate damage to life or limb of patients. But, do we

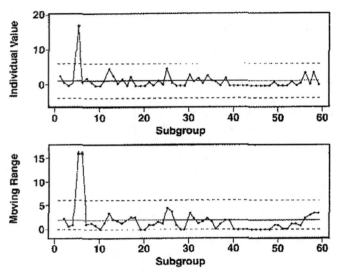

FIGURE1.—Control-chart violation for ionized calcium at Ohio State University Medical Center, Columbus. Individual and moving range (I/MR) for high ionized calcium (ICA). For I values, upper control limit (UCL), 6.152; mean, 1.264; and lower control limit (LCL), 3.625; for MR, UCL, 6.005; R = 1,838; and LCL, 0. Asterisks, test 1, 1 point more than 3.00 σ from center line; test failed at point 5. (Reprinted from Jenkins II JJ, Crawford JM, Bissell MG. Studying critical values: adverse event identification following a critical laboratory values study at the ohio state university medical center. *Am J Clin Pathol* 2007;128:604-609, with permission from American Society for Clinical Pathology.)

know how they were derived in the first place, or how to define new ones? Possibly not, as the scientific literature on this topic has been somewhat surprisingly sparse up until now. In carrying out the research that led to this article we realized that the existence of large, continuously-updated databases of clinical information, including laboratory values, is making possible a new way of possibly using critical values. Plotting the frequency of such critical values on time series, Fig 1, such as control charts, by hospital location, may allow an assessment of the overall critical value health of individual hospital units over time.

M. G. Bissell, MD, PhD, MPH

Accuracy of Send-Out Test Ordering: A College of American Pathologists Q-Probes Study of Ordering Accuracy in 97 Clinical Laboratories

Valenstein PN, Walsh MK, Stankovic AK (St. Joseph Mercy Hospital; College of American Pathologists, Northfield, IL; et al)
Archiv Pathol Lab Med 132:206-210, 2008

Context.—Errors entering orders for send-out laboratory tests into computer systems waste health care resources and can delay patient evaluation and management.

Objectives.—To determine (1) the accuracy of send-out test order entry under "real world" conditions and (2) whether any of several practices are associated with improved order accuracy.

Design.—Representatives from 97 clinical laboratories provided information about the processes they use to send tests to reference facilities and their order entry and specimen routing error rates.

Results.—In aggregate, 98% of send-out tests were correctly ordered and 99.4% of send-out tests were routed to the proper reference laboratory. There was wide variation among laboratories in the rate of send-out test order entry errors. In the bottom fourth of laboratories, more than 5% of send-out tests were ordered incorrectly, while in the top fourth of laboratories fewer than 0.3% of tests were ordered incorrectly. Order entry errors were less frequent when a miscellaneous test code was used than when a specific test code was used (3.9% vs 5.6%; $P = .003$).

Conclusions.—Computer order entry errors for send-out tests occur approximately twice as frequently as order entry errors for other types of tests. Filing more specific test codes in a referring institution's information system is unlikely to reduce order entry errors and may make error rates worse.

▶ Virtually all clinical laboratories send out some of their tests to other laboratories. This includes commercial reference laboratories themselves. For a typical hospital clinical laboratory, the list of orderable test codes available to clinicians only on a send-out basis is longer (sometimes much longer) than the list of tests provided by the laboratory in-house. The authors of this article make several observations about some of the aspects of this common circumstance that make it a more fertile ground for errors than is the case with routine in-house test ordering. These observations include (1) use of more than one reference laboratory (not an uncommon circumstance) may lead to tests being sent to the wrong laboratory; (2) the long list of available send-out tests may lead to confusion of names and other details; (3) ordering physicians may often have less familiarity with the more esoteric tests being ordered through send-out, leading to ambiguity in the orders themselves.

M. G. Bissell, MD, PhD, MPH

What is a significant difference between sequential laboratory results?
Smellie WSA (Clinical Laboratory, General Hosp, Bishop Auckland, County Durham)
J Clin Pathol 61:419-425, 2008

The uncertainty of a numerical laboratory result can be masked by the fact that the laboratory reports an absolute number, whereas users have limited knowledge of the confidence interval of the result. Interpretation of laboratory tests is in reality therefore an inexact science, a balance between clinical context and the likely relevance of a laboratory result.

This review considers the factors which contribute to result variability and examines the implications for interpreting differences between sequential laboratory results. It offers suggestions to deal with a problem which has not yet been much addressed in routine practice. The examples used are restricted to the discipline of clinical biochemistry, although the issues and principles apply to numerical (and indeed qualitative) results in other disciplines.

Laboratories could provide more guidance on the likelihood of a result being significant to assist users. There is a need for discussion about how this is best done, and compatible with electronic result delivery. Options for providing this information are considered.

▶ Clinicians receiving test results from the clinical laboratory are faced with several important challenges of interpretation. These depend on the clinician's purpose in ordering the test. In the case of tests ordered to help establish a diagnosis, these challenges include: determining whether a given result lying outside a population-based reference interval represents an indication of an abnormal state in the particular patient from whom it was sampled; and determining which probabilities on the patient's working differential diagnosis may need to be revised because of the result (given the degree of apparent abnormality it may represent). In the case of tests ordered to monitor a patient's physiological state and/or response to therapy, another challenge is determining whether, and to what degree, a newly repeated laboratory value represents a real change in patient state. Dealing with this issue requires the development of standards for the statistical assessment of the degree of significance of a given change. This, in turn, requires incorporation of knowledge of the components of variability underlying sequential differences.

M. G. Bissell, MD, PhD, MPH

19 Clinical Chemistry

Clinical Application of C-Reactive Protein Across the Spectrum of Acute Coronary Syndromes
Scirica BM, for the Thrombolysis in Myocardial Infarction (TIMI) Study Group (Brigham and Women's Hosp, Boston)
Clin Chem 53:1800-1807, 2007

Background.—High-sensitivity C-reactive protein (hsCRP) is associated with adverse cardiovascular outcomes in acute coronary syndromes (ACS). The ability to formulate recommendations regarding clinical use of hsCRP is limited by a paucity of data regarding several key issues. The purpose of this study was to evaluate hsCRP across the spectrum of ACS.

Methods.—hsCRP was measured on admission in 3225 patients with ACS. hsCRP concentrations were compared in patients who suffered an adverse cardiac outcome within 10 months of study entry and in patients who had no adverse event. Because of heterogeneity in the relationship between hsCRP and clinical outcomes, evaluation was limited to patients from whom samples were collected within 48 h of symptom onset.

Results.—Patients in the highest quartile of hsCRP compared to those in the lowest quartile were at increased risk of death at 30 days [adjusted hazard ratio (adjHR) 4.6, P <0.001] and 10 months (adjHR 3.9, P <0.001). In patients with unstable angina/non–ST-elevation myocardial infarction (STEMI), hsCRP >3 mg/L was associated with increased 10-month mortality (adjHR 2.3, $P = 0.002$), whereas in STEMI a relationship with mortality was seen at hsCRP >10 mg/L (adjHR 3.0, $P = 0.008$). Increased concentrations of hsCRP were strongly associated with the development of heart failure at 30 days (adjHR 8.2, $P = 0.001$) and 10 months (adjHR 2.6, $P = 0.014$).

Conclusion.—Increased baseline concentrations of hsCRP are strongly associated with mortality and heart failure across the ACS spectrum. hsCRP measurement should be performed early after presentation and index diagnosis-specific cutpoints should be used.

▶ Although it has been known for some time now that elevations of high-sensitivity C-reactive protein (hs-CRP) are generally associated with poorer outcomes in acute coronary syndrome (ACS), a number of practical interpretive issues have made it difficult to implement the universal use of this marker. These issues include such things as the optimal timing of hs-CRP measurements vis-à-vis presentation, the most appropriate decision limits to use, the implications for treatment, the prognostic relevance of hs-CRP in patients with ST-segment elevation myocardial infarction (STEMI), and relationship to risk of congestive heart failure (CHF). What has been needed is the inclusion of this marker in a large-scale clinical trial. This article describes such work, in the context of the Orbofiban in Patients with Unstable Coronary Syndromes (OPUS)-Thrombolysis in Myocardial Infarction (TIMI) 16 trial of patients with unstable angina (UA), nonSTEMI (NSTEMI), and STEMI. The findings strongly support the use of the hs-CRP marker in the context of ACS.

M. G. Bissell, MD, PhD, MPH

Novel Serum Biomarker Candidates for Liver Fibrosis in Hepatitis C Patients
Gangadharan B, Antrobus R, Dwek RA, et al (Univ of Oxford, England)
Clin Chem 53:1792-1799, 2007

Background.—Liver biopsy is currently the gold standard for assessing liver fibrosis, and no reliable noninvasive diagnostic approach is available. Therefore a suitable serologic biomarker of liver fibrosis is urgently needed.

Methods.—We used a proteomics method based on 2-dimensional gel electrophoresis to identify potential fibrosis biomarkers. Serum samples from patients with varying degrees of hepatic scarring induced by infection with the hepatitis C virus (HCV) were analyzed and compared with serum from healthy controls.

Results.—We observed the most prominent differences when we compared serum samples from cirrhotic patients with healthy control serum. Inter-α-trypsin inhibitor heavy chain H4 (ITIH4) fragments, $\alpha1$ antichymotrypsin, apolipoprotein L1 (Apo L1), prealbumin, albumin, paraoxonase/arylesterase 1, and zinc-$\alpha2$-glycoprotein were decreased in cirrhotic serum, whereas CD5 antigen-like protein (CD5L) and $\beta2$ glycoprotein I ($\beta2$GPI) were increased. In general, $\alpha2$ macroglobulin (a2M) and immunoglobulin components increased with hepatic fibrosis, whereas haptoglobin and complement components (C3, C4, and factor H-related protein 1) decreased. Novel proteins associated with HCV-induced fibrosis included ITIH4 fragments, complement factor H-related protein 1, CD5L, Apo L1, $\beta2$GPI, and thioester-cleaved products of a2M.

Conclusions.—Assessment of hepatic scarring may be performed with a combination of these novel fibrosis biomarkers, thus eliminating the need for liver biopsy. Further evaluation of these candidate markers needs to be performed in larger patient populations. Diagnosis of fibrosis during early stages will allow early treatment, thereby preventing fibrosis progression (Table 1).

▶ One of the leading causes of hepatic fibrosis and cirrhosis is hepatitis C viral infection (HCV). It has been a great irony of medical practice in this area that

TABLE 1.—Summary of Selected Differentially Expressed Proteins Identified in Serum Samples of Healthy Controls vs The Different Stages of Hepatic scarring.[a]

Classification	Protein name	Changes in Relation to Controls			Protein function
		Mild	Moderate	Cirrhosis	
Plasmin-associated	a2M	↑	⇑	↑ ⇑	Inhibits plasmin
	ITIH4	–	–	↓ ⇓	Can be cleaved by kallikrein (leads to plasmin activation)
Decreased because of compromise in hepatic synthetic function	Albumin	–	–	↓	Liver synthesized protein, most abundant protein of serum
	Prealbumin (transthyretin)	–	–	↓	Liver synthesized protein; carries vitamin A
	Complement C3, C4 and factor H-related protein 1	⇓	↓	↓ ⇓	Liver synthesized protein; involved in complement cascade
HGF-related	α1 antichymotrypsin	–	–	↓	HGF decreases α1 antichymotrypsin
	Haptoglobin	↓	↓	↓ ⇓	HGF decreases haptoglobin synthesis
Lipid metabolism	Apo L1	–	–	⇓	Concentrations correlate with triglycerides and cholesterol
	β2GP1	–	–	⇑	Binds to chylomicrons and HDLs
	Paraoxonase/arylesterase 1	–	–	↓	Degrades oxidized lipids in lipoproteins and cells
	Zinc-α2-glycoprotein	–	–	↓	Stimulated lipolysis in adipocytes
Immune system related	CD5 antigen-like	–	–	⇑	Possible immune system regulation role; IgM related
	IgA1 + IgG2 heavy chain and Ig light chain regions	–	↑	↑ ⇑	Imunoglobulin fragments

⇑, Present only in serum from hepatic scarring patients.
↑, Present in serum from both control and hepatic scarring patients but expressed to a higher extent in hepatic scarring.
–, No significant change.
↓, Present in serum from both control and hepatic scarring patients but expressed to a higher extent in control serum.
⇓, Present only in serum from healthy controls.
[a] Proteins shown were differentially expressed by 2-fold or more when comparing serum gels from healthy controls with the different stages of hepatic fibrosis.
(Reprinted from Gangadharan B, Antrobus R, Dwek RA, et al. Novel serum biomarker candidates for liver fibrosis in hepatitis C patients. *Clin Chem.* 2007;53:1792-1799.)

liver biopsies, the only practical method for diagnosing fibrosis until now, are especially complicated (by bleeding, pain, etc) in the context of cirrhosis. The search for serum biomarkers of hepatic fibrosis has been underway therefore for some time. For example, a panel of 5 biomarkers (α2-macroglobulin, haptoglobin, apoplipoprotein A1, γ-glutamyl transpeptidase, and bilirubin) has been used clinically, but unfortunately has not proven particularly accurate, eliminating the need for biopsies only about 26% of the time. All of which is why an approach based on the new field of proteomics would seem to hold great promise in this area. The authors' use of 2-dimensional gel electrophoresis patterns in normal versus HCV patients provides a potential new window on this practical diagnostic problem.

M. G. Bissell, MD, PhD, MPH

Usefulness of Preoperative Oral Glucose Tolerance Testing for Perioperative Risk Stratification in Patients Scheduled for Elective Vascular Surgery
Dunkelgrun M, Schreiner F, Schockman DB, et al (Erasmus Med Ctr, Rotterdam, The Netherlands)
Am J Cardiol 101:526-529, 2008

Patients scheduled for major vascular surgery are screened for cardiac risk factors using standardized risk indexes, including diabetes mellitus (DM). Screening in patients without a history of DM includes fasting glucose measurement. However, an oral glucose tolerance test (OGTT) could significantly improve the detection of DM and impaired glucose tolerance (IGT) and the prediction of perioperative cardiac events. In a prospective study, 404 consecutive patients without signs or histories of IGT or DM were included and subjected to OGTT. The primary study end point was the composite of perioperative myocardial ischemia, assessed by 72-hour Holter monitoring using ST-segment analysis and troponin release. The primary end point was noted in 21% of the patients. IGT was diagnosed in 104 patients (25.7%), and new-onset DM was detected in 43 patients (10.6%). The OGTT detected 75% of the patients with IGT and 72% of the patients with DM. Preoperative glucose levels significantly predicted the risk for perioperative cardiac ischemia; odds ratios for DM and IGT were, respectively, 3.2 (95% confidence interval 1.3 to 8.1) and 1.4 (95% confidence interval 0.7 to 3.0). In conclusion, the prevalence of undiagnosed IGT and DM is high in vascular patients and is associated with perioperative myocardial ischemia. Therefore, an OGTT should be considered for all patients who undergo elective vascular surgery.

▶ Because diabetes mellitus is a widely recognized major risk factor for cardiovascular disease, it is certainly appropriate that patients scheduled for vascular surgery be screened for diabetes or the prediabetic state of impaired glucose tolerance (IGT). Such patients without the history of either of these conditions are typically screened with a fasting blood glucose (FBG) measurement. It is of some interest to know whether or not a full oral glucose tolerance test (OGTT) would provide any incremental improvement in diagnostic performance over the FBG and thus be a better predictor of clinical outcomes of vascular surgery. The major advantage of OGTT over FBG is in the detection of impaired glucose tolerance, which can only be assessed by the OGTT, and which is associated with a highly increased risk of developing type 2 diabetes mellitus. Of course, an OGTT is a more expensive test than an FBG, and therefore a cost-benefit estimation has some relevance here.

M. G. Bissell, MD, PhD, MPH

A First-Generation Multiplex Biomarker Analysis of Urine For The Early Detection of Prostate Cancer

Laxman B, Morris DS, Yu J, et al (Univ of Michigan Med School, Ann Arbor, MI)

Cancer Res 68:645-649, 2008

Although prostate-specific antigen (PSA) serum level is currently the standard of care for prostate cancer screening in the United States, it lacks ideal specificity and additional biomarkers are needed to supplement or potentially replace serum PSA testing. Emerging evidence suggests that monitoring the noncoding RNA transcript *PCA3* in urine may be useful in detecting prostate cancer in patients with elevated PSA levels. Here, we show that a multiplex panel of urine transcripts outperforms *PCA3* transcript alone for the detection of prostate cancer. We measured the expression of seven putative prostate cancer biomarkers, including *PCA3*, in sedimented urine using quantitative PCR on a cohort of 234 patients presenting for biopsy or radical prostatectomy. By univariate analysis, we found that increased *GOLPH2*, *SPINK1*, and *PCA3* transcript expression and *TMPRSS2:ERG* fusion status were significant predictors of prostate cancer. Multivariate regression analysis showed that a multiplexed model, including these biomarkers, outperformed serum PSA or *PCA3* alone in detecting prostate cancer. The area under the receiver-operating characteristic curve was 0.758 for the multiplexed model versus 0.662 for *PCA3* alone ($P = 0.003$). The sensitivity and specificity for the multiplexed model were 65.9% and 76.0%, respectively, and the positive and negative predictive values were 79.8% and 60.8%, respectively. Taken together, these results provide the framework for the development of highly optimized, multiplex urine biomarker tests for more accurate detection of prostate cancer.

▶ Prostate specific antigen (PSA), a serine protease found in seminal fluid, is the only traditional serum tumor marker to find FDA approval for use as a general population screen for cancer. Its widespread use in this way has led directly to a significant increase in the rate of prostate cancer detection. In spite of this, however, more is needed. The clinical spectrum of PSA positivity includes many benign conditions (like benign prostatic hyperplasia, BPH, and prostatitis), the cutoff in common use (< 4 ng/mL) has been associated with a false negative rate of up to 15%, and a number of refinements for the test have been advocated (free PSA, PSA load, etc) but have sometimes proven complex to implement in practice. This work demonstrates the potential advantages of multiplexing a combination of the newer generation of biomarkers for prostate cancer, and compares their performance directly with that of PSA.

M. G. Bissell, MD, PhD, MPH

Lipoprotein(a) and Cardiovascular Disease in Ethnic Chinese: The Chin-Shan Community Cardiovascular Cohort Study

Chien K-L, Hsu H-C, Su T-C, et al (Natl Taiwan Univ, Taipei; Natl Taiwan Univ Hosp, Taipei; et al)
Clin Chem 54:285-291, 2008

Background.—Little is known about lipoprotein(a) [Lp(a)] as a predictor of vascular events among ethnic Chinese. We prospectively investigated the association of Lp(a) with cardiovascular disease and all-cause death in a community-based cohort.

Methods.—We conducted a community-based prospective cohort study of 3484 participants (53% women; age range, 35–97 years) who had complete lipid measurements and were free of a cardiovascular disease history at the time of recruitment. Over a median follow-up of 13.8-years, we documented 210 cases of stroke, 122 cases of coronary heart disease (CHD), and 781 deaths.

Results.—The incidences for each event increased appreciably with Lp(a) quartile for stroke and all-cause death, but not for CHD. Baseline Lp(a) concentration by quartile was not significantly associated with stroke, all-cause death, and CHD in multivariate analyses. The multivariate relative risk was significant for stroke at the 90th and 95th percentiles and for total death at the 95th and 99th percentiles.

Conclusions.—Our findings suggest a threshold relationship with little gradient of risk across lower Lp(a) values for stroke and all-cause death in Chinese adults.

▶ Lipoprotein (a) [Lp(a)] is an LDL particle with pre-beta electrophoretic mobility carrying principally cholesteryl esters and phospholipids and containing both apolipoprotein B-100 and the carbohydrate-rich apolipoprotein (a), which is a homologue of plasminogen, and therefore potentially prothrombotic in its effects. Hospital-based studies have shown that elevations of Lp(a) are consistently associated with various vascular diseases, however, these have not been consistently confirmed in population-based prospective cohort studies of cardiovascular risk. Most such studies have been confined to 1 sex or age group, and most have been focused on a single vascular outcome as endpoint— either coronary heart disease or stroke, or all-cause cardiovascular mortality. Cardiovascular disease risk patterns differ among various racial groups, and to date there have been no studies specifically of the ethnic Chinese population with regard to Lp(a) and specific cardiovascular outcomes.

These authors undertook a long-term community-based prospective study of this question.

M. G. Bissell, MD, PhD, MPH

The impact of circulating total homocysteine levels on long-term cardiovascular mortality in patients with acute coronary syndromes
Foussas SG, Zairis MN, Makrygiannis SS, et al (Tzanio Hospital, Piraeus, Greece)
Int J Cardiol 124:312-318, 2008

Background.—To evaluate the possible independent impact of circulating total homocysteine (tHcy) levels on long-term cardiovascular mortality, in patients with either ST-segment elevation myocardial infarction (STEMI), or non-ST-segment elevation acute coronary syndromes (NSTE-ACS).

Methods.—A total of 458 STEMI and 476 NSTE-ACS patients who presented consecutively, within the first 12 and 24 h of index pain respectively were studied. Each cohort was divided according to tertiles of circulating tHcy levels upon presentation. Early (30 days) and late (31 days through 5 years) cardiovascular mortality was the predefined study endpoint.

Results.—There was no difference in the risk of 30-day cardiovascular death among the tertiles of tHcy in patients with STEMI (7.2%, 8.5% and 12.4% for the first, second and third tertiles respectively; $p_{trend}=0.3$) or NSTE-ACS (3.1%, 3.8% and 5.7% for the first, second and third tertiles respectively; $p_{trend}=0.5$). Patients in the upper tHcy tertile were at significantly higher unadjusted risk of late (from 31 days through 5 years) cardiovascular death than those in the other two tertiles in STEMI (23.4%, 27.9% and 41.8% for the first, second and third tertiles respectively; $p_{trend}<0.001$), and NSTE-ACS (24.7%, 28.1% and 45.6% for the first, second and third tertiles respectively; $p_{trend}<0.001$) cohorts. However, after adjustment for baseline differences, there was no significant difference in the risk of late cardiovascular death among tHcy tertiles in either cohort. When circulating tHcy levels were treated as a continuous variable, they were significantly associated with late cardiovascular death ($p<0.001$ for both cohorts) by univariate Cox regression analysis, but not by multivariate Cox regression analysis ($p=0.8$, and $p=1$ for STEMI and NSTE-ACS cohorts, respectively).

Conclusions.—Based on the present data circulating tHcy levels determined upon admission do not serve as an independent predictor of long-term cardiovascular mortality in patients with either STEMI or NSTE-ACS.

▶ Homocysteine is a derivative of methionine in amino acid metabolism, and significantly elevated levels of total homocysteine (tHcy) levels are observed in the genetically inherited enzyme defect homocystinuria. These have been shown to be associated with early and severe atherosclerotic vascular disease. These findings have led to the supposition that lower levels of circulating total homocysteine in individuals not necessarily affected by the genetic defect might nonetheless be associated with increased risk for coronary artery disease. This has not been unequivocally established, however, and the whole concept remains controversial. Pathophysiology that might underlie such an association is unclear and, therefore, the question is whether or not homocysteine level can be regarded as an independent risk factor, or whether the association might just be due to confounding. The current authors undertook a modestly powered 5-year prospective outcomes study of total homocysteine levels and acute coronary syndrome. Their negative findings are important.

M. G. Bissell, MD, PhD, MPH

Active B12: A Rapid, Automated Assay for Holotranscobalamin on the Abbott AxSYM Analyzer
Brady J, Wilson L, McGregor L, et al (Axis-Shield Diagnostics, Ltd., Dundee, Scotland, UK)
Clin Chem 54:567-573, 2008

Background.—Conventional tests for vitamin B_{12} deficiency measure total serum vitamin B_{12}, whereas only that portion of vitamin B_{12} carried by transcobalamin (holotranscobalamin) is metabolically active. Measurement of holotranscobalamin (holoTC) may be more diagnostically accurate for detecting B_{12} deficiency that requires therapy. We developed an automated assay for holoTC that can be used on the Abbott AxSYM immunoassay analyzer.

Methods.—AxSYM Active B12 is a 2-step sandwich microparticle enzyme immunoassay. In step 1, a holoTC-specific antibody immobilized onto latex microparticles captures holoTC in samples of serum or plasma. In step 2, the captured holoTC is detected with a conjugate of alkaline phosphatase and antiTC antibody.

Results.—Neither apoTC nor haptocorrin exhibited detectable cross-reactivity. The detection limit was ≤0.1 pmol/L. Within-run and total imprecision (CV ranges) were 3.4%–5.1% and 6.3%–8.5%, respectively. Assay CVs were <20% from at least 3 pmol/L to 107 pmol/L. With diluted serum samples, measured concentrations were 104%–114% of the expected values in the working range of the assay. No interference from bilirubin, hemoglobin, triglycerides, erythrocytes, rheumatoid factor, or total protein was detected at expected (abnormal) concentrations. A comparison of the AxSYM Active B12 assay with a commercial RIA for holoTC yielded the regression equation: $AxSYM = 0.98RIA + 4.7$ pmol/L ($S_{y\ x}$, 11.4 pmol/L; n = 204). Assay throughput was 45 tests/h. A 95% reference interval of 19–134 pmol/L holoTC was established with samples from 292 healthy individuals.

Conclusions.—The AxSYM Active B12 assay allows rapid, precise, sensitive, specific, and automated measurement of human holoTC in serum and plasma.

▶ Vitamin B12 is an essential cofactor in the pathways of 1-carbon metabolism and the regulation of cell division. The deficiency state is a major public health issue, involving the occurrence of megaloblastic anemia, and progressive disease involving the central and peripheral nervous system. The assay for total B12 is the current standard clinical test for vitamin B12 deficiency, but misclassifications based on these results alone do occur; some individuals with measured low levels of B12 have no signs or symptoms of the deficiency state, and on the other hand, clinical neuropsychiatric and metabolic abnormalities can occur among those with total vitamin B12 levels within reference range. The total vitamin B12 assay measures all the vitamin B12 bound to both of the carrier proteins it is principally associated with, namely, transcobalamin (TC) and haptocorrin (HC). B12 bound to TC has a shorter serum half-life than does B12 bound to HC, and because most of the B12 measured in the total B12 assay is bound to HC, this makes it less responsive to changes than an assay of holotranscobalamin would be.

M. G. Bissell, MD, PhD, MPH

Urinary biomarkers in the early diagnosis of acute kidney injury
Han WK, Waikar SS, Johnson A, et al (Harvard Med School, Boston, MA; et al)
Kidney Int 73:863-869, 2008

A change in the serum creatinine is not sensitive for an early diagnosis of acute kidney injury. We evaluated urinary levels of matrix metalloproteinase-9 (MMP-9), N-acetyl-β-D-glucosaminidase (NAG), and kidney injury molecule-1 (KIM-1) as biomarkers for the detection of acute kidney injury. Urine samples were collected from 44 patients with various acute and chronic kidney diseases, and from 30 normal subjects in a cross-sectional study. A case–control study of children undergoing cardio-pulmonary bypass surgery included urine specimens from each of 20 patients without and with acute kidney injury. Injury was defined as a greater than 50% increase in the serum creatinine within the first 48 h after surgery. The biomarkers were normalized to the urinary creatinine concentration at 12, 24, and 36 h after surgery with the areas under the receiver-operating characteristic curve compared for performance. In the cross-sectional study, the area under the curve for MMP-9 was least sensitive followed by KIM-1 and NAG. Combining all three biomarkers achieved a perfect score diagnosing acute kidney injury. In the case–control study, KIM-1 was better than NAG at all time points, but combining both was no better than KIM-1 alone. Urinary MMP-9 was not a sensitive marker in the

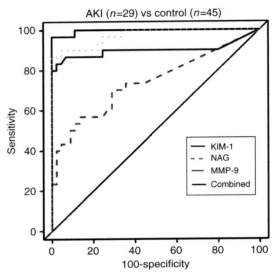

FIGURE 2.—ROC analysis for normalized urinary biomarkers in cross-sectional study. ROC curves of normalized MMP-9, NAG, and KIM-1 as a single test and in combination were plotted. The greater the displacement above and to the left of the line identified, the greater the likelihood that raised values of the test will identify AKI. (Reprinted from Han WK, Waikar SS, Johnson A, et al. Urinary biomarkers in the early diagnosis of acute kidney injury. *Kidney Int.* 2008;73:863-869, with permission from Macmillan Publishers Ltd: Kidney International, copyright 2008.)

case–control study. Our results suggest that urinary biomarkers allow diagnosis of acute kidney injury earlier than a rise in serum creatinine (Fig 2).

▶ Acute kidney injury (AKI) is a category including many different disease entities often seen in the context of multiple organ failure and sepsis. Truly sensitive and specific biomarkers for early AKI are lacking. Traditional blood (creatinine and blood urea nitrogen) and urine (urinary casts and fractional excretion of sodium) markers of kidney injury are insensitive for this purpose. It may be that a panel of newer biomarkers may be required. Such molecules include matrix metalloproteinase-9 (MMP-9), *N*-acetyl-β-D-glucosaminidase (NAG), kidney injury molecule-1 (KIM-1). KIM-1 is a type 1 transmembrane protein not found in normal kidney tissue or urine, but elevated in AKI. NAG is a lysosomal enzyme found in proximal tubular cells, sensitive to a wide variety of tubular injuries. MMP-9 has been seen elevated in animal models of kidney injury. The authors undertook to investigate the correlation of increases in these biomarkers with early AKI in both a cross-sectional study design and a case–control study. See Fig 2 for receiver operating characteristic (ROC) analysis of results.

M. G. Bissell, MD, PhD, MPH

Variation in Thyroid Function Tests in Patients with Stable Untreated Subclinical Hypothyroidism

Karmisholt J, Andersen S, Laurberg P (Aarhus Univ Hosp, Aalborg, Denmark)
Thyroid 18:303-308, 2008

Objective.—Knowledge of variation in thyroid function is important for interpretation of thyroid function tests. We aimed to describe intra-individual variation in thyroid function in patients with stable, untreated subclinical hypothyroidism (SCH) compared to euthyroid individuals to assess the importance of monitoring SCH patients.

Design.—We measured thyrotropin (TSH), free thyroxine (fT_4), and free triiodothyronine (fT_3) monthly for 1 year in a longitudinal study of 15 untreated SCH patients with initial TSH 5–12 mU/L, without trends in TSH, and compared findings with results from 15 euthyroid individuals.

Main outcome.—CV% was 17.0, 6.1, and 6.2 for TSH, fT_4, and fT_3, respectively. Overall CV% for TSH was lower in SCH patients than in controls. Contrary to euthyroid individuals, CV% in SCH patients increased with rising mean TSH ($r^2 = 0.29$, $p = 0.04$). Individual disease set points were established with 45, 6, and 6 tests for TSH, fT_4, and fT_3, with 95% confidence. Differences required between two test results were 40%, 15%, and 15%, respectively, with 90% confidence.

Conclusion.—Percent variation in TSH was lower in SCH than in euthyroid controls, but increased with higher mean TSH. The number of tests needed to establish disease set points was high. The difference required between two tests to be truly different was 40% for TSH and 15% for fT_4 and fT_3.

▶ In a clinical state like that of subclinical hypothyroidism, defined as an elevated thyroid stimulating hormone (TSH) accompanied by a "normal" serum thyroxine (T_4) estimate, the details of biological and analytical intra-individual variation in thyroid function test measurements take on important significance. Subclinical hypothyroidism is frequently a stable situation over time, progressing to thyroid failure in only a subset of cases. It would be of considerable theoretical and practical interest to know if or how such variation in the context of subclinical hypothyroidism differs from that seen in the truly euthyroid individual. Likewise, it would be of value to know what kind of a sampling interval is necessary to predict progression, and how much of a nominal difference in successive values is necessary for demonstrating a real change. The authors undertook to address these issues by using careful pre-analytical technique in systematically repeating TSH, free T4, and free T3 measurements on a series of subclinical hypothyroid patients and comparing coefficients of variation with those on euthyroid controls.

M. G. Bissell, MD, PhD, MPH

Value of Intraoperative Parathyroid Hormone Monitoring

Sharma J, Milas M, Berber E, et al (Emory Univ School of Medicine, Atlanta, GA, USA; Cleveland Clinic, OH, USA)
Ann Surg Oncol 15:493-498, 2008

Background.—Routine use of intraoperative parathyroid hormone (IOPTH) has been challenged in both unilateral/limited (LE) and bilateral exploration (BE). To investigate this, we assessed the usefulness of IOPTH in surgical management of primary hyperparathyroidism and parathyroid carcinoma (PC).

Methods.—Between 1998 and 2006, 1133 patients were explored for hyperparathyroidism: 185 LE, 743 BE with IOPTH, 95 BE without IOPTH, 110 reoperations, and 4 PCs. IOPTH patterns were correlated with parathyroid pathology (single adenoma [SA] or multigland disease [MGD]) and operative success.

Results.—In LE, IOPTH returned to normal in 78% of patients; all patients had SA, and 99% were cured at a mean ± SEM of 1.2 ± .24 years; 22% of LE patients (n = 41) whose IOPTH did not return to normal were converted to BE, and all had MGD. BE with and without IOPTH was equally successful 97% and 98% ($P = NS$) of the time, respectively. In BE in which IOPTH did not return to normal, 9% of patients remained hypercalcemic; tumor distribution mirrored other BE patients (75% SA, 25% MGD). In reoperations, a normal final IOPTH correlated with cure in 99%; otherwise, 59% had persistent disease. Differential bilateral internal jugular vein IOPTH sampling lateralized disease in 77% of reoperations.

Conclusions.—IOPTH is an important adjunct for successful LE by identifying the presence of MGD and avoiding operative failure. IOPTH adds little to BE; however, final IOPTH values may predict persistent disease in BE, reoperations, and PCs.

▶ Intraoperative determination of intact parathyroid hormone (PTH) has been considered useful for the assessment of completeness of parathyroidectomy and as an important adjunct to minimally invasive parathyroid surgery, potentially facilitating cost-effectiveness and the cosmetics of the outcomes. Typically, PTH is measured just before the incision and then again at 10 minutes post resection of the suspect parathyroid tissue. Generally, a decrease of 50% or more in PTH concentration is considered to be an evidence of successful removal. Interpretation of these results in patients with multiglandular disease is generally more complex than is that in cases of solitary parathyroid adenomas. Preoperative or intraoperative PTH levels may also have a use in localizing hyperfunctioning glandular tissue by sampling multiple regional cervical and mediastinal veins. Controversy about these approaches in the context of bilateral explorations and/or unilateral/limited explorations led the authors to reassess the usefulness of the intraoperative approach to measuring PTH.

M. G. Bissell, MD, PhD, MPH

A study to establish gestation-specific reference intervals for thyroid function tests in normal singleton pregnancy

Cotzias C, Wong S-J, Taylor E, et al (West Middlesex Univ Hosp, England, UK; Brondesbury Med Centre, London, UK; Quest Diagnostics, Heston, UK; et al)
Eur J Obstet Gynecol Reprod Biol 137:61-66, 2008

Objective.—To establish gestation-specific reference intervals for thyroid function tests in normal singleton pregnancy.

Study design.—Cross-sectional observational study performed in the Obstetric and Gynaecology department, West Middlesex University Hospital. A single blood sample from 335 pregnant women at various gestations of pregnancy was analysed for thyroid function. FT4, fT3, TSH values at each gestation of pregnancy were calculated.

Results.—From the fT3, fT4 and TSH results, a 95% reference interval was calculated for each hormone for each week of pregnancy.

Conclusion.—We calculated gestation-specific reference intervals for thyroid function tests throughout pregnancy to facilitate clinical management of thyroid disease in pregnancy.

▶ Reliable, relevant, and clinically useful reference ranges for thyroid function tests during pregnancy are not currently available, despite the potentially very great significance of these results for both mother and fetus. Thyroid disease complicates between 1% and 2% of pregnancies. The hypermetabolic state that normal pregnancy represents makes it difficult to assess the state of thyroid status clinically. The understanding of thyroid physiology in pregnancy has been aided by the newer generations of testing available for free thyroxine (fT4), free triiodothyronine (fT3), and thyroid stimulating hormone (TSH), allowing the generalization that fT4 and fT3 levels decrease and TSH levels increase during the advance of pregnancy. The reference ranges cited in the studies on which these generalizations are based have been doubted on critical reappraisal for a variety of important reasons. These facts led the authors to undertake the documentation and cataloguing of week-by-week reference intervals for weeks 6 through 40 of pregnancy, an extremely valuable set of observational data.

M. G. Bissell, MD, PhD, MPH

Clinical Significance of Low Level Human Chorionic Gonadotropin in the Management of Testicular Germ Cell Tumor

Takizawa A, Kishida T, Miura T, et al (Yokohama City Univ Med Ctr, Japan; et al)
J Urol 179:930-935, 2008

Purpose.—The finding of an unexplainable persistent low level of serum human chorionic gonadotropin in the management of testicular cancer sometimes misleads physicians. To avoid unnecessary treatment we suggest a new classification and algorithm for testicular germ cell tumors to discriminate real human chorionic gonadotropin from false-positive results.

Materials and Methods.—A total of 24 patients who seemed to have no cancer with an increased but low level of serum human chorionic gonadotropin were evaluated. They included 17 patients with testicular germ cell tumors and 7 with no evidence of germ cell tumor. In these cases parallel serum and urine human chorionic gonadotropin were measured with the same assay and serum human chorionic gonadotropin was measured with a different assay. False-positive cases were identified by critical criteria according to the classification of gestational trophoblastic disease.

Results.—Of 17 cases of testicular germ cell tumor 12 were classified as false-positive and 5 were classified as true-positive. All of the other 7 cases with no evidence of cancer were classified as phantom cases. Of the 7 patients with phantom human chorionic gonadotropin who had a history of germ cell tumor unnecessary treatments had been performed in 3. After the discrimination was implemented no unnecessary treatments or intensive examinations were performed.

Conclusions.—Appropriate management is possible based on a good understanding of the causes of low human chorionic gonadotropin. Our algorithm for classifying low human chorionic gonadotropin may help avoid unnecessary treatment in these patients (Fig 1).

▶ Serum human chorionic gonadotropin (hCG) levels are, of course, examples of clinical laboratory test results with very different meanings in different clinical

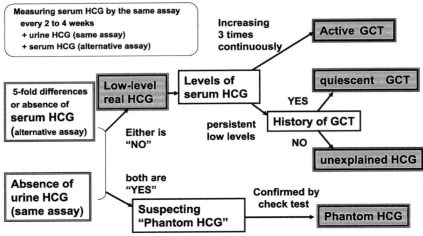

FIGURE 1.—Algorithm for differentiating low level HCG in males. (Reprinted from Takizawa A, Kishida T, Miura T, et al. Clinical significance of low level human chorionic gonadotropin in the management of testicular germ cell tumor. *J Urol.* 2008;179:930-935, with permission from the American Urological Association.)

contexts. As a tumor marker, hCG is important in the detection and management of testicular germ cell tumor, but in this context hCG results that are at low levels, but nonetheless in the positive range, can give rise to concerns about misclassification. Such low level positive hCGs have been classified as: (1) false positives, usually due to an analytical interference from heterophilic antibody in the specimen, (2) true positives in patients with documented previous histories of the tumor, or (3) unexplained positives in patients without either analytical issues or documented tumor history. The goal in sorting all this out, of course, is to avoid unnecessary treatment of false positive cases to the extent possible. The authors have undertaken to develop an empirical algorithm (Fig 1) to aid in the classification of low-level positive hCG results in this context.

M. G. Bissell, MD, PhD, MPH

20 Clinical Microbiology

Prospective Comparison of the Tuberculin Skin Test and 2 Whole-Blood Interferon-γ Release Assays in Persons with Suspected Tuberculosis
Mazurek GH, Weis SE, Moonan PK, et al (Ctrs for Disease Control and Prevention, Atlanta, GA; Univ of North Texas Health Science Ctr, Fort Worth, TX; et al)
Clin Infect Dis 45:837-845, 2007

Background.—Interferon-γ release assays (IGRAs) are attractive alternatives to the tuberculin skin test (TST) for detecting *Mycobacterium tuberculosis* infection. However, the inability to definitively confirm the presence of most *M. tuberculosis* infections hampers assessment of IGRA accuracy. Although IGRAs are primarily indicated for the detection of latent tuberculosis infection, we sought to determine the sensitivity of the TST and 2 whole-blood IGRAs (QuantiFERON-TB assay [QFT] and QuantiFERON-TB Gold assay [QFT-G]) in situations in which infection is confirmed by recovery of *M. tuberculosis* by culture.

Methods.—We conducted a prospective, multicenter, cross-sectional comparison study in which 148 persons suspected to have tuberculosis were tested simultaneously with the TST, QFT, and QFT-G.

Results.—*M. tuberculosis* was cultured from samples from 69 (47%) of 148 persons suspected to have tuberculosis; the TST induration was ≥5 mm for 51 (73.9%) of the 69 subjects (95% confidence interval [CI], 62.5%–82.8%). The QFT indicated tuberculosis infection for 48 (69.6%) of the 69 subjects (95% CI, 57.9%–79.2%) and was indeterminate for 7 (10.1%). The QFT-G yielded positive results for 46 (66.7%) of the 69 subjects (95% CI, 54.9%–76.7%) and indeterminate results for 9 subjects (13.0%). If subjects with indeterminate QFT-G results were excluded, 46 (76.7%) of 60 subjects (95% CI, 64.6%–85.6%) had positive TST results, and the same number of subjects had positive QFT-G results. HIV infection was associated with false-negative TST results but not with false-negative QFT-G results.

Conclusions.—The TST, QFT, and QFT-G have similar sensitivity in persons with culture-confirmed infection. As with the TST, negative QFT and QFT-G results should not be used to exclude the diagnosis of tuberculosis in persons with suggestive signs or symptoms.

▶ The tuberculin skin test has been one of the mainstays of population screening for tuberculosis (TB) for a great many years. The test, of course, uses a gross visual assessment of cell-mediated dermal hypersensitivity reactions to the injection of tuberculin purified protein derivative (PPD), which is derived from cultures of *Mycobacterium tuberculosis*. The sources of diagnostic inaccuracy with the test are well known. False positives occur in persons exposed to nontuberculous mycobacteria, and those who have been vaccinated with the BCG vaccine. False negatives occur in anergic individuals and those infected with human immunodeficiency virus (HIV), as well as those recently vaccinated with live attenuated viral vaccines. In recent years, efforts to develop in vitro diagnostic tests for TB have focused on the role of interferon-γ as a major cytokine in the immune response to *M. tuberculosis* infection. A prospective evaluation of 2 of the new generation of interferon-γ release assays (IGRAs) versus the tuberculin skin test is reported here.

M. G. Bissell, MD, PhD, MPH

Evaluation of the Nitrite and Leukocyte Esterase Activity Tests for the Diagnosis of Acute Symptomatic Urinary Tract Infection in Men

Koeijers JJ, Kessels AGH, Nys S, et al (Univ Hosp Maastricht, the Netherlands; et al)
Clin Infect Dis 45:894-896, 2007

For 422 male patients with symptoms indicative of a urinary tract infection, nitrite and leukocyte esterase activity dipstick test results were compared with results of culture of urine samples. The positive predictive value of a positive nitrite test result was 96%. Addition of results of the leukocyte esterase test did not improve the diagnostic accuracy of the nitrite test.

▶ In recent years the extreme importance of gender bias in subject recruitment for clinical research has been well and famously illustrated by the case of coronary heart disease in women. Our understanding of the acute coronary syndrome and cardiac risk were conditioned by studies conducted on men in such a way that incorrect generalizations of these results to the diagnosis and treatment of female patients led to unintended harm. The current article undertakes to correct a similar problem, although in this case it is a less deadly condition, and this time the gender bias is in the other direction. The guidelines for diagnosis and treatment of urinary tract infection (UTI) in adults have been developed, for the most part, based on clinical experience with women. Men also suffer from this condition. This study corrects some ideas regarding the use of dipstick testing in the context of male UTIs.

M. G. Bissell, MD, PhD, MPH

Multiplexed Reverse Transcriptase PCR Assay for Identification of Viral Respiratory Pathogens at the Point of Care

Létant SE, Ortiz JI, Tammero LFB, et al (Lawrence Livermore Natl Laboratory, CA; et al)
J Clin Microbiol 45:3498-3505, 2007

We have developed a nucleic acid-based assay that is rapid, sensitive, and specific and can be used for the simultaneous detection of five common human respiratory pathogens, including influenza virus A, influenza virus B, parainfluenza virus types 1 and 3, respiratory syncytial virus (RSV), and adenovirus groups B, C, and E. Typically, diagnosis on an unextracted clinical sample can be provided in less than 3 h, including sample collection, preparation, and processing, as well as data analysis. Such a multiplexed panel would enable rapid broad-spectrum pathogen testing on nasal swabs and therefore allow implementation of infection control measures and the timely administration of antiviral therapies. We present here a summary of the assay performance in terms of sensitivity and specificity. The limits of detection are provided for each targeted respiratory pathogen, and result comparisons were performed on clinical samples, our goal being to compare the sensitivity and specificity of the multiplexed assay to the combination of immunofluorescence and shell vial culture currently implemented at the University of California-Davis Medical Center hospital. Overall, the use of the multiplexed reverse transcription-PCR assay reduced the rate of false-negative results by 4% and reduced the rate of false-positive results by up to 10%. The assay correctly identified 99.3% of the clinical negatives and 97% of the adenovirus, 95% of the RSV, 92% of the influenza virus B, and 77% of the influenza virus A samples without any extraction performed on the clinical samples. The data also showed that extraction will be needed for parainfluenza virus, which was only identified correctly 24% of the time on unextracted samples.

▶ Rapid diagnostics for influenza and flu-like illnesses are in great demand during flu season every year. Hospitalizations during this period (October to March of every year) are estimated to range from 50 000 to 400 000 per year. The use of point-of-care diagnostics in emergency departments to classify these patients has been shown to have the potential to reduce hospital stay and antibiotic use significantly. The most prevalent test in use for classifying these patients remains viral culture, which is laborious and time-consuming. More rapid respiratory virus identification technologies have been developed, including immunofluorescence and other rapid antigen detection systems, but such systems suffer from very low sensitivity. Recent studies have shown that immunofluorescence assays detect only 19% of respiratory viruses at viral loads below 106 copies/mL and typical false negative rates for rapid test kits average 30%. For all these reasons, rapid molecular point-of-care tests, like the one described here, are being developed.

M. G. Bissell, MD, PhD, MPH

Testing Strategy To Identify Cases of Acute Hepatitis C Virus (HCV) Infection and To Project HCV Incidence Rates

Page-Shafer K, Pappalardo BL, Tobler LH, et al (Univ of California, San Francisco, CA; Blood Systems Research Inst, San Francisco, CA)
J Clin Microbiol 46:499-506, 2008

Surveillance for hepatitis C virus (HCV) is limited by the challenge of differentiating between acute and chronic infections. In this study, we evaluate a cross-sectional testing strategy that identifies individuals with acute HCV infection and we estimate HCV incidence. Anti-HCV-negative persons from four populations with various risks, i.e., blood donors, Veterans Administration (VA) patients, young injection drug users (IDU), and older IDU, were screened for HCV RNA by minipool or individual sample nucleic acid testing (NAT). The number of detected viremic seronegative infections was combined with the duration of the preseroconversion NAT-positive window period (derived from analysis of frequent serial samples from plasma donors followed from NAT detection to seroconversion) to estimate annual HCV incidence rates. Projected incidence rates were compared to observed incidence rates. Projected HCV incidence rates per 100 person-years were 0.0042 (95% confidence interval [95% CI], 0.0025 to 0.007) for blood donors, 0.86 (95% CI, 0.02 to 0.71) for VA patients, 39.8 (95% CI, 25.9 to 53.7) for young IDU, and 53.7 (95% CI, 23.4 to 108.8) for older IDU. Projected rates were most similar to observed incidence rates for young IDU (33.4; 95% CI, 28.0 to 39.9). This study demonstrates the value of applying a cross-sectional screening strategy to detect acute HCV infections and to estimate HCV incidence.

▶ Hepatitis C virus (HCV) infection represents a significant burden of disease in the population with nearly 4 million cases in the United States and 130 million cases worldwide. In this country, hepatitis C is the primary cause of end-stage liver failure resulting in liver transplantation. Although HVC has been virtually eliminated from the blood donor population as a result of minipool nucleic acid testing (NAT), it nonetheless continues to increase in other populations, specifically among injection drug users, with worldwide prevalences ranging from 25% to 80% and incidences from 9% to 38% per year. Most (60%-80%) acutely infected individuals will progress to a chronic carrier state, but an average of 26% shows resolution of viremia. There is relatively little epidemiological data on the rate of acute HCV infection (ie, incidence of anti-HCV-negative, HCV RNA-positive infections) in different population groups, but such information would be potentially of great value in designing surveillance efforts. The authors offer a testing paradigm to address this need.

M. G. Bissell, MD, PhD, MPH

Utility of Real-Time PCR for Diagnosis of Legionnaires' Disease in Routine Clinical Practice

Diederen BMW, Kluytmans JAJW, Vandenbroucke-Grauls CM, et al (St. Elisabeth Hosp, Tilburg, The Netherlands; Amphia Hosp, Breda, The Netherlands; et al)
J Clin Microbiol 46:671-677, 2008

The main aim of our study was to determine the added value of PCR for the diagnosis of Legionnaires' disease (LD) in routine clinical practice. The specimens were samples submitted for routine diagnosis of pneumonia from December 2002 to November 2005. Patients were evaluated if, in addition to PCR, the results of at least one of the following diagnostic tests were available: (i) culture for *Legionella* spp. on buffered charcoal yeast extract agar or (ii) detection of *Legionella pneumophila* antigen in urine specimens. Of the 151 evaluated patients, 37 (25%) fulfilled the European Working Group on Legionella Infections criteria for a confirmed case of LD (the "gold standard"). An estimated sensitivity, specificity, and overall percent agreement of 86% (32 of 37; 95% confidence interval [CI] = 72 to 95%), 95% (107 of 112; 95% CI = 90 to 98%), and 93% (139 of 149), respectively, were found for 16S rRNA-based PCR, and corresponding values of 92% (34 of 37; 95% CI = 78 to 98%), 98% (110 of 112; 95% CI = 93 to 100%), and 97% (144 of 149), respectively, were found for the *mip* gene-based PCR. A total of 35 patients were diagnosed by using the urinary antigen test, and 34 were diagnosed by the 16S rRNA-based PCR. With the *mip* gene PCR one more case of LD ($n = 36$; not significant) was detected. By combining urinary antigen test and the *mip* gene PCR, LD was diagnosed in an additional 4 (11%) patients versus the use of the urinary antigen test alone. The addition of a *L. pneumophila*-specific *mip* gene PCR to a urinary antigen test is useful in patients with suspected LD who produce sputum and might allow the early detection of a significant number of additional patients.

▶ Legionellae are slow-growing fastidious microorganisms whose successful culture requires selective media and prolonged incubation. Considerable variation has been recorded in the ability of actual laboratories to do this. *Legionella* species are estimated to be responsible for anywhere from 1% to 5% percent of cases of community-acquired pneumonia (CAP). Some 19 *Legionella* species have been associated with human disease, but *Legionella pneumophila* accounts for about 92% of clinical cases. Serological diagnosis is available, but is necessarily an ex post facto phenomenon (4-fold immunoglobulin G or immunoglobulin M titre increase). There is, therefore, a real need for other types of testing to diagnose the disease in earlier stages of illness. Urinary antigen tests and nucleic acid amplification tests (NAAT), most often by polymerase chain reaction (PCR) are useful in this regard. These authors undertook to determine the added value of real time PCR for diagnosis of Legionnaire's disease in routine clinical practice.

M. G. Bissell, MD, PhD, MPH

A New Arenavirus in a Cluster of Fatal Transplant-Associated Diseases

Palacios G, Druce J, Du L (Columbia Univ, NY; Victorian Infectious Diseases Reference Laboratory, Australia; 454 Life Sciences, Branford, CT; et al)
New Engl J Med 358:991-998, 2008

Background.—Three patients who received visceral-organ transplants from a single donor on the same day died of a febrile illness 4 to 6 weeks after transplantation. Culture, polymerase-chain-reaction (PCR) and serologic assays, and oligonucleotide microarray analysis for a wide range of infectious agents were not informative.

Methods.—We evaluated RNA obtained from the liver and kidney transplant recipients. Unbiased high-throughput sequencing was used to identify microbial sequences not found by means of other methods. The specificity of sequences for a new candidate pathogen was confirmed by

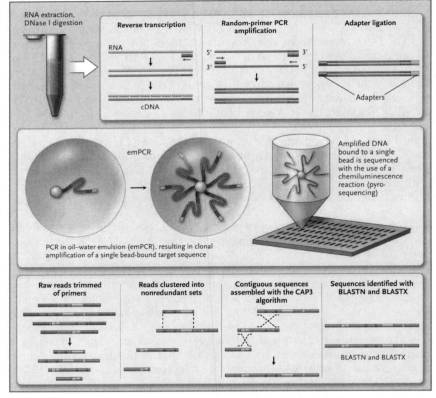

FIGURE 1.—High-Throughput Sequencing Method. PCR denotes polymerase chain reaction. (Reprinted from Palacios G, Druce J, Du L, et al. A new arenavirus in a cluster of fatal transplant-associated diseases. *New Engl J Med.* 2008;358:991-998, with permission from the Massachusetts Medical Society. All Rights Reserved.)

means of culture and by means of PCR, immunohistochemical, and serologic analyses.

Results.—High-throughput sequencing yielded 103,632 sequences, of which 14 represented an Old World arenavirus. Additional sequence analysis showed that this new arenavirus was related to lymphocytic choriomeningitis viruses. Specific PCR assays based on a unique sequence confirmed the presence of the virus in the kidneys, liver, blood, and cerebrospinal fluid of the recipients. Immunohistochemical analysis revealed arenavirus antigen in the liver and kidney transplants in the recipients. IgM and IgG antiviral antibodies were detected in the serum of the donor. Seroconversion was evident in serum specimens obtained from one recipient at two time points.

Conclusions.—Unbiased high-throughput sequencing is a powerful tool for the discovery of pathogens. The use of this method during an outbreak of disease facilitated the identification of a new arenavirus transmitted through solid-organ transplantation (Fig 1).

▶ Surveillance for and discovery of new pathogens is an activity that is greatly facilitated by the advent of methods for the cloning of microbial nucleic acids directly from clinical specimens. Molecular techniques have been useful in the initial characterization of a variety of infectious agents, including the Borna disease virus, hepatitis C virus, Sin Nombre virus, human herpesviruses 6 and 8, *Bartonella henselae*, *Tropheryma whipplei*, West Nile virus, and the SARS coronavirus. Here the authors used the technique of unbiased high throughput sequencing (Fig 1) to characterize specimens from a cluster of 3 Australian visceral organ transplant recipients who received their organs on the same day and died with fever 6 to 8 weeks later. The agent proved to be a newly described arenavirus related to lymphocytic choriomeningitis virus (LCMV). Virions were identified postmortem in brain, cerebrospinal fluid, serum, kidney, and liver. This is a powerful new method.

M. G. Bissell, MD, PhD, MPH

Universal Screening for Methicillin-Resistant *Staphylococcus aureus* at Hospital Admission and Nosocomial Infection in Surgical Patients

Harbarth S, Fankhauser C, Schrenzel J, et al (Univ of Geneva Hosps and Med School, Geneva, Switzerland)
JAMA 299:1149-1157, 2008

Context.—Experts and policy makers have repeatedly called for universal screening at hospital admission to reduce nosocomial methicillin-resistant *Staphylococcus aureus* (MRSA) infection.

Objective.—To determine the effect of an early MRSA detection strategy on nosocomial MRSA infection rates in surgical patients.

Design, Setting, and Patients.—Prospective, interventional cohort study conducted between July 2004 and May 2006 among 21 754 surgical patients at a Swiss teaching hospital using a crossover design to compare 2 MRSA control strategies (rapid screening on admission plus standard infection control measures vs standard infection control alone). Twelve surgical wards including different surgical specialties were enrolled according to a prespecified agenda, assigned to either the control or intervention group for a 9-month period, then switched over to the other group for a further 9 months.

Interventions.—During the rapid screening intervention periods, patients admitted to the intervention wards for more than 24 hours were screened before or on admission by rapid, multiplex polymerase chain reaction. For both intervention (n = 10 844) and control (n = 10 910) periods, standard infection control measures were used for patients with MRSA in all wards and consisted of contact isolation of MRSA carriers, use of dedicated material (eg, gown, gloves, mask if indicated), adjustment of perioperative antibiotic prophylaxis of MRSA

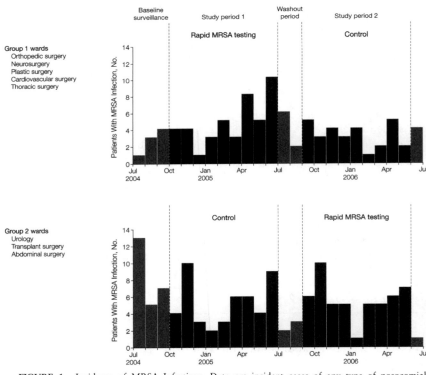

FIGURE 1.—Incidence of MRSA Infections. Data are incident cases of any type of nosocomial methicillin-resistant *Staphylococcus aureus* (MRSA) infection, stratified by period and intervention group. The total number of admissions in the control periods was 10 910 and in the intervention periods was 10 844. (Reprinted from Harbarth S, Fankhauser C, Schrenzel J, et al. Universal screening for methicillin-resistant *Staphylococcus aureus* at hospital admission and nosocomial infection in surgical patients. *JAMA.* 2008;299:1149-1157, with permission from the American Medical Association.)

carriers, computerized MRSA alert system, and topical decolonization (nasal mupirocin ointment and chlorhexidine body washing) for 5 days.

Main Outcome Measures.—Incidence of nosocomial MRSA infection, MRSA surgical site infection, and rates of nosocomial acquisition of MRSA.

Results.—Overall, 10 193 of 10 844 patients (94%) were screened during the intervention periods. Screening identified 515 MRSA-positive patients (5.1%), including 337 previously unknown MRSA carriers. Median time from screening to notification of test results was 22.5 hours (interquartile range, 12.2-28.2 hours). In the intervention periods, 93 patients (1.11 per 1000 patient-days) developed nosocomial MRSA infection compared with 76 in the control periods (0.91 per 1000 patient-days; adjusted incidence rate ratio, 1.20; 95% confidence interval, 0.85-1.69; $P = .29$). The rate of MRSA surgical site infection and nosocomial MRSA acquisition did not change significantly. Fifty-three of 93 infected patients (57%) in the intervention wards were MRSA-free on admission and developed MRSA infection during hospitalization.

Conclusion.—A universal, rapid MRSA admission screening strategy did not reduce nosocomial MRSA infection in a surgical department with endemic MRSA prevalence but relatively low rates of MRSA infection.

Trial Registration.—isrctn.org Identifier: ISRCTN06603006 (Figs 1 and 2).

▶ Exposure to the carriage of antibiotic-resistant organisms like methicillin-resistant *Staphylococcus aureus* (MRSA) is a major hazard of hospitalization.

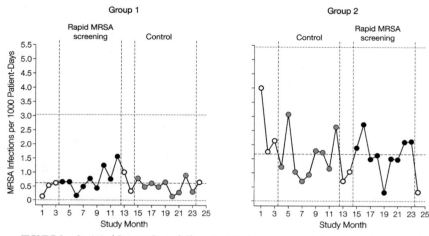

FIGURE 2.—Statistical Process Control Chart. Statistical process control chart shows the nosocomial methicillin-resistant *Staphylococcus aureus* (MRSA) infection rate for each month of the study. The upper and lower control limits (dotted lines) represent 3 SDs from the mean (dashed line). (Reprinted from Harbarth S, Fankhauser C, Schrenzel J, et al. Universal screening for methicillin-resistant *Staphylococcus aureus* at hospital admission and nosocomial infection in surgical patients. *JAMA*. 2008;299:1149-1157, with permission from the American Medical Association.)

Rapid identification of these organisms in hospital inpatients, coupled with interventions to prevent patient-to-patient spread and rapid screening of surgical patients, have long seemed to be logical strategies for prevention of outbreaks of nosocomial infections with these agents. Although policy makers have advocated universal admission screening, there has never been a controlled trial to test the hypothesis that rapid MRSA screening may have a positive impact on patient outcome in this setting. The authors undertook a very large version of such a study. Using a prospective, interventional cohort study design, they looked at 21 754 surgical patients at a Swiss teaching hospital. Their results are important, showing no significant impact of universal MRSA screening on overall nosocomial MRSA infection rates (Figs 1 and 2). More aggressive preemptive isolation may need to be coupled with early detection to affect outcome.

M. G. Bissell, MD, PhD, MPH

Multiplex, Bead-Based Suspension Array for Molecular Determination of Common *Salmonella* Serogroups
Fitzgerald C, Collins M, Van Duyne S, et al (Natl Ctr for Zoonotic, Atlanta, GA)
J Clin Microbiol 45:3323-3334, 2007

We report the development and evaluation of a *Salmonella* O-group-specific Bio-Plex assay to detect the six most common serogroups in the United States (B, C_1, C_2, D, E, and O13) plus serotype Paratyphi A. The assay is based on *rfb* gene targets directly involved in O-antigen biosynthesis; it can be completed 45 min post-PCR amplification. The assay correctly and specifically identified 362 of 384 (94.3%) isolates tested in comparison to traditional serotyping. Seventeen isolates (4.4%) produced results consistent with what is known about the molecular basis for serotypes but different from the results of traditional serotyping, and five isolates (1.3%) generated false-negative results. Molecular determination of the serogroup for rough isolates was consistent with a common serotype in most instances, indicating that this approach has the potential to provide O-group information for isolates that do not express an O antigen. We also report the sequence of the O-antigen-encoding *rfb* gene cluster from *Salmonella enterica* serotype Poona (serogroup O13). Compared with other, previously characterized *rfb* regions, the O13 *rfb* gene cluster was most closely related to *Escherichia coli* O127 and O86. The O-group Bio-Plex assay described here provides an easy-to-use, high-throughput system for rapid detection of common *Salmonella* serogroups.

▶ Tracking food-borne outbreaks of infections with *Salmonella* species requires phenotypic subtyping as a necessary identification tool. *Salmonella* species are serotyped using the Kauffmann-White scheme according to the composition of their O, H, and Vi antigens. There are 46 subtype O serogroups altogether in this scheme and the genetics of their antigenic variations have been determined to be largely because of variation in *rfb* gene clusters. Molecular approaches to serotyping have many potential advantages over serological methods that are subject to vagaries of antiserum production and isolates for which no serotype antigen can be detected. These authors have developed a sevenplex, Luminex bead-based suspension array to detect serogroups B, C1, C2, D, E, and O13, plus serotype Paratyphi A, the most commonly occurring serogroups in the United States. In the course of accomplishing this, the authors actually characterized the *rfb* gene cluster from serogroup O13 for the first time.

M. G. Bissell, MD, PhD, MPH

Analysis of Typing Methods for Epidemiological Surveillance of both Methicillin-Resistant and Methicillin-Susceptible *Staphylococcus aureus* Strains

Faria NA, Carrico JA, Oliveira DC, et al (Instituto de Tecnologia Química e Biológica, Oeiras, Portugal; Instituto de Engenharia de Sistemas e Computadores: Investigação e Desenvolvimento (INESC-ID), Lisboa, Portugal; et al)
J Clin Microbiol 46:136-144, 2008

Sequence-based methods for typing *Staphylococcus aureus*, such as multilocus sequence typing (MLST) and *spa* typing, have increased interlaboratory reproducibility, portability, and speed in obtaining results, but pulsed-field gel electrophoresis (PFGE), remains the method of choice in many laboratories due to the extensive experience with this methodology and the large body of data accumulated using the technique. Comparisons between typing methods have been overwhelmingly based on a qualitative assessment of the overall agreement of results and the relative discriminatory indexes. In this study, we quantitatively assess the congruence of the major typing methods for *S. aureus*, using a diverse collection of 198 *S. aureus* strains previously characterized by PFGE, *spa* typing, MLST, and, in the case of methicillin-resistant *S. aureus* (MRSA), SCC*mec* typing in order to establish the quantitative congruence between the typing methods. The results of most typing methods agree in that MRSA and methicillin-susceptible *S. aureus* (MSSA) differ in terms of diversity of genetic backgrounds, with MSSA being more diverse. Our results show that *spa* typing has a very good predictive power over the clonal relationships defined by eBURST, while PFGE is less accurate for that purpose but nevertheless provides better typeability and discriminatory power. The combination of PFGE and *spa* typing provided even better results. Based on these observations, we suggest the use of the conjugation of *spa* typing and PFGE typing for epidemiological surveillance studies, since this combination provides the ability to infer long-term relationships while maintaining the discriminatory power and typeability needed in short-term studies.

▶ *Staphylococcus aureus* is a major human pathogen with worldwide distribution and a major impact on morbidity and mortality. With the emergence of community-acquired methicillin-resistant *S. aureus* (MRSA), in addition to the existing worldwide difficulties with hospital-acquired MRSA, the ability to accurately type strains of this organism becomes even more essential to both therapeutic and preventative interventions, as well as to geographic tracking of outbreaks and dissemination. Pulsed-field gel electrophoresis (PFGE) of total bacterial DNA after digestion with the restriction enzyme *Sma*I is the current de facto gold standard for such typing. DNA-sequencing technology has become more practical for such work in recent years, however, and has theoretical advantages. The authors used a diverse collection of 198 *S. aureus* strains to compare the performance of several sequence-based methods with PFGE. For optimal use in epidemiological surveillance, they end up recommending a combination of PGFE and sequence-based *spa* typing.

M. G. Bissell, MD, PhD, MPH

Application of a Microsphere-Based Array for Rapid Identification of *Acinetobacter* spp. with Distinct Antimicrobial Susceptibilities

Chen Y-C, Sheng W-H, Chang S-C, et al (Res Diagnostic Ctr, Ctrs Dis Control, Taipei; Natl Taiwan Univ Hosp)
J Clin Microbiol 46:612-617, 2008

Acinetobacter spp. have emerged as important nosocomial and multi-drug-resistant pathogens in the last decade. *A. calcoaceticus*, *A. baumannii*, *Acinetobacter* genospecies 3, and *Acinetobacter* genospecies 13TU are genetically closely related and are referred to as the *A. calcoaceticus-A. baumannii* complex (ACB complex). Distinct *Acinetobacter* spp. may be associated with differences in antimicrobial susceptibility, so it is important to identify *Acinetobacter* spp. at the species level. We developed a microsphere-based array that combines an allele-specific primer extension assay and microsphere hybridization for the identification of *Acinetobacter* spp. This assay can discriminate the 13 different *Acinetobacter* spp. in less than 8.5 h, and it has high specificity without causing cross-reactivity with 14 other common nosocomial bacterial species. The sensitivity of this assay was 100 *A. baumannii* cells per ml of blood, and it could discriminate multiple species in various mixture ratios. The developed assay could differentiate clinical *Acinetobacter* spp. isolates with a 90% identification rate. The antimicrobial susceptibility test showed that *A. baumannii* isolates were resistant to most antimicrobial agents other than imipenem, while the genospecies 3 and 13TU isolates were more susceptible to most antimicrobial agents, especially ciprofloxacin and ampicillin-sulbactam. These results supported the idea that this assay possibly could be applied to clinical samples and provide accurate species identification, which might be helpful for clinicians when they are treating infections caused by *Acinetobacter* spp.

▶ *Acinetobacter* species are important organisms in causing nosocomial infections, and multidrug resistant (MDR) *Acinetobacter* spp. are beginning to emerge. Of the 32 different named and unnamed *Acinetobacter* spp. that have been described, 4 (genospecies 1, 2, 4, and 13TU) are closely related genetically and are known as the *A. calcoaceticus-A. baumannii* complex (ACB complex). The authors make a good case for the value of being able to differentiate these organisms at the species level, namely that differential efficacy of antimicrobial agents against strains of the different ACB species has been demonstrated, and 3 of the 4 ACB species (genospecies 2, 3, and 13TU) have been specifically identified in nosocomial outbreaks. In this article, they demonstrate the usefulness of molecular speciation methods in accomplishing this task. In particular, they developed a microsphere-based hybridization assay and showed that it has robust enough performance to be applied to clinical specimens.

M. G. Bissell, MD, PhD, MPH

Test Characteristics and Interpretation of Cerebrospinal Fluid Gram Stain in Children

Neuman MI, Tolford S, Harper MB (Children's Hosp, Harvard Med School)
Pediatr Infect Dis J 27:309-313, 2008

Background.—Few data exist regarding the test characteristics of cerebrospinal fluid (CSF) Gram stain among children at risk for bacterial meningitis, especially the rate of false positive Gram stain.

Methods.—We conducted a retrospective cohort study of children seen in the emergency department of Children's Hospital Boston who had CSF obtained between December 1992 and September 2005. Patients who had ventricular shunts, as well as those who received antibiotics before CSF was obtained were excluded. Test characteristics of CSF Gram stain were assessed using CSF culture as the criterion standard. Patients were considered to have bacterial meningitis if there was either: (1) growth of a pathogen, or (2) growth of a possible pathogen noted on the final CSF culture report and the patient was treated with a course of parenteral antibiotics for 7 days or more without other indication.

Results.—A total of 17,569 eligible CSF specimens were collected among 16,036 patients during the 13-year study period. The median age of study subjects was 74 days. Seventy CSF specimens (0.4%) had organisms detected on Gram stain. The overall sensitivity of Gram stain to detect bacterial meningitis was 67% [42 of 63; 95% confidence interval (CI): 54–78] with a positive predictive value of 60% (42 of 70; 95% CI: 48–71). Most patients without bacterial meningitis have negative Gram stain [specificity 99.9% (17,478 of 17,506; 95% CI: 99.8–99.9)] with a negative predictive value of 99.9 (17,478 of 17,499; 95% CI: 99.8–99.9).

Conclusions.—CSF Gram stain is appropriately used by physicians in risk stratification for the diagnosis and empiric treatment of bacterial meningitis in children. Although a positive Gram stain result greatly increases the likelihood of bacterial meningitis; the result may be because of contamination or misinterpretation in 40% of cases and should not, by itself, result in a full treatment course for bacterial meningitis.

▶ In the context of possible bacterial meningitis in the pediatric population, culturing cerebrospinal fluid (CSF) for 24 hours or longer is typically an unacceptably long period of time. Decisions to empirically treat and or admit such patients to the hospital are frequently made in the absence of these definitive findings. Various laboratory determinations on CSF are typically used in such cases, including CSF Gram stain, cell count, glucose, and protein. Gram stain positive CSFs are commonly regarded as indicative of high risk for bacterial meningitis. Much hinges on the false-positive and false-negative rates associated with the CSF Gram stain, and it is therefore surprising that there is very little outcomes data in the medical literature dealing with the diagnostic performance of the CSF Gram stain in the context of ruling out bacterial meningitis in children. The authors undertook a retrospective cohort study in 16 000 patients over 13 years at Boston Children's Hospital.

M. G. Bissell, MD, PhD, MPH

Unlabeled Probes for the Detection and Typing of Herpes Simplex Virus
Dames S, Pattison DC, Bromley LK, et al (ARUP Institute for Clinical and Experimental Pathology, Salt Lake City, UT; et al)
Clin Chem 53:1847-1854, 2007

Background.—Unlabeled probe detection with a double-stranded DNA (dsDNA) binding dye is one method to detect and confirm target amplification after PCR. Unlabeled probes and amplicon melting have been used to detect small deletions and single-nucleotide polymorphisms in assays where template is in abundance. Unlabeled probes have not been applied to low-level target detection, however.

Methods.—Herpes simplex virus (HSV) was chosen as a model to compare the unlabeled probe method to an in-house reference assay using dual-labeled, minor groove binding probes. A saturating dsDNA dye (LCGreen® Plus) was used for real-time PCR. HSV-1, HSV-2, and an internal control were differentiated by PCR amplicon and unlabeled probe melting analysis after PCR.

Results.—The unlabeled probe technique displayed 98% concordance with the reference assay for the detection of HSV from a variety of archived clinical samples (n = 182). HSV typing using unlabeled probes was 99% concordant (n = 104) to sequenced clinical samples and allowed for the detection of sequence polymorphisms in the amplicon and under the probe.

Conclusions.—Unlabeled probes and amplicon melting can be used to detect and genotype as few as 10 copies of target per reaction, restricted only by stochastic limitations. The use of unlabeled probes provides an attractive alternative to conventional fluorescence-labeled, probe-based assays for genotyping and detection of HSV and might be useful for other low-copy targets where typing is informative.

▶ Real-time polymerase chain reaction (RT-PCR) has greatly facilitated the automation of assays for the detection, amplification, and quantitation of nucleic acids in patient specimens, both viral and human; this is because it allows for the performance of all these in a single tube. In these reactions the target can be detected using synthetic oligonucleotide probes, a double stranded DNA binding dye, or by the use of an unlabeled probe combined with asymmetric amplification of copies. Unlabeled probes contain no fluorescent moiety, but rather are quantitated by comparison of postamplification DNA melting curves between the dissociation of the probe off of single stranded DNA (ssDNA) resulting from asymmetric PCR and that from the homozygous double stranded DNA amplicon. The authors were interested in exploring the limits of the unlabeled probe technique in terms of copy number detection, typing accuracy, and reproducibility of melting curves in an assay for Herpes Simplex virus (HSV).

M. G. Bissell, MD, PhD, MPH

21 Hematology and Immunology

Arterial carboxyhemoglobin level and outcome in critically ill patients
Melley DD, Finney SJ, Elia A, et al (Imperial College School of Medicine, London)
Crit Care Med 35:1882-1887, 2007

Objective.—Arterial carboxyhemoglobin is elevated in patients with critical illness. It is an indicator of the endogenous production of carbon monoxide by the enzyme heme oxygenase, which modulates the response to oxidant stress. The objective was to explore the hypothesis that arterial carboxyhemoglobin level is associated with inflammation and survival in patients requiring cardiothoracic intensive care.

Design.—Prospective, observational study.

Setting.—A cardiothoracic intensive care unit.

Patients.—All patients admitted over a 15-month period.

Interventions.—None.

Measurements and Main Results.—Arterial carboxyhemoglobin, bilirubin, and standard biochemical, hematologic, and physiologic markers of inflammation were measured in 1,267 patients. Associations were sought between levels of arterial carboxyhemoglobin, markers of the inflammatory response, and clinical outcome. Intensive care unit mortality was associated with lower minimum and greater maximal carboxyhemoglobin levels ($p < .0001$ and $p < .001$, respectively). After adjustment for age, gender, illness severity, and other relevant variables, a lower minimum arterial carboxyhemoglobin was associated with an increased risk of death from all causes (odds risk of death, 0.391; 95% confidence interval, 0.190–0.807; $p = .011$). Arterial carboxyhemoglobin correlated with markers of the inflammatory response.

Conclusions.—Both low minimum and high maximum levels of arterial carboxyhemoglobin were associated with increased intensive care mortality. Although the heme oxygenase system is protective, excessive induction may be deleterious. This suggests that there may be an optimal range for heme oxygenase-1 induction.

▶ The range of conditions known as the systemic inflammatory response syndrome (SIRS), namely sepsis, severe sepsis, and septic shock, are collectively the largest category of mortality in intensive care unit (ICU) patients.

These conditions represent major oxidative stress, which in turn induces the enzyme heme oxygenase (HO-1). Some investigators postulate that the induction of this enzyme may be beneficial to the patient in this context because some of its downstream products (carbon monoxide, biliverdin, and bilirubin) show some anti-inflammatory and antioxidant properties. It has even been suggested that carbon monoxide may have use as a therapeutic agent in the treatment of SIRS. Other investigators note that excessive induction of HO-1 may be deleterious because of release of molecular iron, a pro-oxidant. This altogether suggests that there may be middle range of HO-1 induction that is optimal for survival of SIRS. The current study was undertaken in an attempt to better understand this possibility.

M. G. Bissell, MD, PhD, MPH

Predictors of Endoscopic and Laboratory Evaluation of Iron Deficiency Anemia in Hospitalized Patients

Ioannou GN, Spector J, Rockey DC (Veterans Affairs Puget Sound Health Care System, Seattle, WA; Duke Univ Med Ctr, Durham, NC; Univ of Texas Southwestern Med Ctr, Dallas, TX)
South Med J 100:976-984, 2007

Background.—Many hospitalized anemic patients do not undergo appropriate evaluation. We hypothesized that specific clinical variables were likely to be important in triggering evaluation for iron deficiency anemia.

Methods.—We prospectively identified 637 consecutive anemic patients without acute gastrointestinal bleeding admitted over a three-month period to medical inpatient teams of two teaching hospitals and examined clinical variables that predicted diagnostic evaluation.

Results.—Serum ferritin or serum transferrin saturation (TS) were measured in 43% (271/637) of subjects and were low in 38% (102/271). Predictors of serum ferritin or TS measurement included low hemoglobin concentration and a history of iron supplementation. Predictors of iron deficiency included low hemoglobin concentration (OR 1.9, 95% CI 1.06–3.5) and low mean cell volume (OR 4.6, 95% CI 2.5–8.6). Of 102 patients with iron deficiency anemia, 31% underwent endoscopic evaluation, and 39% had serious gastrointestinal lesions. The only significant predictor of having an endoscopic evaluation was a positive fecal occult blood test (FOBT) (OR 5.2, 95% CI 1.7–16.2).

Conclusions.—In patients with anemia, tests to ascertain iron status are not appropriately performed in hospitalized patients. Patients found to have iron deficiency anemia who are FOBT-positive undergo endoscopic evaluation more frequently than FOBT-negative patients.

▶ Surprisingly few hospitalized patients with anemia undergo any workup for iron deficiency, one of the most common causes of this condition. This is in spite of the fact that testing for iron deficiency is readily available and inexpensive. Furthermore, even when iron deficiency is detected, a large proportion of such patients are not further worked up endoscopically for possible occult blood loss, the most frequent cause of iron deficiency anemia. The authors undertook to discover whether these facts were because of the requirement for identifying the presence of ceratin specific clinical features. This was a prospective study design in which all anemic patients at 2 hospitals (a Veterans' Affairs [VA] hospital and an academic medical center) were followed. Patients admitted with a diagnosis of acute gastrointestinal bleeding were excluded. They find that current practice in this area leaves a great deal to be desired and that new guidelines need to be designed and implemented.

M. G. Bissell, MD, PhD, MPH

Evaluation of Pretransplant Serum Cytokine Levels in Renal Transplant Recipients

Berber İ, Yiğit B, Işitmangil G, et al (Haydarpaşa Numune Education and Res Hosp, Istanbul, Turkey)
Transplant Proc 40:92-93, 2008

Aim.—Cytokines are early predictors of graft dysfunction. In this study we evaluated pretransplant cytokine levels and graft outcomes among renal transplant recipients.

Patients and Methods.—Donor selection was based on results of blood group matching and negative crossmatches. A panel of 35 human serum samples from patients (female/male = 0.4) awaiting renal transplantation and 15 healty control sera were analyzed for interleukin (IL) 1α, IL-2, IL-6, IL-10, tumor necrosis factor-α, interferon-γ, transforming growth factor-β concentrations by enzyme-linked immunosorbent assay. The average age of the patients was 34.5 ± 10.1 years (range 15 to 60). The average duration of renal replacement therapy before renal transplantation was 42.1 ± 57.9 months (range 0 to 288). The types of renal replacement therapy were; hemodialysis ($n = 27$) and CAPD ($n = 8$).

Results.—Pretransplant IL-6 levels were higher among recipients who displayed acute rejection episodes compared with those fact of this complications ($P < .05$) or control sera ($P < .05$). Pretransplant IL-6 levels were higher among recipients with graft failure than those with a functioning graft ($P < .05$). Pretransplant IL-10 levels were higher among recipients with acute rejection episodes and graft failure than those without acute rejection or control subjects, but the difference did not reach significance. There was no correlation between pretransplant cytokine levels and age, gender, type, or duration of renal replacement therapy ($P > .05$).

Conclusion.—High pretransplant serum IL-6 levels are associated with an increased risk of acute rejection episodes and graft failure. IL-10 might contribute an anti-inflammatory action to patients with high serum IL-6 levels.

▶ Cytokines are effector molecules for cellular and humoral immune responses and include the interleukins (ILs), the tumor necrosis factors (TNFs), the interferons (IFNs), and the colony-stimulating factors (CSFs). They are responsible for diverse biological activities but share a number of common characteristics: all are pleiotropic (ie, they can interact with a variety of cellular targets). Cell binding of cytokines in all cases gives rise to activation of signaling pathways and new RNA and protein synthesis. Cytokine assays are becoming an ever more significant part of the clinical laboratory workup for a number of immune-related disease conditions. In the field of solid organ transplantation, acute rejection episodes (AREs) represent a major cause of graft loss among adult renal transplant patients and morbidity among renal transplant recipients overall. They appear to be early indicators of graft dysfunction and thus may provide some mechanistic insight into these incidents. This work proposes the hypothesis that the pretransplant cytokine profile may be associated with graft outcomes in these patients.

M. G. Bissell, MD, PhD, MPH

Noninvasive Optical, Electrical, and Acoustic Methods of Total Hemoglobin Determination

McMurdy JW, Jay GD, Suner S, et al (Brown Univ, Providence, RI; et al)
Clin Chem 54:264-272, 2008

Background.—Anemia is an underdiagnosed, significant public health concern afflicting >2 billion people worldwide. The detrimental effects of tissue oxygen deficiency on the cardiovascular system and concurrent appearance of anemia with numerous high-risk disorders highlight the importance of clinical screening. Currently there is no universally accepted, clinically applicable, noninvasive hemoglobin/hematocrit screening tool. The need for such a device has prompted an investigation into a breadth of techniques.

Methods.—A synopsis of the literature and current directions of research in noninvasive total hemoglobin measurement was collected. Contributions highlighted in this review are limited to those studies conducted with a clinical aspect, and most include in vivo patient studies.

Results.—The review of potential techniques presented here includes optoacoustic spectroscopy, spectrophotometric imaging, diffuse reflectance spectroscopy, transcutaneous illumination, electrical admittance plethysmography, and photoplethysmography. The technological performance, relative benefits of each approach, potential instrumentation design considerations, and future directions are discussed in each subcategory.

Conclusions.—Many techniques reviewed here have shown excellent accuracy, sensitivity, and specificity in measuring hemoglobin/hematocrit, thus in the near future a new clinically viable tool for noninvasive hemoglobin/hematocrit monitoring will likely be widely used for patient care. Limiting factors in clinical adoption will likely involve technology integration into the current standard of care in each field routinely dealing with anemia.

▶ Anemia is a highly important and highly prevalent condition in the world population predisposing to a variety of other morbidities. The World Health Organization (WHO) estimates that there may be as many as 2 billion people with anemia worldwide. The condition is defined in terms of the measured hemoglobin concentration as being present when this analyte is below 12 g/dL for females or below 13 g/dL for males. Screening for anemia involves physical examination findings, in particular, visual inspection of the palpebral conjunctiva, a complete blood cell count (CBC), or use of a small-volume hemoglobin meter. The first of these is notably inaccurate because of interobserver variation, and the latter 2 involve blood sampling. The quest for noninvasive alternatives that can be used directly in the context of routine physical exams continues, and is summarized in this review. The types of technologies covered include the following: conductance methods, imaging and spectrophotometric methods, near infrared (NIR) transmission spectroscopy, reflectance spectroscopy, ultrasound, and optoacoustic spectroscopy.

M. G. Bissell, MD, PhD, MPH

A Novel Hemoglobin, Bonn, Causes Falsely Decreased Oxygen Saturation Measurements in Pulse Oximetry

Zur B, Hornung A, Breuer J, et al (Univ of Bonn, Germany)

Clin Chem 54:594-596, 2008

Background.—A 4-year-old boy and his father exhibited low oxygen saturation measured transcutaneously by pulse oximetry, a finding that could not be confirmed by arterial blood gas analysis. Both patients exhibited slight hemolysis in their blood, and the boy had a microcytic anemia. There was no evidence of hypoxemia or methemoglobinemia. Despite the normal results from the arterial blood gas analysis, a right-to-left-shunt was assumed in the boy until a cardiology examination excluded this diagnosis. Sleep apnea syndrome was suspected in the father and treated with nocturnal positive pressure respiration based on the low oxygen saturation values obtained with pulse oximetry. Only after consultation with our laboratory was a hemoglobin variant suspected and investigated.

Methods.—We performed hemoglobin protein analysis by HPLC, electrophoretic separation, and spectrophotometry and DNA sequence analysis of the α-globin gene.

Results.—Both HPLC chromatographic separation and alkaline electrophoresis revealed a unique hemoglobin peak. In both patients, α-globin gene sequencing revealed amutation resulting in a histidine-to–aspartatic acid substitution at position $\alpha 87$. The low oxygen saturation measurement by pulse oximetry was due to hemoglobin Bonn oxyhemoglobin having an absorption peak at 668 nm, near the 660 nm measured by pulse oximeters.

Conclusion.—Hemoglobin Bonn is a novel hemoglobin variant of the proximal α-globin that results in falsely low oxygen saturation measurements with pulse oximetry.

▶ Transcutaneous monitoring of pO_2 by pulse oximetry is a noninvasive continuous monitoring approach that has been successfully applied for decades. The technique has found much use in neonatal care and in monitoring during surgery. The devices measure the saturated oxyhemoglobin concentration SO_2Hb spectrophotometrically using transcutaneous light-emitting diode technology. They are subject to some variability, but generally correlate quite well with arterial blood gas measurements. This is a curious case history of a father and son who exhibited anomalously low oxygen saturation measured transcutaneously by pulse oximetry. The 2 clinical situations were different based on the low oxygen saturation; the boy was suspected of having a right-to-left shunt and the father was suspected of having sleep apnea. Both of these were ruled out. The laboratory undertook an investigation as to whether a variant hemoglobin was present that might account for the results and ended up discovering a new hemoglobin variant with an absorption maximum at 668 nm, near the 660 nm peak measured by pulse oximeters.

M. G. Bissell, MD, PhD, MPH

The autoantibody rheumatoid factor may be an independent risk factor for ischaemic heart disease in men
Edwards CJ, Syddall H, Goswami R, et al (Southampton Gen Hosp, UK; Univ of Southampton, UK)
Heart 93:1263-1267, 2007

Background.—Subjects with rheumatoid arthritis have an increased prevalence of ischaemic heart disease (IHD). This is most likely in those people with the autoantibody rheumatoid factor (RF). RF is strongly associated with rheumatoid arthritis (RA) but is also present in up to 15% of all adults.

Objective.—To determine whether RF might identify people in a general population who also share an increased likelihood of developing IHD.

Methods.—Subjects from the Hertfordshire Cohort Study were investigated for the presence of RF. Subjects completed a questionnaire and attended a clinic where a history of IHD was recorded (ECG, coronary artery bypass grafting, Rose chest pain). Associations between the presence of RF, antinuclear antibodies (ANA), anticardiolipin antibodies

(ACA) and IHD in 567 men and 589 women were investigated and compared with traditional risk factors for IHD.

Results.—RF was associated with an increased likelihood of IHD in men (odds ratio (OR) = 3.1, 95% CI 1.7 to 5.4, p<0.001). This increased risk could not be explained by traditional risk factors for IHD (mutually adjusted OR for RF 2.9 (95% CI 1.6 to 5.3), p<0.001). There was no significant association between RF in women or between ANA or ACA with IHD in men or women.

Conclusion.—This work suggests that RF is an independent risk factor for IHD in the general population. It lends support to the importance of inflammation in atherosclerosis and suggests that autoimmune processes may be involved. In addition, it raises the intriguing possibility that RF may have a direct role in the pathogenesis of IHD in some subjects.

▶ Rheumatoid factors (RF) are defined as human autoantibodies with specificity for Immunoglobulin G (IgG) molecules, specifically the Fc portion. It is because of their ability to form immune complexes that rheumatoid factors likely contribute to the pathogenesis of rheumatoid arthritis (RA), with which they are most closely associated. But these molecules are also seen in a variety of other autoimmune conditions including Sjogren's syndrome, vasculitides, infections, and lymphoproliferative disorders. They are also seen in as many as 15% of normal adults. Recently, they have also been associated with an increase in risk for ischemic heart disease in patients with autoimmune polyarthritis. Based on the known association of C-reactive protein (cRP) levels with increased cardiac risk, the authors hypothesize that rheumatoid factors may have a role in cardiovascular risk assessment as well. Subjects with chronic inflammatory diseases such as rheumatoid arthritis and systemic lupus erythematosus (SLE) have been found to have increased risk.

M. G. Bissell, MD, PhD, MPH

Quantification of ZAP70 mRNA in B Cells by Real-Time PCR Is a Powerful Prognostic Factor in Chronic Lymphocytic Leukemia

Stamatopoulos B, Meuleman N, Haibe-Kains B, et al (Institut Jules Bordet, Université Libre de Bruxelles (ULB), Brussels, Belgium)
Clin Chem 53:1757-1766, 2007

Background.—Chronic lymphocytic leukemia (CLL) is heterogeneous with respect to prognosis and clinical outcome. The mutational status of the immunoglobulin variable heavy chain region (IGHV) has been used to classify patients into 2 groups in terms of overall survival (OS) and clinical characteristics, but the laborintensive nature and the cost of this time-consuming analysis has prompted investigations of surrogate markers.

Methods.—We developed a standardized quantitative real-time reverse transcription-PCR (qPCR) method to measure zeta-chain (TCR)-associated protein kinase (ZAP70) mRNA in purified CD19+ cells. We evaluated

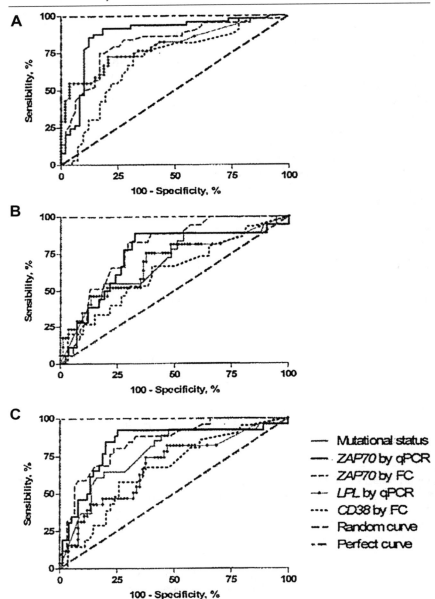

FIGURE 2.—ROC curve analysis of the different prognostic factors vs IGHV mutational status and time-dependent ROC curves. (A), AUC values are in Table 2 AUC values calculated for all markers were compared with a nonparametric test. The qPCR-measured *ZAP70* AUC was significantly different from the *LPL* AUC ($P = 0.014$) and the *CD38* AUC ($P = 0.007$). The AUC for FC-measured *ZAP70* was not significantly different from the AUCs for qPCR-measured *ZAP70* and *LPL* ($P = 0.424$ and 0.165, respectively). (B), time-dependent ROC curves at 1 year after diagnosis. (C) time-dependent ROC curves at 2 years after diagnosis. (Reprinted from Stamatopoulos B, Meuleman N, Haibe-Kains B, et al. Quantification of ZAP70 mRNA in B cells by real-time PCR is a powerful prognostic factor in chronic lymphocytic leukemia. *Clin Chem*. 2007;53:1757-1766.)

this and other methods (flow cytometry analyses of ZAP70 and CD38 proteins and qPCR analysis of lipoprotein lipase mRNA) in a cohort of 108 patients (median follow-up, 82 months) to evaluate any associations with IGHV mutational status, OS, and treatment-free survival (TFS).

Results.—The association between qPCR-measured ZAP70 and IGHV mutational status was statistically significant [χ^2 (1) = 50.95; P<0.0001], and the value of Cramer's V statistic (0.72) indicated a very strong relation. This method also demonstrated sensitivity, specificity, and positive and negative predictive values of 87.8%, 85.7%, 87.5%, and 86%, respectively. ZAP70 expression was significantly associated with OS ($P = 0.0021$) and TFS (P <0.0001). ZAP70$^+$ patients had significantly shorter median TFS (24 months) than ZAP70$^-$ patients (157 months) (P <0.0001). Moreover, qPCR-measured ZAP70 expression has greater prognostic power than IGHV mutational status and the other prognostic markers tested.

Conclusions.—ZAP70 mRNA quantification via qPCR is a strong surrogate marker of IGHV mutational status and a powerful prognostic factor (Fig 2).

▶ Chronic lymphocytic leukemia (CLL) is the most common leukemia in Western countries, affecting primarily the elderly and exhibiting an extremely variable course, with survivals ranging from months to decades. Clinical staging systems are thus needed to help stratify risk of progression in this disease. Systems based on purely clinical findings have not performed well in prognosis. This has led to a search for genetic biomarkers. The best performing of these to date has been the assessment of the mutational status of the immunoglobulin variable heavy chain region (IGHV), but this has not been easily adaptable to practical clinical laboratory assays. Surrogate markers for IGHV have thus become emphasized more recently. Among these have been CD38, lipoprotein lipase (LPL), and the zeta-chain (TCR)-associated protein kinase (ZAP70) expression, found in T lymphocytes and natural killer cells. This latter marker has shown the most promise, and these authors undertook to evaluate ZAP70 mRNA quantitation by real-time PCR. The receiver operating curve (ROC) analyses reflecting these results are shown in Fig 2.

M. G. Bissell, MD, PhD, MPH

New serological markers in inflammatory bowel disease are associated with complicated disease behaviour
Ferrante M, Henckaerts L, Joossens M, et al (Univ Hosp Gasthuisberg, Leuven, Belgium; et al)
Gut 56:1394-1403, 2007

Background and Aims.—Several antibodies have been associated with Crohn's disease and are associated with distinct clinical phenotypes. The aim of this study was to determine whether a panel of new antibodies against bacterial peptides and glycans could help in differentiating inflammatory bowel disease (IBD), and whether they were associated with particular clinical manifestations.

Methods.—Antibodies against a mannan epitope of *Saccharomyces cerevisiae* (gASCA), laminaribioside (ALCA), chitobioside (ACCA), mannobioside (AMCA), outer membrane porins (Omp) and the atypical perinuclear antineutrophilic cytoplasmic antibody (pANCA) were tested in serum samples of 1225 IBD patients, 200 healthy controls and 113 patients with non-IBD gastrointestinal inflammation. Antibody responses were correlated with the type of disease and clinical characteristics.

Results.—76% of Crohn's disease patients had at least one of the tested antibodies. For differentiation between Crohn's disease and ulcerative colitis, the combination of gASCA and pANCA was most accurate. For differentiation between IBD, healthy controls and non-IBD gastrointestinal inflammation, the combination of gASCA, pANCA and ALCA had the best accuracy. Increasing amounts and levels of antibody responses against gASCA, ALCA, ACCA, AMCA and Omp were associated with more complicated disease behaviour (44.7% versus 53.6% versus 71.1% versus 82.0%, $p < 0.001$), and a higher frequency of Crohn's disease-related abdominal surgery (38.5% versus 48.8% versus 60.7% versus 75.4%, $p < 0.001$).

Conclusions.—Using this new panel of serological markers, the number and magnitude of immune responses to different microbial antigens were shown to be associated with the severity of the disease. With regard to the predictive role of serological markers, further prospective longitudinal studies are necessary.

▶ Crohn's disease and ulcerative colitis are subtypes of inflammatory bowel disease (IBD) involving chronic and recurrent inflammation of the GI tract. Current thinking about the pathophysiology of these conditions is that they may arise from overgrowth by specific components of the bowel flora, in turn leading to an aberrant immune response in a susceptible host. Autoantibodies associated with inflammatory bowel disease include atypical perinuclear antineutrophil cytoplasmic antibodies (pANCA), antimannose antibodies on yeast *Saccharomyces cerevisiae* (ASCA), and antibodies against laminaribioside (ALCA), chitobioside (ACCA), mannobioside (AMCA), and outer membrane porins (Omp). These serological markers have been only modestly successful in initially diagnosing inflammatory bowel disease. However, it is possible that combinations of the individual markers within the whole collection may be useful in differentiating Crohn's disease from ulcerative colitis and/or be predictive of disease severity in terms of their patterning over time. It is this hypothesis that these authors set out to investigate.

M. G. Bissell, MD, PhD, MPH

Usefulness of Cell Counter–Based Parameters and Formulas in Detection of β-Thalassemia Trait in Areas of High Prevalence

Rathod DA, Kaur A, Patel V, et al (Smt NHL Municipal Med College, Ahmedabad, India; Greencross Voluntary Blood Bank, Pathology and RIA Laboratory, Ahmedabad, India; et al)
Am J Clin Pathol 128:585-589, 2007

The present study aimed to retrospectively evaluate the usefulness of cell counter–based parameters and formulas in β-thalassemia trait (BTT) detection. The study included 170 BTT cases (hemoglobin [Hb]A_2 >4.0% [0.04]) and 30 non-BTT cases (HbA_2, 2.3%-3.5% [0.02-0.04]). Depending on the hemoglobin level and iron deficiency, the BTT group was further classified into classic BTT (n = 112) and BTT with iron deficiency anemia (n = 58). The RBC count, MCH, MCV, RDW, and Shine and Lal, Mentzler, Srivastava, England and Fraser, Ricerca, and Green indexes were applied. For the first time in the population of India, these 10 cell counter parameters and manual formulas were compared with high-performance liquid chromatography–derived HbA_2 levels for deriving a cost-effective alternative method; and receiver operating characteristic curves were applied. We found that the Shine and Lal, Srivastava, and Mentzler indexes, MCV, and MCH have better discriminative function than the RBC count and red cell distribution width and their related formulas.

▶ Thalassemia is a genetic defect in the synthesis of hemoglobin that affects some 1.5% of the world's population (between 80 and 90 million people, with about 60 000 new carriers born annually). About half of the affected population is found in southeast Asia (India, Thailand, Indonesia, etc). The prevalence of the beta thalassemia trait is about 3.3% in India (varying as high as 8.4% in some regions, and 10-15% in certain communities). Most of these individuals are asymptomatic and, therefore, may not be aware of their carrier status, but it is only through effective screening that the homozygous condition can be prevented. The beta thalassemia trait is associated with mild or no anemia, but nonetheless certain abnormal red cell indices, including a reduced mean corpuscular volume (MCV), mean corpuscular hemoglobin (MCH), and an elevated hemoglobin A2 (HbA2) level. This study was undertaken to systematically compare the diagnostic performance of 10 different cell counter-based indices with HPLC-based hemoglobin methods in mass screening.

M. G. Bissell, MD, PhD, MPH

Preoperative neutrophil-lymphocyte ratio and outcome from coronary artery bypass grafting

Gibson PH, Croal BL, Cuthbertson BH, et al (Univ of Aberdeen, UK)
Am Heart J 154:995-1002, 2007

Background.—An elevated preoperative white blood cell count has been associated with a worse outcome after coronary artery bypass grafting (CABG). Leukocyte subtypes, and particularly the neutrophil-lymphocyte (N/L) ratio, may however, convey superior prognostic information. We hypothesized that the N/L ratio would predict the outcome of patients undergoing surgical revascularization.

Methods.—Baseline clinical details were obtained prospectively in 1938 patients undergoing CABG. The differential leukocyte was measured before surgery, and patients were followed-up 3.6 years later. The primary end point was all-cause mortality.

Results.—The preoperative N/L ratio was a powerful univariable predictor of mortality (hazard ratio [HR] 1.13 per unit, $P < .001$). In a backward conditional model, including all study variables, it remained

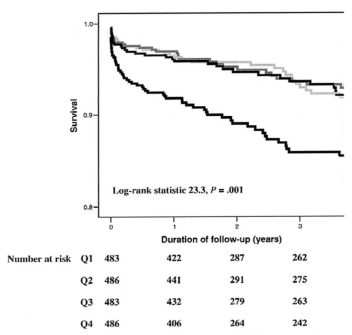

Number at risk		0	1	2	3
	Q1	483	422	287	262
	Q2	486	441	291	275
	Q3	483	432	279	263
	Q4	486	406	264	242

FIGURE 1.—Relationship between quartiles of N/L ratio and all-cause mortality. ▬▬▬▬, Neutrophil-lymphocyte ratio quartile 1. ▬▬▬▬, Neutrophil-lymphocyte ratio quartile 2. ▬▬▬▬, Neutrophil-lymphocyte ratio quartile 3. ▬▬▬▬, Neutrophil-lymphocyte ratio quartile 4. (Reprinted from Gibson PH, Croal BL, Cuthbertson BH, et al. Preoperative neutrophil-lymphocyte ratio and outcome from coronary artery bypass grafting. *Am Heart J.* 2007;154:995-1002. Copyright 2007, with permission from Elsevier.)

a strong predictor (HR 1.09 per unit, $P = .004$). In a further model, including the European system for cardiac operative risk evaluation, the N/L ratio remained an independent predictor (HR 1.08 per unit, $P = .008$). Likewise, it was an independent predictor of cardiovascular mortality and predicted death in the subgroup of patients with a normal white blood cell count. This excess hazard was concentrated in patients with an N/L ratio in the upper quartile (>3.36).

Conclusion.—An elevated N/L ratio is associated with a poorer survival after CABG. This prognostic utility is independent of other recognized risk factors (Fig 1).

▶ That low-grade inflammation probably has an important role in the pathogenesis of atherosclerosis is now well recognized, and several biomarkers of inflammation have been used to predict risk in this context. Coronary artery bypass grafting (CABG) is a procedure in which improvements in stratification of outcome still have value. The total leukocyte count, one of the most readily available markers of inflammation, has been shown to have predictive value for cardiac events in the general population in patients with stable angina and acute coronary syndromes, and being able to predict mortality after CABG. The relationship of total leukocyte count to outcome is complex and nonlinear: It is the neutrophil count that contains much of the predictive power. Also, a low lymphocyte count has been associated with poorer prognosis. The authors undertook a prospective evaluation of the predictive value of the ratio of the preoperative neutrophil and lymphocyte counts. The survival curve analysis in Fig 1 shows the results.

M. G. Bissell, MD, PhD, MPH

Baseline BAL Neutrophilia Predicts Early Mortality in Idiopathic Pulmonary Fibrosis

Kinder BW, Brown KK, Schwarz MI, et al (Univ of Cincinnatti College of Medicine, OH; Natl Jewish Med Ctr, Denver, CO)
Chest 133:226-232, 2008

Background.—The prognostic value of BAL fluid cell count differential in patients with idiopathic pulmonary fibrosis (IPF) is unknown. We hypothesized that baseline BAL fluid cell count differential (*ie*, elevated levels of neutrophils and eosinophils, or reduced levels of lymphocytes) would predict higher mortality among persons with IPF.

Methods.—We evaluated the association of BAL fluid cell count differential and mortality among 156 persons with surgical lung biopsy-proven IPF who underwent bronchoscopy with BAL and cell count differential measurements at presentation. Vital status was obtained among all participants. Cox regression analysis evaluated the association of BAL fluid cell count differential and mortality.

Results.—After controlling for known clinical predictors of mortality, we found that each doubling of baseline BAL fluid neutrophil percentage was associated with a 30% increased risk of mortality (adjusted hazard ratio [HR], 1.28; 95% confidence interval [CI], 1.01 to 1.62; adjusted $p = 0.04$) in the first year after presentation. We observed no association with BAL fluid lymphocyte percentage and mortality (adjusted HR per doubling, 0.99; 95% CI, 0.76 to 1.29; $p = 0.93$) or eosinophil percentage and mortality (adjusted HR per doubling, 0.99; 95% CI, 0.69 to 1.40; $p = 0.95$).

Conclusions.—Increased BAL fluid neutrophil percentage is an independent predictor of early mortality among persons with IPF. Alternatively, BAL fluid lymphocyte and eosinophil percentages were not associated with mortality. The clinical utility of BAL at the time of diagnosis of IPF should be reconsidered.

▶ Prognostic classification of idiopathic pulmonary fibrosis (IPF), the chronic, progressive, and fibrosing form of interstitial lung disease (ILD), is difficult. Overall, 5-year survival in this condition is only 20% to 40%, and important therapeutic decisions about the use of potentially cytotoxic therapies are a necessary part of its treatment. These have been complicated historically by a lack of precision in predicting prognosis. Bronchoalveolar lavage (BAL) is a procedure frequently used in these patients, and the differential cell counts on BAL fluid samples have been considered useful by some authors in characterizing the inflammatory cell populations involved in IPF, although the overall usefulness of BAL in prognosticating IPF has remained controversial because of the lack of well-designed studies. The authors addressed this need by prospectively examining associations between components of BAL fluid differential cell counts (combined with other demographic and clinical data) at the time of diagnosis and mortality.

M. G. Bissell, MD, PhD, MPH

Alternative Complement Pathway in the Pathogenesis of Disease Mediated by Anti-Neutrophil Cytoplasmic Autoantibodies
Xiao H, Schreiber A, Heeringa P, et al (Univ of North Carolina; Univ Med Ctr Groningen, The Netherlands)
Am J Pathol 170:52-64, 2007

Clinical and experimental data indicate that anti-neutrophil cytoplasmic autoantibodies (ANCAs) cause glomerulonephritis and vasculitis. Here we report the first evidence that complement is an important mediator of ANCA disease. Transfer of anti-myeloperoxidase (MPO) IgG into wild-type mice or anti-MPO splenocytes into immune-deficient mice caused crescentic glomerulonephritis that could be completely blocked by complement depletion. The role of specific complement activation pathways was investigated using mice with knockout of the common pathway component C5, classic and lectin binding pathway component C4, and alternative pathway component factor B. After injection of anti-MPO IgG, $C4^{-/-}$ mice developed disease comparable with wildtype disease; however, $C5^{-/-}$ and factor $B^{-/-}$ mice developed no disease. To substantiate a role for complement in human ANCA disease, IgG was isolated from patients with myeloperoxidase ANCA (MPO-ANCA) or proteinase 3 ANCA (PR3-ANCA) and from controls. Incubation of MPO-ANCA or PR3-ANCA IgG with human neutrophils caused release of factors that activated complement. IgG from healthy controls did not produce this effect. The findings suggest that stimulation of neutrophils by ANCA causes release of factors that activate complement via the alternative pathway, thus initiating an inflammatory amplification loop that mediates the severe necrotizing inflammation of ANCA disease.

▶ Circulating autoantibodies directed against myeloperoxidase (MPO) and proteinase 3 (PR3) within the cytoplasm of neutrophils and monocytes are frequently encountered in patients with vasculitis and glomerulonephritis. These antineutrophil cytoplasmic antibodies (ANCA) characterize a large percentage (> 80%) of patients with active Wegener's granulomatosis, microscopic polyangiitis, and crescentic glomerulonephritis of the pauci-immune variety. ANCA IgG is known to be causative of these ANCA-associated cases of vasculitis and glomerulonephritis. The pathogenic effects of these antibodies are apparently augmented by the release of various proinflammatory cytokines, such as tumor necrosis factor (TNF)-α. A variety of intercellular effects have been described upon interaction of ANCA IgG Fc receptor engagement and Fab'2 binding, but the potential involvement of the complement system in any of these had not been postulated previously. This is because complement is not prominent among the substances that are easily demonstrable histochemically in tissue in these cases.

M. G. Bissell, MD, PhD, MPH

22 Transfusion Medicine and Coagulation

A functional coagulation test to identify anti-β_2-glycoprotein I dependent lupus anticoagulants
Devreese KMJ (Ghent Univ Hosp, Belgium)
Thromb Res 119:753-759, 2007

Introduction.—Lupus Anticoagulants (LAC) activity due to β_2-glycoprotein I (β_2GPI) antibodies shows a high correlation with thrombotic events. Since the binding of β_2GPI antibodies to phospholipids may be influenced by the final calcium chloride ($CaCl_2$) concentration a discrimination between β_2GPI dependent LAC and β_2GPI independent LAC could be possible using clotting tests with various $CaCl_2$ concentrations and making them this way more sensitive to the presence of β_2GPI antibodies.

Materials and Methods.—I evaluated the effect of 5 mM, 8.3 mM, 10.3 mM and 17.9 mM final $CaCl_2$ concentration in a commonly used screening test for LAC, the PTT-LA, on LAC positive patients with and without β_2GPI antibodies.

Results.—Mean coagulation times of LAC patients negative for β_2GPI antibodies were significant shorter with 5 mM $CaCl_2$ in comparison with 8.3 mM and 10 mM ($P < 0.05$ and $P < 0.01$, respectively). In the LAC patients with positive β_2GPI antibodies no significant difference at 5 mM $CaCl_2$, 8.3 mM or 10 mM was observed.

Mean coagulation times at 5 mM $CaCl_2$ were significant higher ($P = 0.003$) in patients positive for β_2GPI antibodies than in patients negative for β_2GPI antibodies.

Conclusion.—The most remarkable observation was that the coagulation time, measured by PTT-LA at low final $CaCl_2$ concentration, is much more prolonged in the LAC positive β_2GPI antibody positive patients than in the LAC positive β_2GPI antibody negative patients. Thus, the competition with clotting factors for binding on phospholipids is stronger for β_2GPI antibodies than for other antibodies and explains the longer coagulation times in the presence of β_2GPI antibodies.

▶ The so-called "antiphospholipid syndrome," associated with increased thrombotic tendency and morbidity in pregnancy, is actually a misnomer. It is now known that the characteristic autoantibodies called "antiphospholipid antibodies" are not actually directed against phospholipids per se, but are instead directed against certain plasma proteins that have high affinity for binding anionic phospholipids. Two of these proteins are found frequently enough in specimens from these patients to suggest a significant pathophysiological role, namely β2-glycoprotein 1 (β2-GP1) and prothrombin. Of these, the association with β2-GP1 is strong enough that it is considered an independent risk factor for the syndrome. The autoantibodies that bind specifically through β2-GP1 are called "anticardiolipin antibodies." Standard approaches to diagnostic testing for the antiphospholipid syndrome are based on the combination of a phospholipid-dependent coagulation assay and an immunosorbent method for anticardiolipin. This author undertook to manipulate calcium chloride concentrations in the assay conditions to better differentiate lupus anticoagulant due to antibodies against β2-GP1 from that due to other antibodies.

M. G. Bissell, MD, PhD, MPH

Prokaryotic versus eukaryotic recombinant Lutheran blood group protein for antibody identification
Seltsam A, Grüger D, Blasczyk R (Hannover Med School, Germany)
Transfusion 47:1630-1636, 2007

Background.—At present, identification of antibodies against high-frequency antigens is limited to reference laboratories having panels of rare red blood cell (RBC) specimens in stock. Antibodies against Lu[b] are among the most frequent clinically relevant antibody specificities directed against high-frequency antigens.

Study Design and Methods.—Soluble recombinant Lu[b] fusion proteins consisting of the first three N-terminal immunoglobulin superfamily domains and a V5-His tag were generated. Eukaryotic recombinant Lu[b] proteins were isolated from cell culture supernatant of stably transfected HEK293 cells with anti-V5 Sepharose. Prokaryotic Lu[b] fusion proteins were expressed in *Escherichia coli*, purified by Ni-NTA, and refolded by chromatographic procedures. Ten anti-Lu[b] serum samples, 6 anti-Lu[a] serum samples, 30 serum samples directed against other blood group antigens, 10 serum samples from patients with RBC autoantibodies, and 100 serum samples from randomly selected donors were used for antibody screening.

Results.—Eukaryotic and prokaryotic recombinant Lu[b] proteins proved to be equally suited for identification of anti-Lu[b]. Recombinant Lu[b] protein–based enzyme-linked immunosorbent assay correctly identified samples containing anti-Lu[b] sera, and the titers were at least two times higher than those measured by the gel agglutination–based indirect antiglobulin test. In hemagglutination inhibition assays, recombinant Lu[b] protein neutralized all anti-Lu[b], but none of the other alloantibodies decreased in reactivity.

Conclusion.—Antibody detection systems based on soluble eukaryotic or prokaryotic recombinant blood group proteins have the potential to replace current systems with rare RBCs for identification of alloantibodies against high- or low-frequency antigens. This innovation could bring routine laboratories one step closer to specialized antibody diagnostics.

▶ There is a subset of red blood cell (RBC) antigens that occur so widely in the general population as to be, in fact, near universal (> 90%) in prevalence. Examples are antigens like antiLub, antiKpb, antiYta, and antiVel. Alloantibodies against these high-frequency RBC antigens are not well characterized by routine antibody identification tests using standard test cell panels. The current usual practice in such cases is to use nonstandard test cell panels based on the use of extremely rare blood specimens from donors lacking the high-frequency antigens. Such panels are available for use almost exclusively in reference laboratories, creating logistical delays in the processing of such units in regular blood banks or transfusion services. This has given rise to an effort to develop a new generation of antibody identification assays based on the use of recombinant high-frequency blood group proteins produced in eukaryotic or prokaryotic expression systems. Because protein expression has been known to differ between these 2 types of expression systems, the authors undertook to examine this.

M. G. Bissell, MD, PhD, MPH

Genotypes and serum concentrations of human alpha-1-antitrypsin "P" protein variants in a clinical population

Bornhorst JA, Calderon FRO, Procter M, et al (Univ of Arkansas for Med Sciences, Little Rock, AR; Laboratories Inst of Clinical and Experimental Pathology, Salt Lake City, UT; et al)
J Clin Pathol 60:1124-1128, 2007

Background.—Alpha-1-antitrypsin (AAT) deficiency is a relatively common genetic disorder that can lead to the development of pulmonary disorders. Diagnosis of AAT deficiency is typically performed by isoelectric focusing (IEF) protein phenotyping in concert with determination of AAT serum concentration levels. The "P" phenotypic variant is associated with several known genetic variants that are found at unknown relative frequencies.

Aims.—To investigate the genetic variation of "P" alleles in patient samples.

Methods.—A DNA sequencing protocol for the full AAT coding region from serum was developed. Additionally, a retrospective evaluation of AAT concentrations in serum samples containing "P" allele IEF phenotype variants was undertaken.

Results.—"P" phenotypic variants are observed in ~ 1 of every 900 samples received in the reference laboratory. Heterozygous "MP" allele samples exhibited a wide range of serum protein concentrations. Genotyping revealed the presence of the deleterious P_{lowell} variant in six heterozygous MP samples, two heterozygous PZ samples, and one homozygous PP

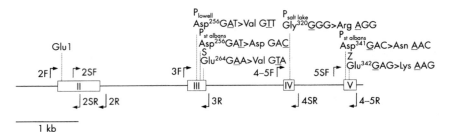

1 kb

FIGURE 1.—Genomic map of the coding regions of the alpha-1-antitrypsin gene. White boxes indicate exons II–V (the first amino acid of the mature protein is depicted in exon II). Black arrows indicate amplicon primer sites and light arrows indicated additional sequencing primers. The locations of the P, S, and Z genetic variants are shown in exons III–V, where they occur. (Reprinted from Bornhorst JA, Calderon FRO, Procter M, et al. Genotypes and serum concentrations of human alpha-1-antitrypsin "P" protein variants in a clinical population. *J Clin Pathol.* 2007;60:1124-1128.)

sample. A non-deleterious $P_{st\ albans}$ variant was observed in a single MP sample. A novel heterozygous AAT M"P" variant, $P_{salt\ lake}$ was identified, that did not exhibit a reduced AAT serum concentration.

Conclusions.—Genetic heterogeneity is present in clinical "P" phenotype variants identified by IEF, and the deleterious P_{lowell} variant appears to be relatively common. Sequencing of "P" phenotype variants can provide useful clinical information, especially when the "P" phenotype variant is paired with a deficiency phenotype allele (Fig 1).

▶ As is well known, $\alpha 1$-antitrypsin (AAT) deficiency is one of the most common genetic abnormalities in Caucasian populations, with prevalence estimates as high as 1 in 3000 individuals. Over 100 genetic variants of AAT have been described. Pulmonary disease resulting from AAT deficiency is most frequently associated with the presence of the S and Z phenotypic variants (Z also causing hepatic cirrhosis) (Fig 1). Pairings of these with the normal M allele are for the most part nondeleterious and do not decrease AAT levels enough to cause pulmonary disease, but when paired with one another do. The phenotypic variants are identified by isoelectric focusing of serum AAT protein. A third category of phenotypic variant, called P, features a mixed array of subtypes, not all of which are deleterious per se. The authors have developed a full gene DNA sequencing protocol for the full AAT coding region that allows an estimate of the frequency of these P variant subtypes.

M. G. Bissell, MD, PhD, MPH

Clinical Testing for Mutations in the *MEN1* Gene in Sweden: A Report on 200 Unrelated Cases

Tham E, Grandell U, Lindgren E, et al (Karolinska Institutet, Stockholm; Karolinska Univ Hosp Solna, Stockholm; Karolinska Univ Hosp Huddinge, Stockholm; et al)

J Clin Endocrinol Metab 92:3389-3395, 2007

Context.—Multiple endocrine neoplasia type 1 (MEN1) is a tumor syndrome of the parathyroid, endocrine pancreas, and anterior pituitary caused by mutations in the *MEN1* gene on 11q13.

Objective.—The goal of this study was to determine the *MEN1* mutation spectrum and detection rate among Swedish patients and identify which patient categories should be tested for *MEN1* mutations.

Design/Setting/Patients.—DNA sequences and referral forms from patients referred to the Department of Clinical Genetics at Karolinska University Hospital, Sweden, for clinical *MEN1* mutation screening were analyzed. The mutation status of 371 patients (including 200 probands) was ascertained, and the multiplex ligation-dependent probe amplification (MLPA) assay was evaluated for the detection of large deletions.

Main Outcome Measure.—The main outcome measure was *MEN1* genotypes.

Results.—Forty-eight of 200 index cases (24%) shared 40 different mutations (18 novel). A total of 69% of all mutations resulted in a truncated protein. Two large deletions were detected by MLPA. A total of 94% of all MEN1 families had a mutation in the coding region of the *MEN1* gene. A total of 6% of sporadic cases had *MEN1* mutations. There was no correlation between severe disease and mutation type or location.

Conclusions.—A total of 4% of all mutations were large deletions, and MLPA is now included in our standard *MEN1* mutation screening. Individuals with at least one typical endocrine tumour and at least one of the following: 1) a first-degree relative with a major endocrine tumor; 2) an age of onset less than 30 yr; and/or 3) multiple pancreatic tumors/parathyroid hyperplasia were most likely to harbor a mutation; thus these patients should be screened for *MEN1* mutations (Fig 2).

▶ An interesting collection of inherited cancers are the multiple endocrine neoplasia (MEN) syndromes (MEN 1, MEN 2A, and MEN 2B). These conditions represent familial disorders inherited as autosomal dominants and presenting with tumors arising histologically from the amine precursor uptake and decarboxylase (APUD) neuroendocrine tissues. The APUD tissues, of course, synthesize a number of polypeptide hormones such as corticotropin, calcitonin, gastrin, glucagon, insulin, melanocyte-stimulating hormone, secretin, and vasoactive intestinal peptide (VIP). The degree to which these hormones are expressed varies among cases. MEN type I (MEN 1) has been mapped cytogenetically to position 11q13 on the long arm of chromosome 11, and involves

A

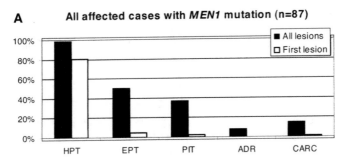

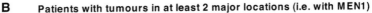

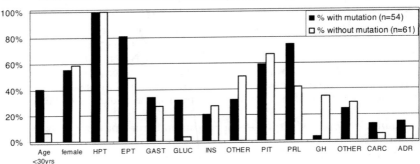

FIGURE 2.—A, Distribution of tumor types in the 87 affected patients with *MEN1* mutations. The *filled columns* represent all lesions present in all affected MEN1 patients, whereas the *white columns* depict their first detected lesion. A total of 86 patients had HPT. Of the 44 patients with EPT tumor, 32% had gastrinoma (GAST), 32% had glucagonoma (GLUC), 39% had panceatic polypeptide-oma, 21% had insulinoma (INS), and 21% were unknown or nonfunctioning. Note that the majority of patients had pancreatic tumors that produced more than one hormone. At least 25% had metastasis, but information on malignancy was not available for 17 patients (39%). Of the 13 patients with carcinoids (CARCs), 46% had metastasis: two with bronchial, three with thymic, and one with gastric carcinoid. HPT was the first detected lesion in 70 patients (81%). Of the remaining 17 patients, four had EPT tumors (4.7%), two had PIT tumors (2.3%), one had a bronchial carcinoid (1.2%), and information on the first lesion was lacking for the remaining 10. B, Tumor types in all patients with MEN1. A total of 115 patients had tumors in at least two major locations, and thus fulfilled the criteria for MEN1. The *filled columns* represent patients with *MEN1* mutations, and the *white columns* represent patients without detected *MEN1* mutations. The EPT and PIT tumors are further subdivided into hormone-producing groups. Cases with a mutation were younger at their first operation, had a higher frequency of EPT tumor (44 of 54 compared with 30 of 61), and more often glucagonoma (14 of 44 compared with one of 30). They also had a higher incidence of prolactinoma (PRL) (24 of 32 compared with 17 of 43) and a lower incidence of GH-producing PIT tumors (one of 32 compared with 14 of 41). ADR, Adrenal tumor; GH, GH-producing pituitary tumor. (Reprinted from Tham E, Grandell U, Lindgren E, et al. Clinical testing for mutations in the *MEN1* gene in Sweden: a report on 200 unrelated cases. *J Clin Endocrinol Metab*. 2007;92:3389-3395. Copyright 2007 The Endocrine Society.)

tumors of the parathyroid, endocrine pancreas or duodenum, and anterior pituitary, among others (Fig 2). The authors have undertaken to demonstrate the feasibility of genetic screening of an at-risk population and study the mutation spectrum and detection rate for MEN 1 mutations. This may have implications for the broader clinical use of such screening.

M. G. Bissell, MD, PhD, MPH

Is flow cytometry accurate enough to screen platelet autoantibodies?

Hézard N, Simon G, Macé C, et al (Laboratoire d'Hématologie, CHU Robert Debré, Reims, France)
Transfusion 48:513-518, 2008

Background.—The diagnosis of immune thrombocytopenic purpura (ITP) is a diagnosis of exclusion, as stated by international guidelines. Nevertheless, the assessment of platelet (PLT) antibodies has been reported as helpful for the diagnosis and the follow-up of ITP patients. PLT antibodies are detected by highly specialized assays, such as monoclonal antibody–specific immobilization of PLT antigen (MAIPA) test. Flow cytometry for PLT-associated immunoglobulin G (PAIgG) detection has been described more recently. This study was meant to evaluate the utility of flow cytometry to screen accurately patients needing further MAIPA testing.

Study Design and Methods.—PAIgG, PAIgM, and PAIgA were determined in 107 consecutive patients and in 147 healthy controls in parallel. MAIPA testing was performed in all patients. The accuracy of flow cytometry was assessed with a receiver operating characteristics (ROC) curve analysis versus MAIPA.

Results.—MAIPA assay found PLT-specific IgG in 27 patients (25%). The ROC curve analysis showed that no false-negative result in flow cytometry was obtained for a mean fluorescence intensity (MFI) cutoff of 0.2. With this cutoff, PAIgG were positive in 61 patients (57%). In this series, MAIPA was unnecessary in 42 percent of patients (corresponding to true-negative results). When MAIPA was positive, PAIgM values ranged from 0.1 to 1.0, and PAIgA from 0.1 to 2.

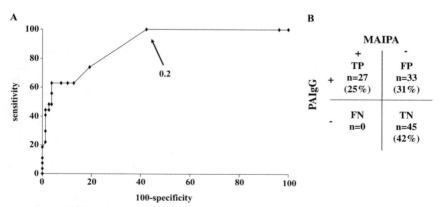

FIGURE 3.—ROC curve and contingency table: flow cytometric PAIgG determination versus MAIPA. For a 100 percent sensitivity, the best specificity (57%) was obtained for an MFI cutoff of 0.2 (A). True negative (TN) indicates that specific PLT testing by MAIPA should be unnecessary in 40 percent of patients (B). TP = true-positive value; FP = false-positive value; FN = false-negative value. (Reprinted from Hézard N, Simon G, Macé C, et al. Is flow cytometry accurate enough to screen platelet autoantibodies? *Transfusion.* 2008;48:513-518.)

Conclusion.—Flow cytometry for PAIgG assessment may be used to accurately decide whether or not MAIPA must be subsequently performed. In this series, MAIPA was unnecessary in 42 percent of patients. Moreover, PAIgM results suggested that its determination combined with PAIgG may be of interest in ITP investigation (Fig 3).

▶ Immune thrombocytopenic purpura (ITP) is an acquired disorder of accelerated platelet (PLT) consumption associated with PLT autoantibodies, either de novo or secondary to another condition. The current diagnostic criteria include history, physical examination, complete blood count (CBC), and peripheral smear interpretation to exclude other causes of thrombocytopenia. It has been suggested that additional clinical laboratory testing could perhaps profitably be incorporated into this definition, namely the detection of PLT-associated immunoglobulins (PAIg) by flow cytometry and the detection and characterization of specific PLT antibodies (ie, those specifically directed against PLT glycoproteins and non-PLT specific antibodies. The latter may be performed using highly specialized assays like the monoclonal antibody-specific immobilization of PLT antigen (MAIPA) test. The question addressed by the authors is the head-to-head comparison of the value of these 2 techniques in aiding diagnosis of ITP. They provide a receiver operating characteristics (ROC) curve of the results (Fig 3).

M. G. Bissell, MD, PhD, MPH

Prothrombin fragment 1 + 2 in urine as an indicator of sustained coagulation activation after total hip arthroplasty
Borris LC, Breindahl M, Ryge C, et al (Århus Univ Hosp, Denmark; BESST-TEST ApS, Kgs. Lyngby, Denmark; Univ of Copenhagen, Hørsholm, Denmark; et al)
Thromb Res 121:369-376, 2007

Purpose.—Prothrombin fragment 1 + 2 measured in spot urine (uF1 + 2) is an indicator of thrombin generation. We examined whether measured levels of uF1 + 2 can be used to differentiate between patients who do and do not acquire sustained coagulation activation after total hip arthroplasty (THA).

Methods.—We performed two separate studies in patients undergoing THA. Study 1 was a prospective pilot study aiming to roughly estimate the extent of pre- and postoperative fluctuations in the uF1 + 2 concentration. Study 2 was a larger prospective cohort study aiming to verify the findings of Study 1 and to examine the association between the uF1 + 2 concentrations and risk of vascular thrombotic complications (VTC) or death. Finally, we sought to define a cut-off concentration value that could be used to identify patients with a sustained uF1 + 2 elevation after the first postoperative week. The urine samples were analysed by ELISA. In both studies thromboprophylaxis was used for at least 7 days after the operation.

Results.—The operative trauma resulted in elevation of the uF1 + 2 level in all patients compared with the preoperative level and levels in the healthy volunteers. Ten out of 113 patients (8.8%) in the second study suffered VTC or death, assumed to be caused by a coagulation problem. Analysis of variance revealed the following statistically significant associations: pre- vs. postoperative log uF1 + 2 levels ($P < 0.0001$), log uF1 + 2 levels comparing patients with and without events ($P = 0.004$); and the individual log uF1 + 2 levels ($P < 0.0001$). A cut-off value of uF1 + 2 concentration between 0.3 and 0.5 nmol/l had a sensitivity and a negative predictive value between 100% and 90%, and specificity between 45% and 63% and overall accuracy between 50% and 65%. This value was obtained by the analysis of a receiver operating characteristic curve with the purpose of identifying patients with sustained coagulation activation on day 5 after operation.

Conclusion.—Our studies suggest that measured levels of uF1 + 2 can be potentially used to assess the individual risk of VTC after THA and to test for non-invasive detection of sustained coagulation activation.

▶ Surgical trauma is associated with a prothrombotic state in which the coagulation cascade is activated, resulting in thrombin generation and formation of fibrin clots. Normally, this state obtains for a matter of days postoperatively, but in some cases it may persist and lead to vascular thrombotic complications like deep vein thrombosis (DVT), pulmonary embolism (PE), acute myocardial infarction (AMI), transient ischemic attacks (TIAs), or stroke. In the case of a total hip arthroplasty procedure, for example, recent practice has included some weeks of coverage with low molecular weight heparin (LMWH) post operatively as a preventive measure. Many surgeons are reluctant to undertake this, as the approach is beset by concerns for balancing risks of hemorrhage versus benefits of prevention. There has, therefore, been a need for a reliable method of surveillance. The authors here present a study of the use of measured levels of urine prothrombin fragments 1 and 2 (uF1 + 2) for such an application.

M. G. Bissell, MD, PhD, MPH

Factor V Leiden mutation: a treatable etiology for sporadic and recurrent pregnancy loss
Glueck CJ, Gogenini S, Munjal J, et al (Cholesterol Ctr, Jewish Hosp, Cincinnati, OH)
Fertil Steril 89:410-416, 2008

Objective.—We hypothesized that the thrombophilic G1691A factor V Leiden (FVL) gene mutation was a common, significant, and treatable cause of sporadic and recurrent pregnancy loss (RPL).

Design.—We compared the frequency of the FVL mutation in 141 women with ≥1 pregnancy and 1 sporadic pregnancy loss (308 live births,

141 pregnancy losses), 44 women with ≥1 pregnancy and ≥3 pregnancy losses (105 live births, 180 pregnancy losses), and 638 women with ≥1 live birth pregnancy and 0 pregnancy loss (1553 live births).

Setting.—Outpatient Clinical Research Center.

Patient(s).—A total of 823 caucasian women with consecutive measures of the FVL mutation.

Main Outcome Measure(s).—We used polymerase chain reaction techniques to characterize the thrombophilic FVL G1691A gene mutation.

Result(s).—Of the 638 controls, 47 (7.4%) had FVL heterozygosity versus 16 heterozygous and 2 homozygous FVL cases (18/141, 12.8%) in 141 women with 1 sporadic pregnancy loss versus 9/44 RPL cases (20.5%, 8 heterozygous and 1 homozygous FVL). The FVL frequency in cases with 1 sporadic pregnancy loss (18/141, 12.8%) did not differ from RPL cases (9/44, 20.45%).

Conclusion(s).—After unexplained sporadic pregnancy loss, as well as after RPL, to provide the option to prospectively optimize subsequent live birth outcomes with low-molecular-weight heparin thromboprophylaxis, we suggest that measurements be done of the FVL mutation, a treatable etiology for sporadic pregnancy loss as well as for RPL.

▶ Pregnancy loss, sporadic and or recurrent, has been associated with thrombophilia in some studies in the obstetric gynecological literature, but not others, and the topic remains highly controversial. Among these studies, factor V Leiden, the inherited thrombophilic factor, has been associated with fetal loss in some studies, again controversially. Thrombophilia mediated by hyperestrogenism of pregnancy is synergistic with factor V Leiden-mediated thrombophilia, potentially promoting thrombus formation in the placental spiral arteries, placental insufficiency, and pregnancy loss. However, there is no uniform agreement on the usefulness of thromboprophylaxis for optimizing pregnancy outcomes in this context. These authors having concluded on the basis of previous work that the thrombophilic factor V Leiden gene mutation G1691A was associated with poor pregnancy outcomes, undertook this re-examination of the question in a prospective study design. They conclude that this mutation is a common, significant, and treatable cause of both sporadic and recurrent pregnancy loss.

M. G. Bissell, MD, PhD, MPH

Overnight or fresh buffy coat–derived platelet concentrates prepared with various platelet pooling systems
Dijkstra-Tiekstra MJ, Kuipers W, Setroikromo AC, et al (Sanquin Blood Bank Northeast Region, Groningen, The Netherlands)
Transfusion 48:723-730, 2008

Background.—For logistic reasons, possibilities to produce both platelet (PLT) concentrates prepared from fresh or overnight-stored whole blood (fresh and o/n PCs, respectively) are convenient. The consequences of both possibilities are not well described. The PLT pooling system used might also influence the condition of PCs. Our aim was to compare fresh and o/n PCs with different PLT pooling systems.

Study Design and Methods.—Fresh and o/n PCs were prepared from buffy coats and plasma in PLT pooling systems of Baxter, Fresenius, Terumo, or Pall (n = 5). PCs were stored for 9 days. The in vitro quality was determined by the PLT count, pH, glucose, lactate, pO_2, pCO_2, CD62P expression, and annexin V binding.

Results.—The o/n PCs showed higher PLT count (approx. 460×10^9/PC vs. approx. 310×10^9/PC), pCO_2, and lactate concentration and lower pH, pO_2, glucose concentration, CD62P expression (until Day 5), and annexin V binding (until Day 7) compared with fresh PCs ($p < 0.05$). Only for o/n PCs in the Baxter and Fresenius systems did the pH and glucose concentration remain higher, and the lactate concentration and CD62P expression remained lower than that of o/n PCs in the Pall and Terumo systems. The pH for fresh PCs in the Baxter and Fresenius systems was more often greater than 7.4 than for fresh PCs in the Terumo or Pall systems.

Conclusion.—The quality of PCs depended on whether PCs were prepared from fresh or overnight-stored whole blood and on the used PLT pooling system. The main difference between fresh and o/n PCs was the PLT count.

▶ The in vitro quality and in vivo effectiveness of platelet concentrates depend on a variety of factors including leukoreduction, storage temperature, gas exchange capabilities of the storage containers, and duration of storage. European standards specify acceptable pH ranges at 22°C at the end of shelf life of 6.4 to 7.4 or 6.8 to 7.4 (Dutch standards). An important logistical question relates to the comparability of platelets prepared from fresh blood with overnight stored whole blood. Studies of these have shown no significant differences between platelet concentrates prepared from single buffy coats and via the platelet rich plasma (PRP) method. There have been no such comparisons for fresh with overnight stored platelet concentrates from prepooled buffy coats. Such prepooled buffy coat platelet concentrates are mostly produced in platelet pooling systems containing an in-line leukoreduction filter. These authors examined and compared the performances of platelet pooling systems of various manufacturers.

M. G. Bissell, MD, PhD, MPH

ADAMTS13 related markers and von Willebrand factor in plasma from patients with thrombotic microangiopathy (TMA)

Kobayashi T, Wada H, Nishioka N, et al (Mie Univ Graduate School of Medicine, Tsu, Japan)
Thromb Res 121:849-854, 2008

The ADAMTS13 (a disintegrin and metalloprotease with a thrombospondin type I domain 13) related markers were measured in the plasma of healthy volunteers and thrombotic microangiopathy (TMA) patients including thrombotic thrombocytopenic purpura (TTP) to examine their efficacy in the diagnosis of TTP.

The plasma levels of the ADAMTS13 antigen and ADAMTS13-factor XI complex were significantly lower in TMA patients with a significant decreased ADAMTS13 activity (and these patients were considered to have TTP) than in the healthy volunteers. The plasma levels of ADAMTS13 antigens closely correlated with those of ADAMTS13-factor XI complex. Autoantibody for ADAMTS 13 was also positive in almost all TTP patients. In addition, the ratio of von Willebrand factor (VWF)/ADAMTS13 activity was significantly high in TTP suggesting that this ratio might be more useful for the differential diagnosis of TTP than the ADAMTS13 assay alone.

These findings suggest that ADAMTS13 related markers are useful for the diagnosis and analysis of TTP (Fig 1).

▶ ADAMTS13 refers to a disintegrin and metalloproteinase with a thrombospondin type 1 domain 13 that was first identified in 2001. It is a zinc metalloproteinase, which specifically cleaves the von Willebrand factor (VWF) multimer at the Tyr (1605)-Met (1606) bond in the A2 region of the molecule.

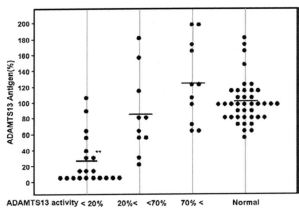

FIGURE 1.—Plasma levels of ADAMTS13 antigen in patients with TMA. (Reprinted from Kobayashi T, Wada H, Nishioka N, et al. ADAMTS13 related markers and von Willebrand factor in plasma from patients with thrombotic microangiopathy (TMA). *Thromb Res.* 2008;121:849-854, Copyright 2007 Elsevier Ltd.)

The von Willebrand multimer, normally produced in and released from vascular endothelial cells, is commonly found in plasma of patients with thrombotic thrombocytopenic purpura (TTP). It probably interacts with circulating platelets to cause clumping due to elevated shear stress. VWF is a large glycoprotein that is necessary for high shear stress platelet adhesion and aggregation. TTP is associated with low plasma levels of ADAMTS13 activity, as is thrombotic microangiopathy (TMA) in general. These authors undertook to assess levels not only of ADAMTS13 but also ADAMTS13-factor XI complex, autoantibody against ADAMTS13, and the ratio of VWF to ADAMTS13 (VWF/ADAMTS13) in patients specifically with TMA (Fig 1).

M. G. Bissell, MD, PhD, MPH

Thrombophilia screening in asymptomatic children
Thornburg CD, Dixon N, Paulyson-Nuñez K, et al (Duke Univ School of Med, Durham; Wake Forest Univ School of Med, Winston-Salem, NC)
Thromb Res 121:597-604, 2008

Children with a family history of thrombophilia and/or thrombosis are often referred to pediatric thrombosis centers for evaluation. This article reviews the risks and benefits of thrombophilia testing in this unique population. The article also reviews an approach to testing including a stepwise evaluation and involvement of a genetic counselor.

▶ Coagulation testing is an extremely commonly ordered investigation in medical practice. One aspect of this is testing for thrombophilia. Parents with thrombosis and /or thrombophilia frequently ask whether their children should also be screened for the disorder and the presence of a positive family history of thrombosis and/or thrombophilia is an indication for such testing. In considering the option of testing children for thrombophilia, the benefits and risks of screening should be considered. Although such testing may help the family understand thrombophilia, it may not be of immediate benefit to the child. It may provide motivation to change lifestyle to reduce thrombosis risk, but is time-consuming and expensive. Testing may not only reduce the occurrence of venous thromboembolism in the general population but also may create a false sense of security; also, testing may not only reduce occurrence of venous thromboembolism in a single family but also may trigger discrimination in obtaining insurance.

M. G. Bissell, MD, PhD, MPH

Usefulness of high-concentration calcium chloride solution for correction of activated partial thromboplastin time (APTT) in patients with high-hematocrit value

Kanahara M, Kai H, Okamura T, et al (Kurume Univ Hosp, Japan; Kurume Univ School of Med, Japan; et al)
Thromb Res 121:781-785, 2008

Introduction.—Pseudoprolongation of activated partial thromboplastin time (APTT) is a serious problem in anticoagulation therapy for patients with high hematocrit, such as cyanotic congenital heart diseases. APTT pseudoprolongation occurs when APTT assay is performed using routinely used vacuum sampling tubes containing citrate. Because the plasma fraction is small in high-hematocrit blood, the prescribed volume of citrate would be excessive for APTT assay, resulting in prolongation of clotting or APTT pseudoprolongation. CLSI – The Clinical and Laboratory Standards Institute (formerly NCCLS) method is the established method to correct the pseudoprolongation. However, the CLSI method needs repeated blood drawings and time-consuming, complicate procedures. Thus, alternative simple method is desired.

Method.—We examined whether APTT pseudoprolongation would be prevented by the increase in free calcium ion concentration by using high-concentration calcium chloride solution for the assay. Blood samples were obtained from 15 patients with high hematocrit ($65 \pm 6\%$) who had cyanotic congenital heart disease.

Result.—Conventional APTT assay using 0.025 mol/L calcium chloride solution gave greater APTT compared with the CLSI method (51.7 ± 11.8 vs. 34.6 ± 4.7 s, $p < 0.001$). However, when 0.035 mol/L calcium chloride solution was used, APTT (36.6 ± 5.8 s) was similar to that obtained from the CLSI method. There was a good correlation in APTT values between high-calcium chloride solution method and the CLSI method (the slope $= 0.57$, $r^2 = 0.49$).

Conclusion.—High-calcium chloride solution method is useful to correct APTT pseudoprolongation. Because of the simplicity and the need of a single blood drawing, this method would reduce the burdens of not only patients but also clinical laboratory.

▶ The activated partial thromboplastin time (APTT) is used in clinical practice as a routine monitor for the effectiveness and safety of heparin anticoagulation. It can also detect abnormalities in clotting factors I, II, V, VIII, IX, X, XI, lupus anticoagulant, prekallikrein, and high molecular weight kininogen. Spuriously, high measured values of the APTT (APTT pseudo prolongation) can occur in patients with unusually high hematocrits, such as with cyanotic congenital heart disease and polycythemia vera. This artifact occurs when standard evacuated specimen sampling tubes containing citrate anticoagulant (3.13% by volume) are used for sample collection. In these tubes, when the specimen is dispersed in the smaller fluid volume present in high hematocrit samples, the citrate reduces the calcium concentration sufficiently to prolong the activated partial thromboplastin time. The authors propose a simple modification of the standard APTT assay involving the use of an increased concentration of calcium chloride (0.035 mol/L instead of 0.025 mol/L).

M. G. Bissell, MD, PhD, MPH

Aprotinin does not prolong the Sonoclot aprotinin-insensitive activated clotting time
Dong Y, Nuttall GA, Oliver WC Jr, et al (Mayo Clinic College of Medicine, Rochester, MN)
J Clin Anesth 19:424-428, 2007

Study Objective.—To determine whether a new Sonoclot-based, aprotinin-insensitive activated clotting time (aiACT) assay yields stable results over a broad range of aprotinin concentrations.

Design.—Prospective trial conducted on in vitro blood samples.

Setting.—Tertiary-care teaching medical center.

Participants.—19 healthy adult volunteers.

Interventions.—Whole blood samples were collected from volunteers. Heparin (2 U/mL) and escalating concentrations of aprotinin of 160 to 500 kallikrein inhibitory units (KIU)/mL were added in vitro.

Measurements and Main Results.—Celite ACT, kaolin ACT, and aiACT assays were completed. The aiACT showed stable activated clotting time (ACT) results on heparinized, noncitrated blood with added aprotinin (P = nonsignificant). In contrast, celite ACT and kaolin ACT were greatly prolonged when aprotinin was added to heparinized, noncitrated, and citrated blood ($P < 0.05$). The aiACT had consistent results at all aprotinin concentrations (P = nonsignificant).

Conclusions.—Aprotinin (160, 320, and 500 KIU/mL) significantly prolongs the ACT value with celite and kaolin activators but not with the aprotinin-insensitive activator.

▶ Anticoagulation is essential for the prevention of thrombosis in patients undergoing cardiopulmonary bypass during cardiac surgery. For many years, the standard form of anticoagulation for this indication was fixed-dose titration and bolus injection of heparin, based on the result of an activated clotting time (ACT) test result. The more nonspecific serine protease inhibitor Aprotinin was introduced into this context as an alternative to heparin about 15 years ago, and has shown considerable success in reducing bleeding and need for transfusion in these patients, but issues have arisen with regard to the ACT measurement. The activated clotting time values obtained in the presence of Aprotinin vary considerably depending on the particular activating substance used in the ACT assay. These biases could create risk of inadequate anticoagulation and subsequent intra- or postoperative thrombosis. The authors examined the effects of varying Aprotinin concentrations on 3 different ACT activators (SonACT, kACT, and aiACT) both in citrated and noncitrated blood.

M. G. Bissell, MD, PhD, MPH

Association between urokinase haplotypes and outcome from infection-associated acute lung injury

Arcaroli J, Sankoff J, Liu N, et al (Univ of Colorado at Denver; Univ of Alabama at Birmingham)

Intensive Care Med 34:300-307, 2008

Objective.—Alterations in coagulation, including elevated pulmonary and systemic concentrations of urokinase, are frequent in patients with acute lung injury (ALI). Urokinase potentiates neutrophil activation and contributes to the severity of pulmonary injury in preclinical models of ALI. The objective of this study was to examine associations between polymorphisms and haplotypes of urokinase with risk for and outcomes from ALI.

Design.—Prospective cohorts of healthy European-American adults and those with infection-associated ALI.

Setting.—Academic medical centers participating in NIH funded studies of low tidal volume ventilation for ALI.

Patients.—Controls were 175 healthy European-American subjects. Patients were 252 individuals with infection-associated ALI, prospectively followed for 60 days for mortality.

Interventions.—Genetic polymorphisms and haplotypes in the urokinase gene were determined.

Measurements and Main results.—Six polymorphisms, rs1916341, rs2227562, rs2227564, rs2227566, rs2227571, and rs4065, defining 98% of all urokinase haplotypes, were analyzed. There were no statistically significant associations between any single urokinase polymorphism or haplotype and risk for developing ALI. In contrast, there was a statistically significant relationship between the CGCCCC haplotype and both 60-day mortality and ventilator-free days that remained present in a multivariate analysis controlling for age and sex ($p = 0.033$ for 60-day mortality and < 0.001 for ventilator-free days).

Conclusions.—These results identify a specific urokinase haplotype as a genetic risk factor for higher mortality and more severe clinical outcome in patients with infection-associated ALI.

► The combination of bilateral infiltrates on chest X-ray with hypoxemia in the absence of evidence for left-sided cardiac failure defines the syndrome known as Acute Lung Injury (ALI). This condition often has an underlying infectious etiology and is characterized histologically by interstitial edema, microvascular thrombi, local neutrophilia, and deposition of fibrin in the alveoli. Changes in the functioning of coagulation and fibrinolysis pathways play an important role in mediating these effects. The serine protease urokinase cleaves plasminogen to produce plasmin, mediating fibrinolysis. In addition, urokinase has also been shown to facilitate neutrophil activation and inflammation. Urokinase concentrations are increased in both serum and bronchoalveolar lavage (BAL) fluid in patients with ALI. Genetic polymorphisms of urokinase show functional differences that could be significant with regard to its role in ALI. The authors undertook a prospective investigation to test this hypothesis, examining urokinase haplotype in a well-characterized cohort of patients with ALI.

M. G. Bissell, MD, PhD, MPH

23 Cytogenetics and Molecular Pathology

A Rapid Polymerase Chain Reaction-Based Screening Method for Identification of All Expanded Alleles of the Fragile X (*FMR1*) Gene in Newborn and High-Risk Populations
Tassone F, Pan R, Amiri K, et al (Univ of California, Davis; School of Medicine, CA; United Arab Emirates, Univ; et al)
J Mol Diagn 10:43-49, 2008

Fragile X syndrome, the most common inherited cause of intellectual impairment and the most common single gene associated with autism, generally occurs for fragile X mental retardation 1 (*FMR1*) alleles that exceed 200 CGG repeats (full-mutation range). Currently, there are no unbiased estimates of the number of full-mutation *FMR1* alleles in the general population; a major obstacle is the lack of an effective screening tool for expanded *FMR1* alleles in large populations. We have developed a rapid polymerase chain reaction (PCR)-based screening tool for expanded *FMR1* alleles. The method utilizes a chimeric PCR primer that targets randomly within the expanded CGG region, such that the presence of a broad distribution of PCR products represents a positive result for an expanded allele. The method is applicable for screening both males and females and for allele sizes throughout the premutation (55 to 200 CGG repeats) and full-mutation ranges. Furthermore , the method is capable of rapid detection of expanded alleles using as little as 1% of the DNA from a single dried blood spot. The methodology presented in this work is suitable for screening large populations of newborn or those at high risk (eg, autism, premature ovarian failure, ataxia, dementia) for expanded *FMR1* alleles. The test described herein costs less than $5 per sample for materials; with suitable scale-up and automation, the cost should approach $1 per sample.

▶ Fragile X syndrome is the most common heritable cause of mental retardation and commonly associated with autism. It is, for the most part, caused by large (> 200) runs of noncoding CGG repeat expansions within the fragile X mental retardation 1 (*FMR1*) gene. These represent the full fragile X mutation. Smaller (55-200) runs of such repeats (premutations) give rise to 4% to 14% of all premature ovarian failure in the general population, as well as a late-onset neurodegenerative disorder and a tremor/ataxia syndrome. It has been estimated that there may be between 1 and 2 million premutation carriers in the United States population, but to date there have been no general population screens carried out to estimate male and female carrier frequencies. Similarly, there have been no good screenings for the full mutation frequency in the general United States population. The authors developed a new PCR-based approach that reliably distinguishes between normal females, females with the full mutation fragile X allele, something which traditional PCR has failed to do.

M. G. Bissell, MD, PhD, MPH

A common 8q24 Variant and the Risk of Colon Cancer: A Population-Based Case-Control Study

Li L, Plummer SJ, Thompson CL, et al (Case Western Reserve Univ, Cleveland, OH; Cleveland Clinic, OH; et al)
Cancer Epidemiol Biomarkers Prev 17:339-342, 2008

Three recent studies identified common variants on 8q24 that confer modestly increased susceptibility to colorectal cancer. Here, we replicate the association in a population-based case-control study of colon cancer, including 561 cases and 721 unrelated controls. The rs6983267 marker was significantly associated with colon cancer risk. Compared with those homozygous for the T allele, the heterozygous and homozygous carriers for the G allele had an age-adjusted odds ratio of 1.39 (95% confidence interval, 1.03-1.88) and 1.68 (95% confidence interval, 1.21-2.33), respectively. An additive model showed strong evidence for a gene-dose response relationship ($P_{trend} = 0.0022$). The association remained statistically significant when restricted to Caucasians only (527 cases and 679 controls; $P_{trend} = 0.0056$). Further adjustment for other known risk factors did not alter the results. Stratified analysis revealed no evidence for effect modification by family history of colorectal cancer, age, or gender. These data replicate the association identified from recent studies, providing additional evidence supporting the rs6983267 genetic polymorphism as a marker predisposing to colon cancer.

▶ Cytogenetic abnormalities of chromosome 8 have been noted to be associated with a number of different solid tumors in examination of FISH in tumor specimens. These include lipoblastoma, infantile fibrosarcoma, osteochondroma, embryonal rhabdomyosarcoma, and pleomorphic adenoma of the salivary gland. A number of relatively common genetic variants of chromosome 8 (gain of 8q and deletion of 8p) have been found to be associated with increased risk for prostate cancer. Two of these in the 8q24 region, namely rs6983267 and rs10505477, have also more recently shown similar associations with risk for colorectal carcinoma and adenoma in several cohort and case-control studies. These studies have been both genome-wide and focused associations. The authors undertook a prospective population-based case-control study design of the Kentucky tumor registry to see if they could reproduce the earlier findings. The study involved 561 newly incident colon cancer cases and 721 population-based controls recruited between July 2003 and March 2007.

M. G. Bissell, MD, PhD, MPH

Noninvasive Prenatal Diagnosis of Fetal Chromosomal Aneuploidies by Maternal Plasma Nucleic Acid Analysis
Lo YMD, Chiu RWK (Chinese Univ of Hong Kong, Prince of Wales Hosp, Shatin, New Territories)
Clin Chem 54:461-466, 2008

Background.—The discovery of circulating cell-free fetal nucleic acids in maternal plasma has opened up new possibilities for noninvasive prenatal diagnosis. The potential application of this technology for the noninvasive prenatal detection of fetal chromosomal aneuploidies is an aspect of this field that is being actively investigated. The main challenge of work in this area is the fact that cell-free fetal nucleic acids represent only a minor fraction of the total nucleic acids in maternal plasma.

Methods and Results.—We performed a review of the literature, which revealed that investigators have applied methods based on the physical and molecular enrichment of fetal nucleic acid targets from maternal plasma. The former includes the use of size fractionation of plasma DNA and the use of the controversial formaldehyde treatment method. The latter has been achieved through the development of fetal epigenetic and fetal RNA markers. The aneuploidy status of the fetus has been explored through the use of allelic ratio analysis of plasma fetal epigenetic and RNA markers. Digital PCR has been shown to offer high precision for allelic ratio and relative chromosome dosage analyses.

Conclusions.—After a decade of work, the theoretical and practical feasibility of prenatal fetal chromosomal aneuploidy detection by plasma nucleic acid analysis has been demonstrated in studies using small sample sets. Larger scale independent studies will be needed to validate these initial observations. If these larger scale studies prove successful, it is expected that with further development of new fetal DNA/RNA markers and new analytical methods, molecular noninvasive prenatal diagnosis of the major chromosomal aneuploidies could become a routine practice in the near future (Figs 1 and 2).

▶ A major indication for prenatal diagnostic testing in pregnant women is for the detection of fetal chromosomal aneuploidies. The invasive methods for this include amniocentesis and chorionic villus sampling. These, of course, are highly invasive and constitute a significant risk to the fetus. Attempts to stratify this risk have led to the use of fetal ultrasonography and maternal serum biochemical screening, but these techniques do not directly measure the core molecular abnormalities involved, and thus lack sensitivity and specificity. Development of new forms of testing is, thus, very much a continuing

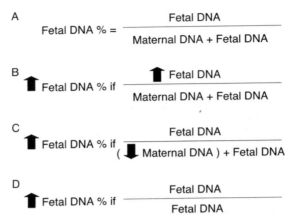

FIGURE 1.—Schematic illustration of the major approaches to increasing the fractional concentration of cell-free fetal DNA. The fractional concentration of fetal DNA in maternal plasma is given by the ratio of the absolute concentration of cell-free fetal DNA to that of the total cell-free DNA in maternal plasma (A). Approaches to increase the fractional concentration of fetal nucleic acids in maternal plasma may involve selective enrichment of fetal DNA (B), suppression of maternal background DNA (C), or elimination of the maternal nucleic acid background by detecting nucleic acids that are virtually completely fetus specific, such as fetal epigenetic or fetal RNA markers (D). (Reprinted from Lo YMD, Chiu RWK. Noninvasive prenatal diagnosis of fetal chromosomal aneuploidies by maternal plasma nucleic acid analysis. *Clin Chem.* 2008;54:461-466, with permission from the 2008 American Association for Clinical Chemistry.)

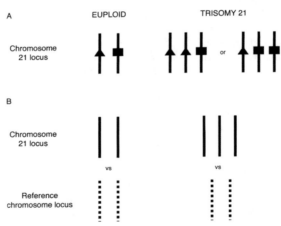

FIGURE 2.—Approaches for determining fetal chromosome dosage in cell-free nucleic acids in maternal plasma using trisomy 21 as an example. (A), allelic ratio analysis involves the assessment of the ratio between alleles at a heterozygous locus located on chromosome 21. The allelic ratio for such a locus would be expected to be 1:1 for a euploid fetus but 2:1 or 1:2 for a trisomic fetus. (B), relative chromosome dosage analysis involves the assessment of the ratio between a chromosome 21 locus and a nonchromosome 21 reference locus. The ratio among fetal-derived nucleic acid molecules would be expected to be 2:2 for a euploid fetus but 3:2 for a trisomic fetus. (Reprinted from Lo YMD, Chiu RWK. Noninvasive prenatal diagnosis of fetal chromosomal aneuploidies by maternal plasma nucleic acid analysis. *Clin Chem.* 2008;54:461-466, with permission from the 2008 American Association for Clinical Chemistry.)

technical need and a challenge in the field. It was discovered in 1997 that cell-free DNA circulates in maternal plasma, and although most of this material (97%) is of maternal origin, nonetheless, fetal cell-free DNA does circulate also. The authors systematically review the recent development of a variety of approaches to enriching the fraction of cell-free fetal DNA (Fig 1) and give work with Trisomy 21 (Fig 2) as an example.

M. G. Bissell, MD, PhD, MPH

Screening and Familial Testing of Patients for α_1-Antitrypsin Deficiency

Hogarth DK, Rachelefsky G (Univ of Chicago, IL; UCLA School of Medicine, Ctr for Asthma, Allergy, and Respiratory Diseases, Los Angeles, CA)
Chest 133:981-988, 2008

α_1-Antitrypsin deficiency (AATD) is an autosomal-codominant genetic disorder that predisposes individuals to the development of liver and lung disease. AATD is greatly underrecognized and underdiagnosed. Early identification allows preventive measures to be taken, the most important of which is the avoidance of smoking (including the inhalation of second-hand smoke) and exposure to environmental pollutants. Early detection also allows careful lung function monitoring and augmentation therapy while the patient still has preserved lung function. Cost factors and controversies have discouraged the initiation of large-scale screening programs of the newborn and adult populations in the United States and Europe (except for Sweden). There are sound medical reasons for targeted screening. Evidence-based recommendations for testing have been published by the American Thoracic Society/European Respiratory Society task force, which take potential social, psychological, and ethical adverse factors into consideration. This review discusses rationales for testing and screening for AATD in asymptomatic individuals, family members, and the general population, weighing benefits against potential psychological, social, and ethical implications of testing. For most, negative issues are outweighed by the benefits of testing. AATD testing should be routine in the management of adults with emphysema, COPD, and asthma with incompletely reversible airflow obstruction.

▶ α_1-Antitrypsin deficiency (AATD) is an autosomal codominant condition involving decreased production or secretion of the serine protease inhibitor AAT. This condition is a major risk factor for the development of liver disease in children, being the most common genetic cause of such disease and the most frequent diagnosis leading to liver transplantation in neonates. It also is an extremely frequent cause of emphysema in adults. This review covers the types and rationales of testing within the general population for this condition. The discussion includes the balancing of benefits and risks associated with psychological, social, and ethical dimensions. The condition is greatly underrecognized and underdiagnosed. Early detection is critical to efforts at prevention, especially avoiding smoking. Cost is great for general population screening programs, but targeted screening is both more feasible and beneficial. The article includes discussion of evidence-based recommendations made by the American Thoracic Society and European Respiratory Society Task force.

M. G. Bissell, MD, PhD, MPH

Technical report: Analysis of citrated blood with thromboelastography: Comparison with fresh blood samples
Wasowicz M, Srinivas C, Meineri M, et al (Univ Health Network, Toronto, Ontario; et al)
Can J Anesth 55:284-289, 2008

Purpose.—Thromboelastography (TEG) evaluates the viscoelastic properties of whole blood to assess clot formation and hemostasis. When blood cannot be analyzed immediately, it is stored in citrated tubes to be analyzed after recalcification. In this study, we evaluated the results of TEG analysis performed on citrated blood and compared these results to values obtained from activated (kaolin and tissue factor) and non activated, fresh blood samples, obtained at various time intervals (one, two, and three hours).

Methods.—Four blood samples were collected from each of ten healthy volunteers. The following TEG analyses were performed on each sample: reaction time (r), k time (k), alpha angle (α), and maximum amplitude (MA). Studies were done using fresh, non citrated blood, obtained within five minutes of collection, and using citrated blood, one, two, and three hours after collection. Samples were analyzed, with and without activation, using kaolin and tissue factor.

Results.—Tissue factor activated and non activated, citrated samples had shorter r and k times ($P = 0.03$, $P = 0.008$, $P < 0.0001$, and

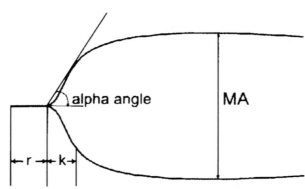

FIGURE 1.—Normal thromboclastogram (TEG) showing the derivation of r time, k time, alpha angle, and maximum amplitude (MA). (Reprinted from Wasowicz M, Srinivas C, Meineri M, et al. Technical report: analysis of citrated blood with thromboelastography: comparison with fresh blood samples. *Can J Anesth* 2008;55:284-289.)

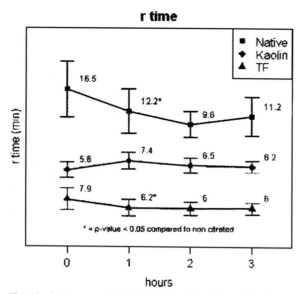

FIGURE 2.—Thromboclastogram results of r time (time = 0) and citrated blood at one, two, and three hours after storage. Blood samples were analyzed without activation (■, native), with tissue factor(TF) activation (▲,TF), and with kaolin activation (♦, kaolin). Values are expressed as mean ± standard derivation. Asterisks indicate results which were statistically significant ($P = 0.008$, $P = 0.03$, and $P = 0.35$ for native, TF, and kaolin measurements, respectively). (Reprinted from Wasowicz M, Srinivas C, Meineri M, et al. Technical report: analysis of citrated blood with thromboelastography: comparison with fresh blood samples. *Can J Anesth* 2008;55:284-289.)

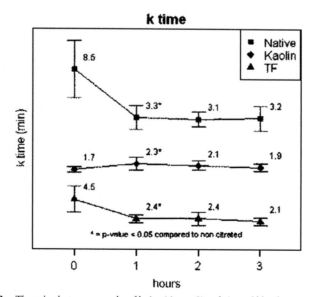

FIGURE 3.—Thromboclastogram results of k time(time = 0) and citrated blood at one, two, and three hours after storage. Blood samples were analyzed without activation (■, native), with tissue factor (TF) activation (▲,TF), and with kaolin activation (♦, kaolin). Values are expressed as mean ± standard deviation. Asterisks indicate results, which were statistically significant ($P < 0.001$, $P < 0.0001$, and $P = 0.03$ for native, TF, and kaolin measurements, respectively). (Reprinted from Wasowicz M, Srinivas C, Meineri M, et al. Technical report: analysis of citrated blood with thromboelastography: comparison with fresh blood samples. *Can J Anesth* 2008;55:284-289.)

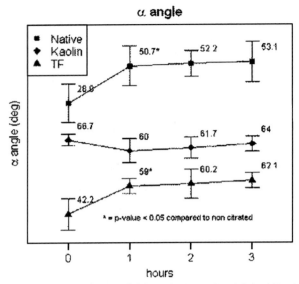

FIGURE 4.—Thromboclastogram results of alpha angle (time = 0) and citrated blood at one, two, and three hours after storage. Blood samples were analyzed without activation (■, native), with tissue factor (TF) activation (▲,TF), and with kaolin activation (◆, kaolin). Values are expressed as mean ± standard deviation. Asterisks indicate results which were statistically significant ($P < 0.0001$, $P < 0.0001$, and $P = 0.08$ for native, tissue factor (TF), and kaolin measurements, respectively). (Reprinted from Wasowicz M, Srinivas C, Meineri M, et al. Technical report: analysis of citrated blood with thromboelastography: comparison with fresh blood samples. *Can J Anesth* 2008;55:284-289.)

$P < 0.0001$, respectively) and higher alpha angle and MA values ($P < 0.0001$, $P < 0.0001$, $P = 0.79$, and $P = 0.03$, respectively) compared to fresh, non citrated samples. These findings were consistent with a hypercoagulable state. Conversely, citrated samples, activated with kaolin, yielded results similar to those obtained from fresh, non citrated samples. The TEG measurements were similar among citrated samples stored from one to three hours.

Conclusions.—Our results demonstrate that TEG measures, performed on citrated blood samples, yield results that are consistent with a hyperocoagulable state. Using kaolin to activate citrated samples, on the other hand, yields results similar to those obtained from non citrated, fresh blood samples (Figs 1-5).

▶ Thromboelastography (TEG) is widely used to monitor coagulation and guide blood transfusion in a variety of different surgeries, trauma, and postpartum hemorrhage. It is a technique based on the rheological properties of blood clotting that uses whole blood and monitors the entire clotting process, including initiation and speed of clot formation, clot strength, and fibrinolysis. In this it differs from the specific clotting assays, prothrombin time (PT), activated partial thromboplastin time (aPTT), fibrinogen level, and platelet count. The assay can use either citrated or noncitrated blood as the specimen. Using

Maximum amplitude (ma)

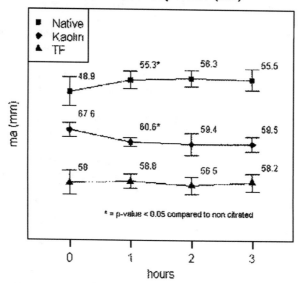

FIGURE 5.—Thromboclastogram results of maximum amplitude (time = 0) and citrated blood at one, two, and three hours after storage. Blood samples were analyzed without activation (■, native), with tissue factor (TF) activation (▲,TF), and with kaolin activation (◆, kaolin). Values are expressed as mean ± standard deviation. Asterisks indicate results which were statistically significant ($P = 0.03$, $P = 0.79$, and $P < 0.001$ for native, TF, and kaolin measurements, respectively). (Reprinted from Wasowicz M, Srinivas C, Meineri M, et al. Technical report: analysis of citrated blood with thromboelastography: comparison with fresh blood samples. *Can J Anesth* 2008;55:284-289.)

noncitrated blood avoids contact activation that can occur during sample storage, but requires that the specimen be run within 5 minutes of sampling, which may not always be practical. Concerns have been articulated regarding the possibility that thromboelastography (TEG) results on citrated blood may differ systematically from those on fresh blood, and that storage time may be a variable affecting TEG results (Figs 1-5).

M. G. Bissell, MD, PhD, MPH

A Simple and Robust Quantitative PCR Assay to Determine *CYP21A2* Gene Dose in the Diagnosis of 21-Hydroxylase Deficiency

Parajes S, Quinterio C, Domínguez F, et al (Fundación Pública Gallega de Medicina Genómica (Unidad de Medicina Molecular), Santiago de Compostela, Spain)
Clin Chem 53:1577-1584, 2007

Background.—Correct diagnosis of 21-hydroxylase deficiency (21OHD) requires the identification of *CYP21A2* gene deletions and

CYP21A1P/CYP21A2 chimeric genes, which are disease-causing alleles, and gene duplications, which can lead to false-positive 21OHD allele results Because lack of suitable *CYP21A2* dosage assessment methods hampers correct 21OHD diagnosis, we developed a new assay based on the relative quantification of the *CYP21A2* gene using the *DSP* gene as a reference.

Methods.—The assay to determine *CYP21A2* copy number is based on real-time PCR. The method also detects the presence of the *CYP21A1P/CYP21A2* chimeric gene. We used a duplex PCR to coamplify the DSP gene, included as an internal control, along with *CYP21A2*. The difference in threshold cycles between *CYP21A2* and *DSP* genes (ΔCt) was used to assess *CYP21A2* copy number.

Results.—The ΔCt values obtained from 24 samples used to set up the method clearly differentiated 3 nonoverlapping intervals, which corresponded to the number of *CYP21A2* copies: -1.35 to -0.25 defined 2 gene copies, $+0.20$ to $+2.00$ defined 1 copy, and -2.50 to -1.50 defined 3 copies. With these intervals we were able to assess the gene copy number in 24 additional samples.

Conclusions.—This new method for gene copy assessment detects homozygous and heterozygous *CYP21A2* gene deletions, *CYP21A1P/CYP21A2* chimeric genes, and gene duplications. Moreover, the method is robust, fast, and easy to use in a molecular diagnosis laboratory. This method together with *CYP21A2* gene sequencing can provide a definitive system for the detection of almost all, common as well as rare, 21OHD alleles.

▶ Congenital adrenal hyperplasia is an autosomal recessive impairment of cortisol synthesis, due in the vast majority of cases to a deficiency in the enzyme 21 hydroxylase. The classical form of the condition occurs with complete absence of the enzyme and the nonclassical form results from a partial absence. The phenotypic expression is variable, including ambiguous genitalia in females and precocious puberty in males. Incidence ranges from 1 in 5000 to 1 in 15 000 live births. The gene encoding for 21 hydroxylase is *CYP21A2* localized to chromosome 6 (6p21.3). Most of the mutations associated with 21 hydroxylase deficiency are intergenic recombinations or deletions or duplications. Assessment of the *CYP21A2* copy number is important with regard to avoiding false positive results. Time-consuming Southern blots can accomplish this reliably, but PCR-based methods would be preferable. The authors' method for real-time PCR more rapidly detects deletions, chimerisms, and duplications in this gene.

M. G. Bissell, MD, PhD, MPH

A Novel Method to Capture Methylated Human DNA from Stool: Implications for Colorectal Cancer Screening

Zou H, Harrington J, Rego RL, et al (Mayo Clinic, Rochester, MN)
Clin Chem 53:1646-1651, 2007

Background.—Assay of methylated DNA markers in stool is a promising approach for colorectal cancer (CRC) screening. A method to capture hypermethylated CpG islands from stool would enrich target analyte and allow optimal assay sensitivity.

Methods.—Methyl-binding domain (MBD) protein was produced using a pET6HMBD plasmid with MBD DNA sequence cloned from rat MeCP2 gene and bound to a column of nickel-agarose resin. We first established the feasibility of using the MBD column to extract methylated human DNA in a high background of fecal bacterial DNA. To explore the impact of MBD enrichment on detection sensitivity, the tumor-associated methylated vimentin gene was assayed with methylation-specific PCR from stools to which low amounts of cancer cell DNA (0–50 ng) were added and from stools from CRC patients and healthy individuals. Stools from cancer patients were selected with low amounts of human DNA (median 7 ng, range 0.5–832 ng).

Results.—With MBD enrichment, methylated vimentin was detected in stools enriched with ≥10 ng of cancer cell DNA and in CRC stool with a range of native human DNA amounts from 4 to 832 ng. Without MBD enrichment, methylated vimentin was not detected in the enriched stools and was detected in only 1 cancer stool with high human DNA (832 ng). In stools from healthy individuals methylated vimentin was not detected, with or without MBD enrichment.

Conclusions.—MBD capture increases assay sensitivity for detecting methylated DNA markers in stool. Applied clinical studies for stool cancer screening are indicated.

▶ Colorectal cancer, one of the most common forms of cancer worldwide, is diagnosed in approximately 150 000 patients per year in the United States, 37% of whom will die of the disease; yet, when detected at early stages, it is curable. Colorectal cancer screening has been either too invasive or insufficiently accurate, which has led to continuing search for useful biomarkers. Currently, the use of molecular markers in stool is an area of emphasis in colorectal cancer screening. Methylated DNA markers occur with high frequency in early stage neoplasia and represent predictable assay targets on gene promoter regions. Using crude stool DNA directly as a PCR template, however, is disadvantageous, in that it consists predominantly of DNA from local flora and of dietary origin. Human DNA represents less than 0.1% of the total. Sampling of human DNA can be facilitated by the use of methyl-binding domain (MBD) protein in purifying CpG islands.

M. G. Bissell, MD, PhD, MPH

Analysis of the T1288R Mutation of the Wilson Disease ATP7B Gene in Four Generations of a Family: Possible Genotype-Phenotype Correlation with Hepatic Onset

Leggio L, Malandrino N, Loudianos G, et al (Catholic Univ of Rome, Italy; Ospedale Regionale per le Microcitemie of Cagliari and CNR Inst of Neurogenetics and Neuropharmacology, Cagliari, Italy)
Dig Dis Sci 52:2570-2575, 2007

Wilson disease, an autosomal recessive disorder due to mutations of the ATP7B gene, is characterized by copper accumulation and toxicity in the liver and subsequently in other organs, mainly the brain and cornea. A new missense mutation (T1288R) of the ATP7B gene has recently been discovered in a Wilson disease patient in our laboratory. The aim of the present study was to analyze clinical and genetic features of more generations of the family of the patient in which the new mutation T1288R was discovered. A total of 19 subjects were studied; in particular, four generations of the patient's family were analyzed. The ATP7B gene was analyzed

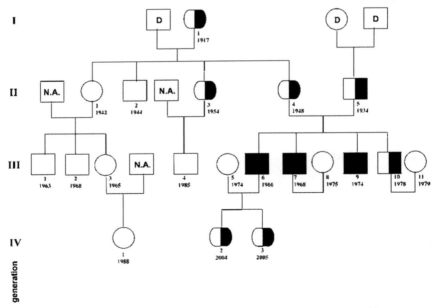

FIGURE 1.—Pedigree of the Wilson disease family analyzed. The subjects are indicated by progressive Arabic numbers according to the four generations: I1, II1–II5, III1–III11, and IV1–IV3. The four-figure number below each subject number indicates the year of birth. Subject III7 represents the patient affected by Wilson disease in whom the new mutation T1288R was previously discovered in our laboratory. D, deceased at the time this study began; NA, not analyzed.□, Male without T1288R mutation.○, Female without T1288R mutation.■, Male with homozygote T1288 mutation.◪, Male with heterozygote T1288 mutation. ◑, Female with heterozygote T1288 mutation. (Reprinted from Leggio L, Malandrino N, Loudianos G, et al. Analysis of the T1288R mutation of the Wilson disease ATP7B gene in four generations of a family: Possible genotype-phenotype correlation with hepatic onset. *Dig Dis Sci.* 2007;52:2570-2575, with permission from the Springer Science+Business Media, LLC 2007.)

by single-strand conformational polymorphism followed by direct sequencing. Two brothers presented a clinical diagnosis of Wilson disease with an hepatic phenotype and a genotype characterized by the homozygotic mutation T1288R. The heterozygotic mutation T1288R was found in seven subjects belonging to all four generations. The present study represents the first screening for a Wilson disease mutation through four generations of a nonconsanguineous family. All the patients with the homozygotic T1288R mutation in the present pedigree presented an hepatic phenotype without a neurological presentation. Consequently, a genotype-phenotype correlation could be hypothesized, although further studies are necessary to clarify this topic (Fig 1).

▶ The autosomal recessive abnormality known as Wilson's disease (WD) results in abnormal copper deposition in the liver, and then subsequently in other organs, principally the brain and cornea. The gene for this condition, known as ATP7B, is localized to the 13q14.1 position on the long arm of chromosome 13 and is some 21 exons in length, encoding for a copper-transporting P-type adenosine triphosphatase (P-type ATPase). This enzyme serves within the liver to transport copper into the secretory pathway where it binds to apoceruloplasmin and out via the bile. Over 250 disease-causing mutations of ATP7B have been described to date. Most affected individuals are compound heterozygotes. The authors describe the discovery of a new missense mutation of the WD gene associated uniquely with a clinical presentation including a Coombs-positive hemolytic anemia. They further describe their genetic analysis of 4 generations of the index patient's pedigree (Fig 1).

M. G. Bissell, MD, PhD, MPH

Variants in the *CRP* Gene as a Measure of Lifelong Differences in Average C-Reactive Protein Levels: The Cardiovascular Risk in Young Finns Study, 1980–2001

Kivimäki M, Lawlor DA, Smith GD, et al (Univ College London, UK; Univ of Bristol, UK; et al)

Am J Epidemiol 166:760-764, 2007

Genetic association studies have used variants in the C-reactive protein (*CRP*) gene to estimate causal effects of lifelong circulating CRP levels on disease endpoints. However, the extent to which the genetic variants are actually associated with lifelong circulating CRP levels has not been demonstrated empirically. In a population-based prospective cohort study (1980–2001) of 1,609 young Finns (768 men and 841 women), the authors genotyped five single nucleotide polymorphisms in the *CRP* gene (−717A/G, −286C/T/A, +1059G/C, +1444T/C, and +1846G/A) and assessed circulating CRP levels at ages 3–18 years and 24–39 years. The haplotypes from the five single nucleotide polymorphisms were associated with circulating CRP levels in childhood and adulthood, with the strongest effect being found for average CRP level across these two measures taken at two time points in the life course. In combination, the haplotype pairs accounted for 3.9%, 3.3%, and 5.0% of the variation in circulating CRP levels in childhood, in adulthood, and for the mean of CRP levels at both time points, respectively. These findings support the assumption that the above genetic variants define groups with long-term differences in circulating CRP levels.

▶ Controversy continues to surround the question of whether observed elevations in C-reactive protein (CRP) levels in the context of cardiovascular disease risk is a part of the causal chain or an incidental marker of other causal factors and preclinical disease only. The notion that it may be noncausal is supported by epidemiological studies that fail to relate variants in the CRP gene to coronary outcomes. Genetic variants associated with higher CRP levels should be associated with greater cardiovascular disease risk if CRP is causal, as long as population stratification did not create confounders of associations between genotypes and CRP levels or cardiovascular disease risk. What is uncertain in this argument, however, is the degree to which the genetic variants are correlated with lifelong differences in CRP levels. These authors undertook to address this question by examining long-term associations between the 2 variables in population-based cohort studies among the Finns.

M. G. Bissell, MD, PhD, MPH

Rationale, Design, and Methodology of the Women's Genome Health Study: A Genome-Wide Association Study of More Than 25 000 Initially Healthy American Women

Ridker PM, Chasman DI, Zee RYL, et al (Brigham and Women's Hospital, Boston, MA; et al)
Clin Chem 54:249-255, 2008

The primary aim of the Women's Genome Health Study (WGHS) is to create a comprehensive, fully searchable genome-wide database of >360 000 single nucleotide polymorphisms among at least 25 000 initially healthy American women participating in the ongoing NIH-funded Women's Health Study (WHS). These women have already been followed over a 12-year period for major incident health events including but not limited to myocardial infarction, stroke, cancer, diabetes, osteoporosis, venous-thromboembolism, cognitive decline, and common visual disorders such as age- related macular degeneration and cataracts. Investigations within the WGHS will seek to identify relevant patterns of genetic polymorphism that predict future disease states in otherwise healthy American women, and to evaluate patterns of genetic polymorphism that relate to multiple intermediate phenotypes including blood-based determinants of disease that were measured at baseline for each study participant. By linking genome-wide data to the existing epidemiologic databank of the parent

WHS, which includes comprehensive dietary, behavioral, and traditional exposure data on each participant since cohort inception in 1992, the WGHS will also allow exploration of gene-environment and gene-gene interactions as they relate to incident disease states. Thus, with continued follow-up of the WHS, the WGHS provides a unique scientific resource— a full-cohort, prospective, genome-wide association study among initially healthy American women.

▶ The principal goal of the Women's Genome Health Study (WGHS), as a subset of the ongoing Women's Health Study (WHS) is to create a genome-wide database of > 360 000 single nucleotide polymorphisms (SNPs) among a group of some 25 000 women participants in the larger study. These are women who already have a 12-year history of follow-up within the study for major health events including myocardial infarction, stroke, cancer, diabetes, osteoporosis, venous thromboembolism, cognitive disorders, age-related macular degeneration, and cataracts. The study is thus a full cohort, prospective, genome-wide association study that will seek to correlate predictive patterns of genetic polymorphism prospectively with disease incidence and with predictive baseline lab measurements. The databank for the Women's Health Study includes comprehensive dietary, behavioral, and exposure data as well as baseline physical assessments. The preferred analytical approach is the genome wide association study (GWAS) comparing genetic variation across the genome between patients with different disease states or different risk factor profiles.

M. G. Bissell, MD, PhD, MPH

Systematic Search for Placental DNA-Methylation Markers on Chromosome 21: Toward a Maternal Plasma-Based Epigenetic Test for Fetal Trisomy 21

Chim SSC, Jin S, Lee TYH, et al (Li Ka Shing Inst of Health Sci, The Chinese Univ of Hong Kong, Shatin, New Territories)
Clin Chem 54:500-511, 2008

Background.—The presence of fetal DNA in maternal plasma represents a source of fetal genetic material for noninvasive prenatal diagnosis; however, the coexisting background maternal DNA complicates the analysis of aneuploidy in such fetal DNA. Recently, the *SERPINB5* gene on chromosome 18 was shown to exhibit different DNA-methylation patterns in the placenta and maternal blood cells, and the allelic ratio for placenta-derived hypomethylated *SERPINB5* in maternal plasma was further shown to be useful for noninvasive detection of fetal trisomy 18.

Methods.—To develop a similar method for the noninvasive detection of trisomy 21, we used methylation-sensitive single nucleotide primer extension and/or bisulfite sequencing to systematically search 114 CpG islands (CGIs)—76% of the 149 CGIs on chromosome 21 identified by bioinformatic criteria—for differentially methylated DNA patterns. The methylation index (MI) of a CpG site was estimated as the proportion of molecules methylated at that site.

Results.—We identified 22 CGIs which were shown to contain CpG sites that were either completely unmethylated (MI = 0.00) in maternal blood cells and methylated in the placenta (MI range, 0.22–0.65), or completely methylated (MI = 1.00) in maternal blood cells and hypomethylated in the placenta (MI range, 0.00–0.75). We detected, for the first time, placental DNA-methylation patterns on chromosome 21 in maternal plasma during pregnancy and observed their postpartum clearance.

Conclusion.—Twenty-two (19%) of the 114 studied CGIs on chromosome 21 showed epigenetic differences between samples of placenta and maternal blood cells; these CGIs may provide a rich source of markers for noninvasive prenatal diagnosis.

▶ Diagnosing Down's syndrome (trisomy 21) currently requires invasive sampling of fetal cells, representing a measurable risk to the fetus. Circulating fetal DNA, representing 3% to 6% of the total DNA in maternal plasma could be used as an alternative specimen, but to date, its use in this way has been complicated by the presence of coexisting background maternal DNA in circulation. Y chromosome or paternally inherited markers have been used to identify fetal DNA but, of course, Y chromosomes cannot be used for female fetuses, and in general, no single paternally inherited marker can be used for all possible fetal maternal pairs. The authors have sought sex- and polymorphism-independent markers of fetal DNA via epigenetic approaches, namely DNA methylation pattern differences between the placenta and maternal blood cells (presumed to be the principal sources of fetal and maternal nucleic acids in maternal plasma, respectively. They found that 22 CpG islands (GGIs) on chromosome 21 showed such epigenetic differences and thus may provide a source of markers furthering this form of noninvasive prenatal diagnosis.

M. G. Bissell, MD, PhD, MPH

Subject Index

Author Index